I.V. Therapy

made Incredibly Easy!®

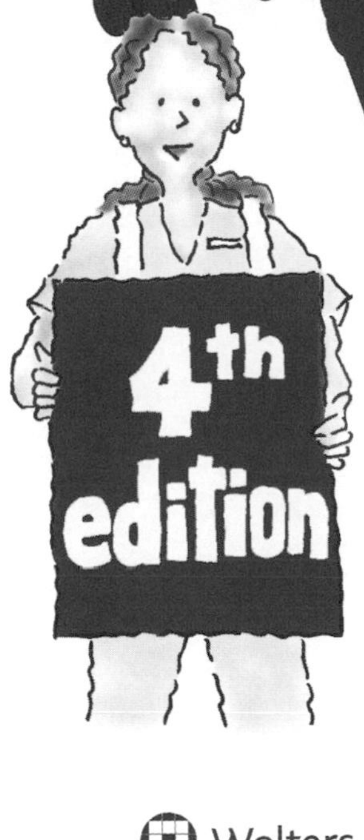

4th edition

Wolters Kluwer Health | Lippincott Williams & Wilkins

Philadelphia • Baltimore • New York • London
Buenos Aires • Hong Kong • Sydney • Tokyo

Staff

Executive Publisher
Judith A. Schilling McCann, RN, MSN

Clinical Director
Joan M. Robinson, RN, MSN

Art Director
Elaine Kasmer

Clinical Project Manager
Jennifer Meyering RN, BSN, MS, CCRN

Editor
Diane Labus

Clinical Editors
Robyn Wang RN, MPH, APRN
Dorothy P. Terry, RN

Illustrator
Bot Roda

Design Assistant
Kate Zulak

Associate Manufacturing Manager
Beth J. Welsh

Editorial Assistants
Karen J. Kirk, Jeri O'Shea, Linda K. Ruhf

The clinical treatments described and recommended in this publication are based on research and consultation with nursing, medical, and legal authorities. To the best of our knowledge, these procedures reflect currently accepted practice. Nevertheless, they can't be considered absolute and universal recommendations. For individual applications, all recommendations must be considered in light of the patient's clinical condition and, before administration of new or infrequently used drugs, in light of the latest package-insert information. The authors and publisher disclaim any responsibility for any adverse effects resulting from the suggested procedures, from any undetected errors, or from the reader's misunderstanding of the text.

© 2010 by Lippincott Williams & Wilkins. All rights reserved. This book is protected by copyright. No part of it may be reproduced, stored in a retrieval system, or transmitted, in any form or by any means — electronic, mechanical, photocopy, recording, or otherwise — without prior written permission of the publisher, except for brief quotations embodied in critical articles and reviews and testing and evaluation materials provided by publisher to instructors whose schools have adopted its accompanying textbook. For information, write Lippincott Williams & Wilkins, 323 Norristown Road, Suite 200, Ambler, PA 19002-2756.

Printed in China

IVMIE4–041012

Library of Congress Cataloging-in-Publication Data

I.V. therapy made incredibly easy!. — 4th ed.
p. ; cm.
Includes bibliographical references and index.
ISBN 978-1-60547-198-3
1. Intravenous therapy. 2. Nursing. I. Lippincott Williams & Wilkins. II. Title: IV therapy made incredibly easy!
[DNLM: 1. Infusions, Intravenous—Nurses' Instruction. 2. Drug Therapy—Nurses' Instruction. WB 354 I93 2009]

RM170.I25 2009
615'.6—dc22
2009009702

RRS1207

Contents

Contributors and consultants

Catherine B. Amero, MSN/Ed, CRNI, LNC
Nurse Educator
Infusion Nurses Society
Norwood, Mass.

Jane Banton, RN, BSN
Oncology Clinic Nurse
University of Wisconsin Hospitals and Clinics
Madison

Sandra J. Hamilton, RN, BSN, MEd, CRNI
Faculty
Great Basin College
Elko, Nev.
Hospice Nurse
Nathan Adelson Hospice
Pahrump, Nev.

Susan K. Poole, RN, BSN, MS, CRNI, CNSN
Senior Director, Accreditation
Walgreens OptionCare
Buffalo Grove, Ill.

Donna Scemons, RN, MSN, MA, FNP-C, CNS
President
Healthcare Systems, Inc.
Castaic, Calif.

Ruth K. Seignemartin, MOL, CRNI, CNAA
Co-owner/Chief Operations Officer
Integrated Health Professionals
Spokane Valley, Wash.

Angelia Sims, RN, CRNI, OCN
Staff Nurse, Infusion Services
Tuality Healthcare
Hillsboro, Ore.

Denise Stefancyk, RN, BSN, CCRC
Staff Nurse
University of Massachusetts Medical Center
Worcester

Allison J. Terry, RN, MSN, PhD
Director, Center for Nursing
Alabama Board of Nursing
Montgomery

Not another boring foreword

If you're like me, you're too busy caring for your patients to have the time to wade through a foreword that uses pretentious terms and umpteen dull paragraphs to get to the point. So let's cut right to the chase! Here's why this book is so terrific:

1. It will teach you all the important things you need to know about I.V. therapy. (And it will leave out all the fluff that wastes your time.)
2. It will help you remember what you've learned.
3. It will make you smile as it enhances your knowledge and skills.

Don't believe me? Try these recurring logos on for size:

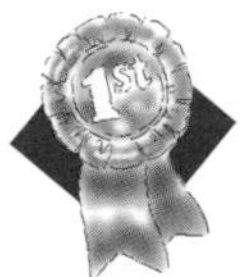

Best practice — Provides evidence-based standards for administering and monitoring I.V. therapy

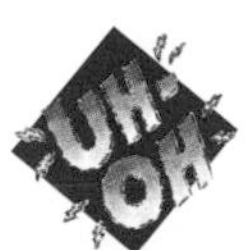

Warning — Alerts about possible risks or complications

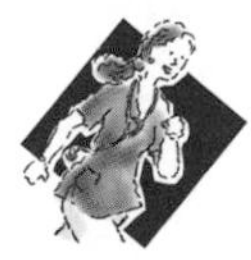

Running smoothly — Offers pointers on how to ensure that the patient and his equipment remain problem-free

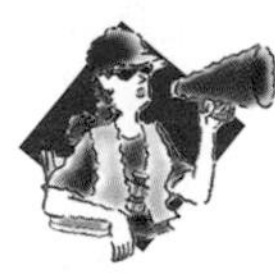

That's a wrap! — Contains a succinct summary of key chapter information for a quick review

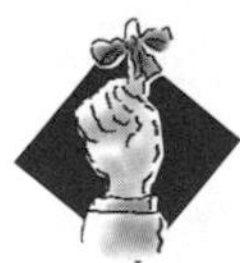

Memory jogger — Reinforces learning through easy-to-remember anecdotes and mnemonics

See? I told you! And that's not all. Look for me and my friends in the margins throughout this book. We'll be there to explain key concepts, provide important care reminders, and offer reassurance. Oh, and if you don't mind, we'll be spicing up the pages with a bit of humor along the way, to teach and entertain in a way that no other resource can.

I hope you find this book helpful. Best of luck throughout your career!

Joy

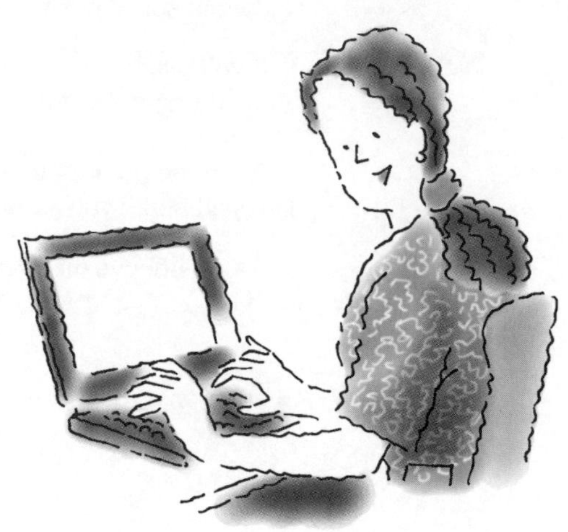

Introduction to I.V. therapy

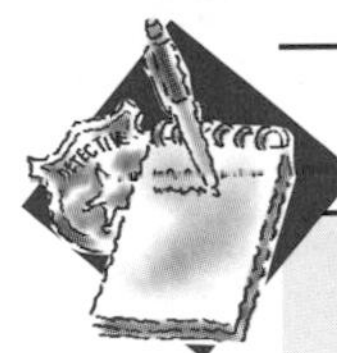

Just the facts

In this chapter, you'll learn:

- ♦ uses of I.V. therapy
- ♦ I.V. delivery methods
- ♦ infusion flow rates
- ♦ legal and professional standards governing use of I.V. therapy
- ♦ patient teaching regarding I.V. therapy
- ♦ the proper way to document I.V. therapy.

A look at I.V. therapy

One of your most important nursing responsibilities is to administer fluids, medications, and blood products to patients. In I.V. therapy, liquid solutions are introduced directly into the bloodstream.

I.V. therapy is used to:

- restore and maintain fluid and electrolyte balance
- provide medications and chemotherapeutic agents
- transfuse blood and blood products
- deliver parenteral nutrients and nutritional supplements.

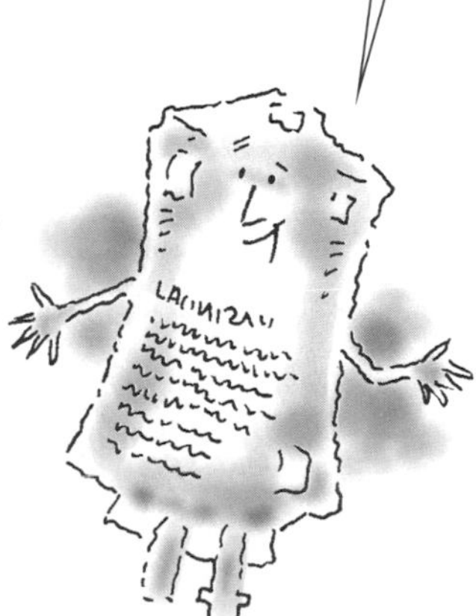

Benefits of I.V. therapy

I.V. therapy has great benefits. For example, it can be used to administer fluids, drugs, nutrients, and other solutions when a patient is unable to take oral substances.

On target and fast

I.V. drug delivery also allows more accurate dosing. Because the entire amount of a drug given I.V. reaches the bloodstream immediately, the drug begins to act almost instantaneously.

Risks of I.V. therapy

Like other invasive procedures, I.V. therapy has its downside. Risks include bleeding, blood vessel damage, fluid overload, infiltration (infusion of the I.V. solution into surrounding tissues rather than the blood vessel), infection, overdose (because response to I.V. drugs is more rapid), incompatibility when drugs and I.V. solutions are mixed, and adverse or allergic responses to infused substances.

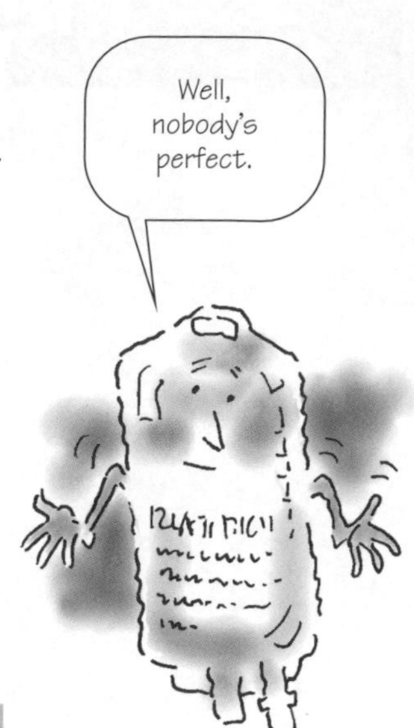

Strings attached

Patient activity can also be problematic. Simple tasks, such as transferring to a chair, ambulating, and washing oneself, can become complicated when the patient must cope with I.V. poles, I.V. lines, and dressings.

No such thing as a free lunch — or I.V.!

Finally, I.V. therapy is more costly than oral, subcutaneous, or intramuscular methods of delivering medications.

Fluids, electrolytes, and I.V. therapy

One of the primary objectives of I.V. therapy is to restore and maintain fluid and electrolyte balance. To understand how I.V. therapy works to restore fluid and electrolyte balance, let's first review some basics of fluids and electrolytes.

We're all wet (well, mostly)

The human body is composed largely of liquid. These fluids account for about 60% of total body weight in an adult who weighs 155 lb (70.5 kg) and about 80% of total body weight in an infant.

Of solvents and solutes

Body fluids are composed of water (a solvent) and dissolved substances (solutes). The solutes in body fluids include electrolytes (such as sodium) and nonelectrolytes (such as proteins).

Fluid functions

What functions do body fluids provide? They:

- help regulate body temperature
- transport nutrients and gases throughout the body
- carry cellular waste products to excretion sites.

Understanding body fluid distribution

Body fluid is distributed between two main compartments—extracellular and intracellular. Extracellular fluid (ECF) has two components—interstitial fluid (ISF) and intravascular fluid (plasma). This illustration shows body fluid distribution for a 155-lb (70.5-kg) adult.

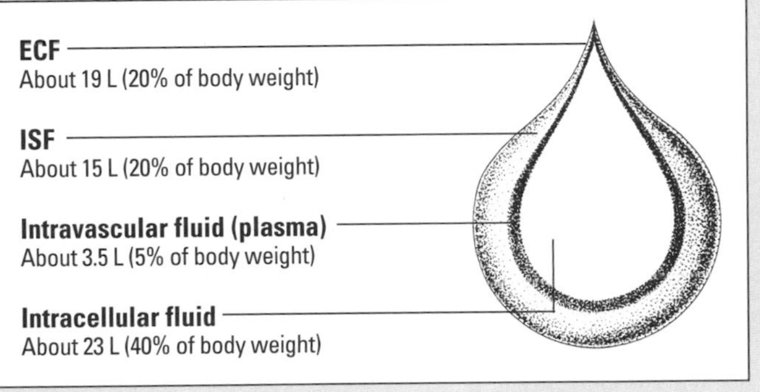

With optimal fluid levels, you're riding a wave of good health!

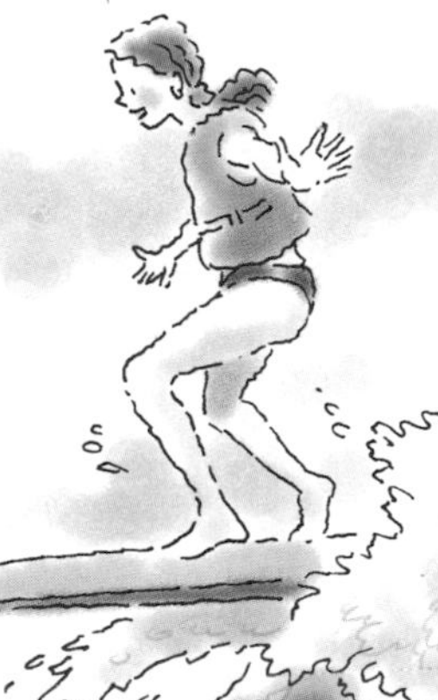

Aim for the optimum

When fluid levels are optimal, the body performs swimmingly; however, when fluid levels deviate from the acceptable range, organs and systems can quickly become congested.

Inside and outside

Body fluids exist in two major compartments: inside the cells and outside the cells. The fluid inside the cells—about 55% of the total body fluid—is called *intracellular fluid* (ICF). The rest is called *extracellular fluid* (ECF). Normally, the distribution of fluids between the two compartments is constant. (See *Understanding body fluid distribution.*)

The ABCs of ECF

ECF occurs in two forms: interstitial fluid (ISF) and intravascular fluid. ISF surrounds each cell of the body; even bone cells are bathed in it. Intravascular fluid is blood plasma, the liquid component of blood. It surrounds red blood cells (RBCs) and accounts for most of the blood volume.

In an adult, about 5% of body fluid is intravascular ECF; about 15% is interstitial ECF. Part of that interstitial ECF is transcellular fluid, which includes cerebrospinal fluid and lymph. Transcellular fluid contains secretions from the salivary glands, pancreas, liver, and sweat glands.

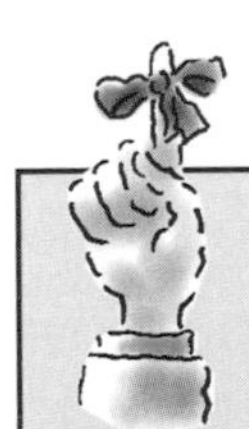

Memory jogger

Remember, when it comes to body fluids, two i's make an e. The two *i's* (intravascular and interstitial fluid) are part of the *e* (extracellular fluid), not the *i* (intracellular fluid).

Daily fluid gains and losses

Each day the body gains and loses fluid through several different processes. The illustration at right shows the main sites involved. The amounts shown apply to adults; infants exchange a greater amount of fluid than adults.

Note: Gastric, intestinal, pancreatic, and biliary secretions total about 8,200 ml. However, because they're almost completely reabsorbed, they aren't usually counted in daily fluid gains and losses.

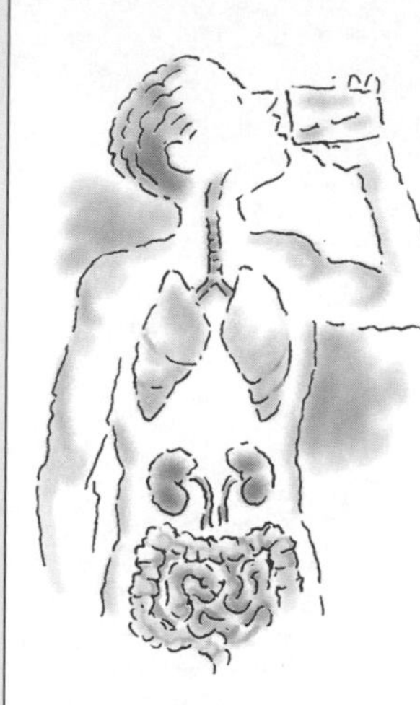

Daily total intake— 2,400 to 3,200 ml
- Liquids—1,400 to 1,800 ml
- Water in foods (solid)— 700 to 1,000 ml
- Water of oxidation (combined water and oxygen in the respiratory system)—300 to 400 ml

Daily total output— 2,400 to 3,200 ml
- Lungs (respiration)— 600 to 800 ml
- Skin (perspiration)— 300 to 500 ml
- Kidneys (urine)— 1,400 to 1,800 ml
- Intestines (feces)— 100 ml

Balancing act

Maintaining fluid balance in the body involves the kidneys, heart, liver, adrenal and pituitary glands, and nervous system. This balancing act is affected by:
- fluid volume
- distribution of fluids in the body
- concentration of solutes in the fluid.

You gain some, you lose some

Every day, the body gains and loses fluid. To maintain fluid balance, the gains must equal the losses. (See *Daily fluid gains and losses.*)

Hormones at work

Fluid volume and concentration are regulated by the interaction of two hormones: antidiuretic hormone (ADH) and aldosterone.

ADH, sometimes referred to as the water-conserving hormone, affects fluid volume and concentration by regulating water retention. It's secreted when plasma osmolarity increases or circulating blood volume decreases and blood pressure drops. Aldosterone acts to retain sodium and water. It's secreted when the serum sodium level is low, the potassium level is high, or the circulating volume of fluid decreases.

Thirst quencher

The thirst mechanism (awareness of the desire to drink) also regulates water volume and participates with hormones in maintaining fluid balance. Thirst is experienced when water loss equals 2% of body weight or when osmolarity (solute concentration) increases. Drinking water restores plasma volume and dilutes ECF osmolarity.

Picking out the baseline

Nurses need to anticipate changes in fluid balance that can occur during I.V. therapy. Therefore, it's important to establish the patient's baseline fluid status before starting fluid replacement therapy. During I.V. therapy, changes in fluid status alert the nurse to impending fluid imbalances. (See *Identifying fluid imbalances*.)

Identifying fluid imbalances

By carefully assessing a patient before and during I.V. therapy, you can identify fluid imbalances early—before serious complications develop. The following assessment findings and test results indicate fluid deficit or excess.

Fluid deficit

- Weight loss
- Increased, thready pulse rate
- Diminished blood pressure, commonly with orthostatic hypotension
- Decreased central venous pressure
- Sunken eyes, dry conjunctivae, decreased tearing
- Poor skin turgor (not a reliable sign in elderly patients)
- Pale, cool skin
- Poor capillary refill (more than 2 seconds)
- Lack of moisture in groin and axillae
- Thirst
- Decreased salivation
- Dry mouth
- Dry, cracked lips
- Furrows in tongue
- Difficulty forming words (patient needs to moisten mouth first)
- Mental status changes
- Weakness
- Diminished urine output
- Increased hematocrit
- Increased serum electrolyte levels
- Increased blood urea nitrogen (BUN) levels
- Increased serum osmolarity

Fluid excess

- Weight gain
- Elevated blood pressure
- Bounding pulse that isn't easily obliterated
- Jugular vein distention
- Increased respiratory rate
- Dyspnea
- Moist crackles or rhonchi on auscultation
- Edema of dependent body parts; sacral edema in patients on bed rest; edema of feet and ankles in ambulatory patients
- Generalized edema
- Puffy eyelids
- Periorbital edema
- Slow emptying of hand veins when the arm is raised
- Decreased hematocrit
- Decreased serum electrolyte levels
- Decreased BUN levels
- Reduced serum osmolarity

Electrolytes

Electrolytes are a major component of body fluids. There are six major electrolytes: sodium, potassium, calcium, chloride, phosphorus, and magnesium.

You'll get a charge outta this

As the name implies, electrolytes are associated with electricity. These vital substances are chemical compounds that dissociate in solution into electrically charged particles called *ions*. Like wiring for the body, the electrical charges of ions conduct current that's necessary for normal cell function. (See *Understanding electrolytes*.)

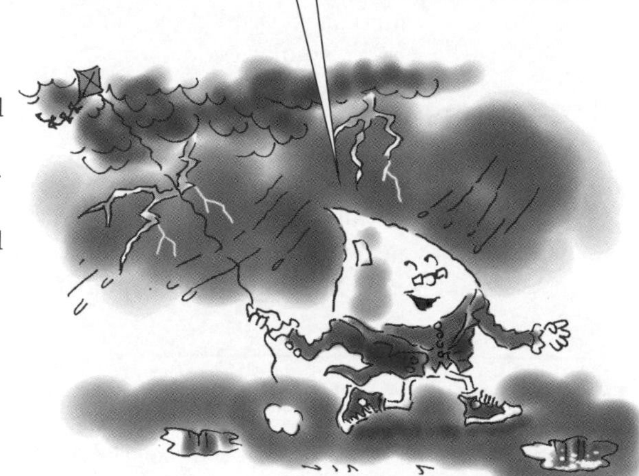

Understanding electrolytes

Six major electrolytes play important roles in maintaining chemical balance: sodium, potassium, calcium, chloride, phosphorus, and magnesium. Electrolyte concentrations are expressed in milliequivalents per liter (mEq/L) and milligrams per deciliter (mg/dl).

Electrolyte	Principal functions	Signs and symptoms of imbalance
Sodium (Na^+) • Major cation in extracellular fluid (ECF) • Normal serum level: 135 to 145 mEq/L	• Maintains appropriate ECF osmolarity • Influences water distribution (with chloride) • Affects concentration, excretion, and absorption of potassium and chloride • Helps regulate acid-base balance • Aids nerve- and muscle-fiber impulse transmission	*Hyponatremia:* fatigue, muscle weakness, muscle twitching, decreased skin turgor, headache, tremor, seizures, coma *Hypernatremia:* thirst, fever, flushed skin, oliguria, disorientation, dry, sticky membranes
Potassium (K^+) • Major cation in intracellular fluid (ICF) • Normal serum level: 3.5 to 5.0 mEq/L	• Maintains cell electroneutrality • Maintains cell osmolarity • Assists in conduction of nerve impulses • Directly affects cardiac muscle contraction • Plays a major role in acid-base balance	*Hypokalemia:* decreased GI, skeletal muscle, and cardiac muscle function; cardiac arrhythmias; decreased reflexes; rapid, weak, irregular pulse; muscle weakness or irritability; fatigue; decreased blood pressure; decreased bowel motility; paralytic ileus *Hyperkalemia:* muscle weakness; nausea; diarrhea; oliguria; paresthesia (altered sensation) of the face, tongue, hands, and feet; cardiac arrhythmias

Understanding electrolytes *(continued)*

Electrolyte	Principal functions	Signs and symptoms of imbalance
Calcium (Ca^{++}) • Major cation found in ECF of teeth and bones • Normal serum level: 8.9 to 10.1 mg/dl	• Enhances bone strength and durability (along with phosphorus) • Helps maintain cell-membrane structure, function, and permeability • Affects activation, excitation, and contraction of cardiac and skeletal muscles • Participates in neurotransmitter release at synapses • Helps activate specific steps in blood coagulation • Activates serum complement in immune system function	*Hypocalcemia:* muscle tremor, muscle cramps, tetany, tonic-clonic seizures, paresthesia, bleeding, arrhythmias, hypotension, numbness or tingling in fingers, toes, and area surrounding the mouth *Hypercalcemia:* lethargy, fatigue, depression, confusion, headache, muscle flaccidity, nausea, vomiting, anorexia, constipation, hypertension, polyuria, cardiac arrhythmias and ECG changes (shortened QT interval and widened T wave)
Chloride (Cl^-) • Major anion found in ECF • Normal serum level: 96 to 106 mEq/L	• Maintains serum osmolarity (along with Na^+) • Combines with major cations to create important compounds, such as sodium chloride (NaCl), hydrogen chloride (HCl), potassium chloride (KCl), and calcium chloride ($CaCl_2$)	*Hypochloremia:* increased muscle excitability, tetany, decreased respirations *Hyperchloremia:* stupor; rapid, deep breathing; muscle weakness
Phosphorus (P) • Major anion found in ICF • Normal serum phosphate level: 2.5 to 4.5 mg/dl	• Helps maintain bones and teeth • Helps maintain cell integrity • Plays a major role in acid-base balance (as a urinary buffer) • Promotes energy transfer to cells • Plays essential role in muscle, red blood cell, and neurologic function	*Hypophosphatemia:* paresthesia (circumoral and peripheral), lethargy, speech defects (such as stuttering or stammering), muscle pain and tenderness *Hyperphosphatemia:* renal failure, vague neuroexcitability to tetany and seizures, arrhythmias and muscle twitching with sudden rise in phosphate level
Magnesium (Mg^{++}) • Major cation found in ICF (closely related to Ca^{++} and P) • Normal serum level: 1.5 to 2.5 mg/dl with 33% bound protein and remainder as free cations	• Activates intracellular enzymes; active in carbohydrate and protein metabolism • Acts on myoneural vasodilation • Facilitates Na^+ and K^+ movement across all membranes • Influences Ca^{++} levels	*Hypomagnesemia:* dizziness, confusion, seizures, tremor, leg and foot cramps, hyperirritability, arrhythmias, vasomotor changes, anorexia, nausea *Hypermagnesemia:* drowsiness, lethargy, coma, arrhythmias, hypotension, vague neuromuscular changes (such as tremor), vague GI symptoms (such as nausea), peripheral vasodilation, facial flushing, sense of warmth, slow, weak pulse

Fluid and electrolyte balance

Fluids and electrolytes are usually discussed in tandem, especially where I.V. therapy is concerned, because fluid balance and electrolyte balance are interdependent. Any change in one alters the other, and any solution given I.V. can affect a patient's fluid and electrolyte balance.

Electrolyte balance

Not all electrolytes are distributed evenly. The major intracellular electrolytes are:

- potassium
- phosphorus.

The major extracellular electrolytes are:

- sodium
- chloride.

ICF and ECF contain different electrolytes because the cell membranes separating the two compartments have selective permeability—that is, only certain ions can cross those membranes. Although ICF and ECF contain different solutes, the concentration levels of the two fluids are about equal when balance is maintained.

I practice selective permeability. Some electrolytes get through my membranes and some don't.

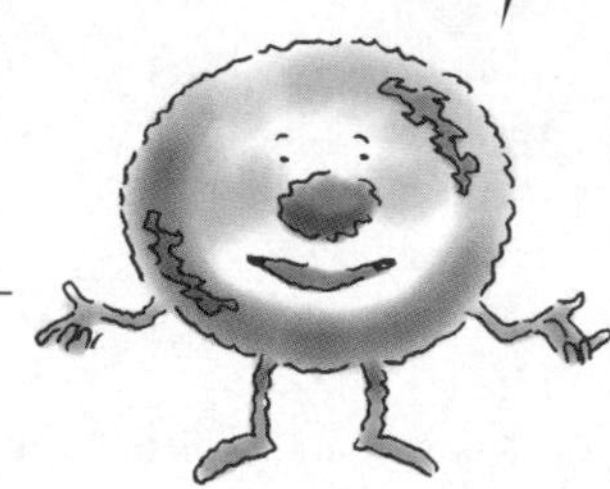

Extra(cellular) credit

The two ECF components—ISF and intravascular fluid (plasma)—have identical electrolyte compositions. Pores in the capillary walls allow electrolytes to move freely between the ISF and plasma, allowing for equal distribution of electrolytes in both substances.

The protein contents of ISF and plasma differ, however. ISF doesn't contain proteins because protein molecules are too large to pass through capillary walls. Plasma has a high concentration of proteins.

Fluid movement

Fluid movement is another mechanism that regulates fluid and electrolyte balance.

Ebb and flow

Body fluids are in constant motion; although separated by membranes, they continually move between the major fluid compartments. In addition to regulating fluid and electrolyte balance, this movement is how nutrients, waste products, and other substances get into and out of cells, organs, and systems.

Fluid movement is influenced by membrane permeability and colloid osmotic and hydrostatic pressures. Balance is maintained when solute and fluid molecules are distributed evenly on each side of the membrane. When this scale is tipped, these molecules are able to restore balance by crossing membranes as needed.

Solute and fluid molecules have several modes for moving through membranes. Solutes move between compartments mainly by:

- diffusion (passive transport)
- active transport.

Fluids (such as water) move between compartments by:

- osmosis
- capillary filtration and reabsorption.

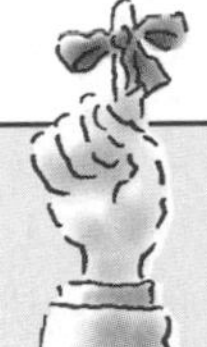

Memory jogger

Remember, diffusion is a descender; active transport is an ascender.

Diffusion descends (high to low)

In **d**iffusion, molecules **descend** the concentration gradient. Movement is from an area of **higher** concentration to one of **lower** concentration.

Active transport ascends (low to high)

In **a**ctive transport, molecules **ascend** against the gradient. Movement is from an area of **lower** concentration to an area of **higher** concentration, as if **a**scending.

Passive is popular

Most solutes move by diffusion—that is, their molecules move from areas of higher concentration to areas of lower concentration. This change is referred to as "moving down the concentration gradient." The result is an equal distribution of solute molecules. Because diffusion doesn't require energy, it's considered a form of passive transport.

Moving against the gradient

By contrast, in active transport, molecules move from areas of lower concentration to areas of higher concentration. This change, referred to as "moving against the concentration gradient," requires energy in the form of adenosine triphosphate.

In active transport, molecules are moved by physiologic pumps. You're probably familiar with one active transport pump—the sodium-potassium pump. It moves sodium ions out of cells to the ECF and potassium ions into cells from the ECF. This pump balances sodium and potassium concentrations.

Oh, osmosis

Fluids (particularly water) move by osmosis. Movement of water is caused by the existence of a concentration gradient. Water flows passively across the membrane, from an area of higher water concentration to an area of lower water concentration. This dilution process stops when the solute concentrations on both sides of the membrane are equal.

Osmosis between ECF and ICF depends on the osmolarity (concentration) of the compartments. Normally, the osmotic (pulling) pressures of ECF and ICF are equal.

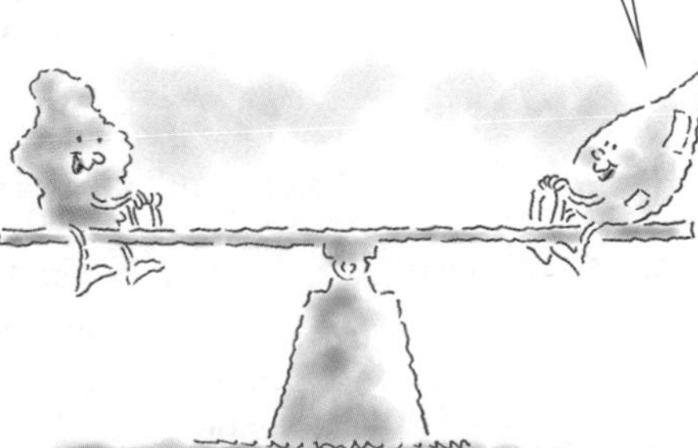

Equal, yet unbalanced

Osmosis can create a fluid imbalance between ECF and ICF compartments, despite equal concentrations of solute, if the concentrations aren't optimal. This imbalance can cause complications such as tissue edema.

Aren't I
special? Only
capillaries like me have
walls thin enough to
let solutes pass.

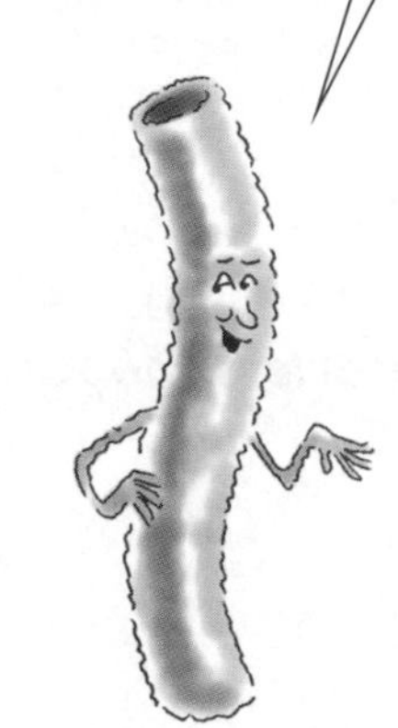

Up against the capillary wall

Of all the vessels in the vascular system, only capillaries have walls thin enough to let solutes pass. Water and solutes move across capillary walls by two opposing processes:

- capillary filtration
- capillary reabsorption.

From high to low

Filtration is the movement of substances from an area of high hydrostatic pressure to an area of lower hydrostatic pressure. (Hydrostatic pressure is the pressure at any level on water at rest due to the weight of water above it.) Capillary filtration forces fluid and solutes through capillary wall pores and into the ISF.

Left unchecked, capillary filtration would cause plasma to move in only one direction — out of the capillaries. This movement would cause severe hypovolemia and shock.

Reabsorption to the rescue

Fortunately, capillary reabsorption keeps capillary filtration in check. During filtration, albumin (a protein that can't pass through capillary walls) remains behind in the diminishing volume of water. As the albumin concentration inside the capillaries increases, the albumin begins to draw water back in by osmosis. Water is thus reabsorbed by capillaries.

May the force be with you

The osmotic, or pulling, force of albumin in capillary reabsorption is called *colloid osmotic pressure* or *oncotic pressure*. As long as capillary blood pressure exceeds colloid osmotic pressure, water and diffusible solutes can leave the capillaries and circulate into the ISF. When capillary blood pressure falls below colloid osmotic pressure, water and diffusible solutes return to the capillaries.

And albumin
like me has a lot of pull
around here in the
capillary system. They
even have a fancy
name for it — colloid
osmotic pressure!

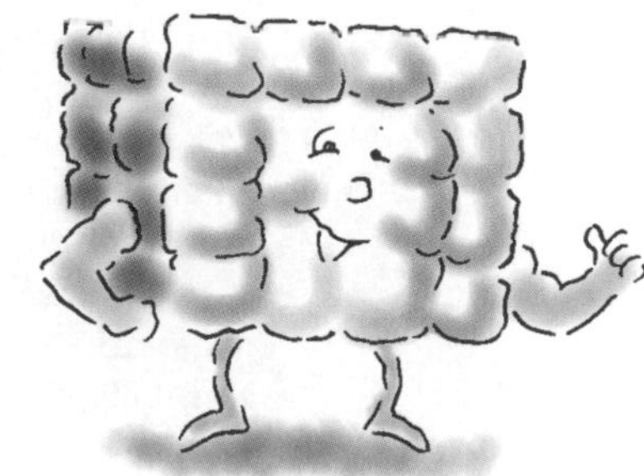

Pressure points

In any capillary, blood pressure normally exceeds colloid osmotic pressure up to the vessel's midpoint, and then falls below colloid osmotic pressure along the rest of the vessel. That's why capillary filtration takes place along the first half of a capillary and reabsorption occurs along the second half. As long as capillary blood pressure and plasma albumin levels remain normal, no net movement of water occurs. Water is equally lost and gained in this process.

Correcting imbalances

The effect an I.V. solution has on fluid compartments depends on the solution's osmolarity compared with serum osmolarity.

Osmolarity at parity?

Osmolarity is the concentration of a solution. It's expressed in milliosmols of solute per liter of solution (mOsm/L). Normally, serum has the same osmolarity as other body fluids, about 300 mOsm/L. A lower serum osmolarity suggests fluid overload; a higher serum osmolarity suggests hemoconcentration and dehydration.

Bringing back the balance

The doctor may order I.V. solutions to maintain or restore fluid balance. There are three basic types of I.V. solutions:

- isotonic
-  hypotonic
- hypertonic. (See *Understanding I.V. solutions*, page 12.)

A few common solutions can be used to illustrate the role of I.V. therapy in restoring and maintaining fluid and electrolyte balance. (See *Quick guide to I.V. solutions*, page 13.)

An isotonic solution stays where it's infused — inside the blood vessel.

Isotonic solutions

An isotonic solution has the same osmolarity (or tonicity) as serum and other body fluids. Because the solution doesn't alter serum osmolarity, it stays where it's infused — inside the blood vessel (the intravascular compartment). The solution expands this compartment without pulling fluid from other compartments.

One indication for an isotonic solution is hypotension due to hypovolemia. Common isotonic solutions include lactated Ringer's and normal saline.

Understanding I.V. solutions

Solutions used for I.V. therapy may be isotonic, hypotonic, or hypertonic. The type you give a patient depends on whether you want to change or maintain his body fluid status.

Isotonic solution

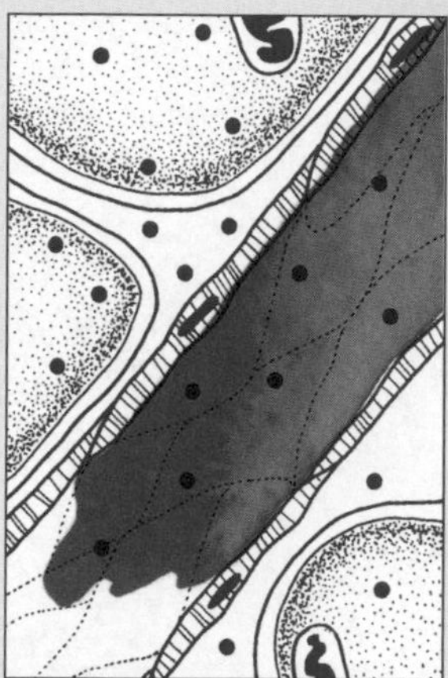

An isotonic solution has an osmolarity about equal to that of serum. Because it stays in the intravascular space, it expands the intravascular compartment.

Hypotonic solution

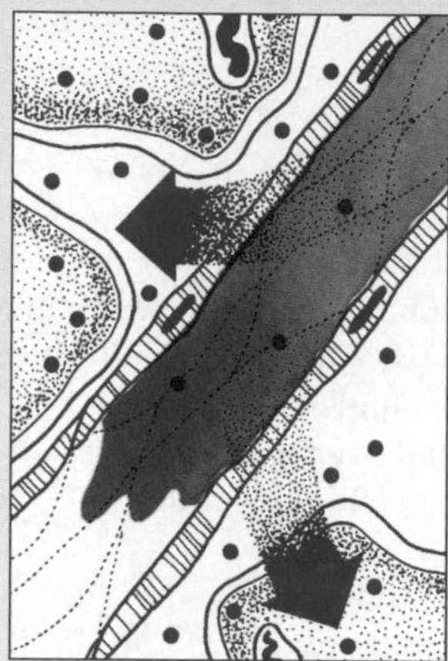

A hypotonic solution has an osmolarity lower than that of serum. It shifts fluid out of the intravascular compartment, hydrating the cells and the interstitial compartments.

Hypertonic solution

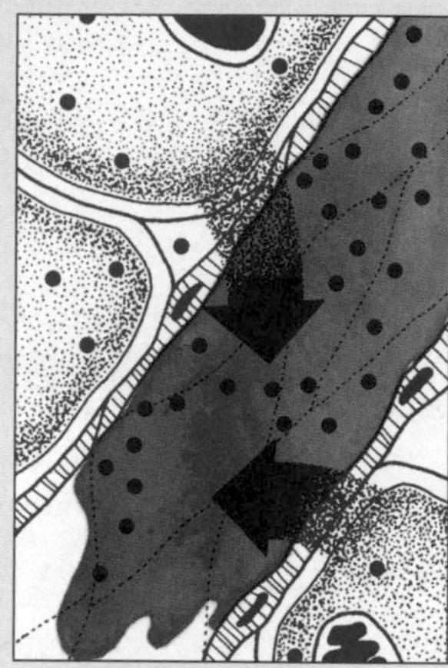

A hypertonic solution has an osmolarity higher than that of serum. It draws fluid into the intravascular compartment from the cells and the interstitial compartments.

Hypertonic solutions

A hypertonic solution has an osmolarity higher than serum osmolarity. When a patient receives a hypertonic I.V. solution, serum osmolarity initially increases, causing fluid to be pulled from the interstitial and intracellular compartments into the blood vessels.

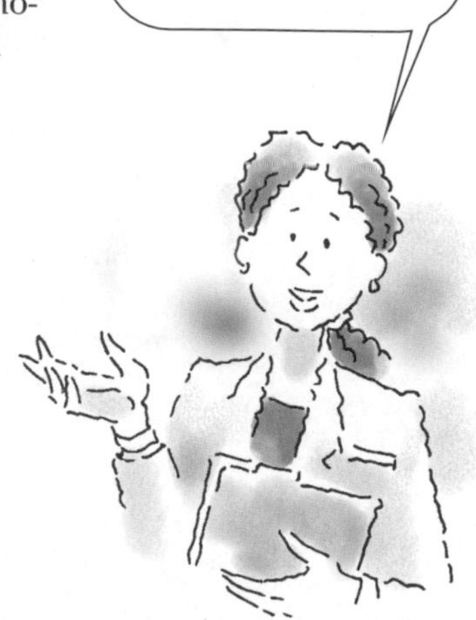

When, why, and how to get hyper

Hypertonic solutions may be ordered for patients postoperatively because the shift of fluid into the blood vessels caused by a hypertonic solution has several beneficial effects for these patients. For example, it:

- reduces the risk of edema
- stabilizes blood pressure
- regulates urine output.

Quick guide to I.V. solutions

A solution is isotonic if its osmolarity falls within (or near) the normal range for serum (240 to 340 mOsm/L). A hypotonic solution has a lower osmolarity; a hypertonic solution, a higher osmolarity. This chart lists common examples of the three types of I.V. solutions and provides key considerations for administering them.

Solution	Examples	Nursing considerations
Isotonic	• Lactated Ringer's (275 mOsm/L) • Ringer's (275 mOsm/L) • Normal saline (308 mOsm/L) • Dextrose 5% in water (D_5W) (260 mOsm/L) • 5% albumin (308 mOsm/L) • Hetastarch (310 mOsm/L) • Normosol (295 mOsm/L)	• Because isotonic solutions expand the intravascular compartment, closely monitor the patient for signs of fluid overload, especially if he has hypertension or heart failure. • Because the liver converts lactate to bicarbonate, don't give lactated Ringer's solution if the patient's blood pH exceeds 7.5. • Avoid giving D_5W to a patient at risk for increased intracranial pressure (ICP) because it acts like a hypotonic solution. (Although usually considered isotonic, D_5W is actually isotonic only in the container. After administration, dextrose is quickly metabolized, leaving only water—a hypotonic fluid.)
Hypotonic	• Half-normal saline (154 mOsm/L) • 0.33% sodium chloride (103 mOsm/L) • Dextrose 2.5% in water (126 mOsm/L)	• Administer cautiously. Hypotonic solutions cause a fluid shift from blood vessels into cells. This shift could cause cardiovascular collapse from intravascular fluid depletion and increased ICP from fluid shift into brain cells. • Don't give hypotonic solutions to patients at risk for increased ICP from stroke, head trauma, or neurosurgery. • Don't give hypotonic solutions to patients at risk for third-space fluid shifts (abnormal fluid shifts into the interstitial compartment or a body cavity)—for example, patients suffering from burns, trauma, or low serum protein levels from malnutrition or liver disease.
Hypertonic	• Dextrose 5% in half-normal saline (406 mOsm/L) • Dextrose 5% in normal saline (560 mOsm/L) • Dextrose 5% in lactated Ringer's (575 mOsm/L) • 3% sodium chloride (1,025 mOsm/L) • 25% albumin (1,500 mOsm/L) • 7.5% sodium chloride (2,400 mOsm/L)	• Because hypertonic solutions greatly expand the intravascular compartment, administer them by I.V. pump and closely monitor the patient for circulatory overload. • Hypertonic solutions pull fluid from the intracellular compartment, so don't give them to a patient with a condition that causes cellular dehydration—for example, diabetic ketoacidosis. • Don't give hypertonic solutions to a patient with impaired heart or kidney function—his system can't handle the extra fluid.

For more information on I.V. solutions, see pages C1 to C4.

Some examples of hypertonic solutions are dextrose 5% in half-normal saline (405 mOsm/L), dextrose 5% in normal saline (560 mOsm/L), and dextrose 5% in lactated Ringer's (527 mOsm/L).

Hypotonic solutions

A hypotonic solution has an osmolarity lower than serum osmolarity. When a patient receives a hypotonic solution, fluid shifts out of the blood vessels and into the cells and interstitial spaces, where osmolarity is higher. A hypotonic solution hydrates cells while reducing fluid in the circulatory system.

Hypotonic solutions may be ordered when diuretic therapy dehydrates cells. Other indications include hyperglycemic conditions, such as diabetic ketoacidosis and hyperosmolar hyperglycemic nonketotic syndrome. In these conditions, high serum glucose levels draw fluid out of cells. Examples of hypotonic solutions include half-normal saline, 0.33% sodium chloride, dextrose 2.5% in water, and dextrose 2.5%.

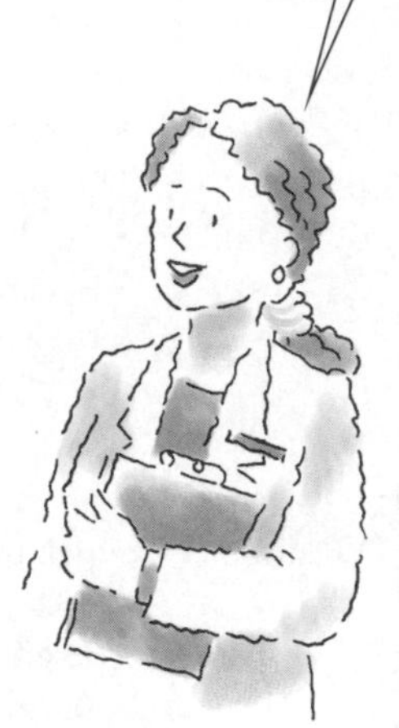

Flood warning

Because hypotonic solutions flood cells, certain patients shouldn't receive them. For example, patients with cerebral edema or increased intracranial pressure shouldn't receive hypotonic solutions because the increased ECF can cause further edema and tissue damage.

Additional uses of I.V. therapy

In addition to restoring and maintaining fluid and electrolyte balance, I.V. therapy is used to administer drugs, transfuse blood and blood products, and deliver parenteral nutrition.

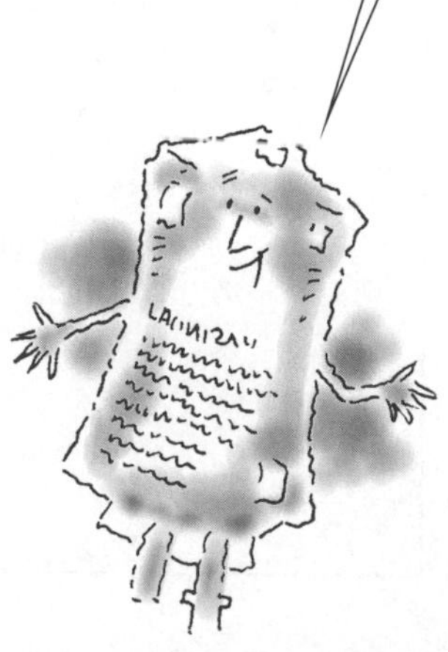

Drug administration

The I.V. route provides a rapid, effective way of administering medications. Commonly infused drugs include antibiotics, thrombolytics, histamine-receptor antagonists, and antineoplastic, cardiovascular, and anticonvulsant drugs.

Drugs may be delivered long-term by continuous infusion, over a short period, or as a single dose.

Blood administration

Your nursing responsibilities may include giving blood and blood components and monitoring patients receiving transfusion therapy. Blood products can be given through a peripheral I.V. catheter or central venous access device. Various blood products are given to:

- restore and maintain adequate circulatory volume
- prevent cardiogenic shock
- increase the blood's oxygen-carrying capacity
- maintain hemostasis.

Parts of the whole

Whole blood is composed of cellular elements and plasma. Cellular elements include:

- erythrocytes, or RBCs
- leukocytes, or white blood cells
- thrombocytes, or platelets.

Each of these elements is packaged separately for transfusion. Plasma may be delivered intact or separated into several components that may be given to correct various deficiencies. Whole blood transfusions are unnecessary unless the patient has lost massive quantities of blood (25% to 30%) in a short period.

Parenteral nutrition

Parenteral nutrition provides essential nutrients to the blood, organs, and cells by the I.V. route. It isn't the same as a seven-course meal in a fine restaurant, but parenteral nutrition can contain the essence of a balanced diet.

TPN is a customized blend that provides all of a patient's energy and nutrient requirements.

It isn't gourmet, but it has all you need...

Total parenteral nutrition (TPN) is customized for each patient. The ingredients in solutions developed for TPN are designed to meet a patient's energy and nutrient requirements:

- proteins
- carbohydrates
- fats
- electrolytes
- vitamins
- trace elements
- water.

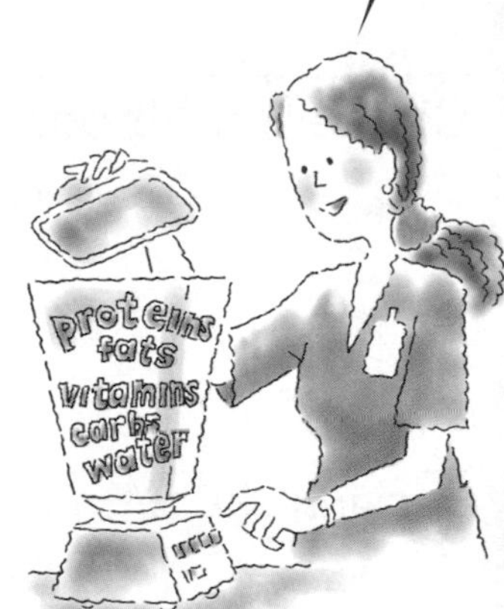

Time for TPN?

TPN should be used only when the gut is unable to absorb nutrients. A patient can receive TPN indefinitely; however, long-term TPN can cause liver damage.

A limited menu

Peripheral parenteral nutrition (PPN) is delivered by peripheral veins. PPN is used in limited nutritional therapy. The solution contains fewer nonprotein calories and lower amino acid concentrations than TPN solutions. It may also include lipid emulsions. A patient can receive PPN for approximately 3 weeks. It can be used to support the nutritional status of a patient who doesn't require total nutritional support. Complications associated with PPN include risk of vein damage, infiltration, and fluid overload.

Tracking changes

When the patient is receiving parenteral nutrition, keep close track of changes in his fluid and electrolyte status and glucose levels. You'll also need to assess his response to the nutrient solution to detect early signs of complications such as alterations in the pancreatic enzymes (lipase, amylase trypsin, and chymotrypsin), triglycerides, or albumin.

I.V. delivery

Depending in part on how concentrated an I.V. solution is, it may be delivered through one of two routes: a peripheral vein or a central vein.

Usually, a low-concentration solution is infused through a peripheral vein in the arm or hand; a more concentrated solution must be given through a central vein. (See *Veins used in I.V. therapy.*) Medications or fluids that may be administered centrally include:

- those with a pH less than 5 or greater than 9
- those with an osmolarity greater than 500 mOsm/L
- parenteral nutrition formulas containing more than 10% dextrose or more than 50% protein
- continuous vesicant chemotherapy (chemotherapy that's toxic to tissues).

Delivery methods

There are three basic methods for delivering I.V. therapy:

 continuous infusion

 intermittent infusion

 direct injection.

Setting the terms

Continuous I.V. therapy allows you to give a carefully regulated amount of fluid over a prolonged period. In intermittent I.V. therapy, a solution (commonly a medication such as an antibiotic) is given for shorter periods at set intervals. Direct injection (sometimes called I.V. push) is used to deliver a single dose (bolus) of a drug.

Veins used in I.V. therapy

This illustration shows the veins commonly used for peripheral and central venous therapy.

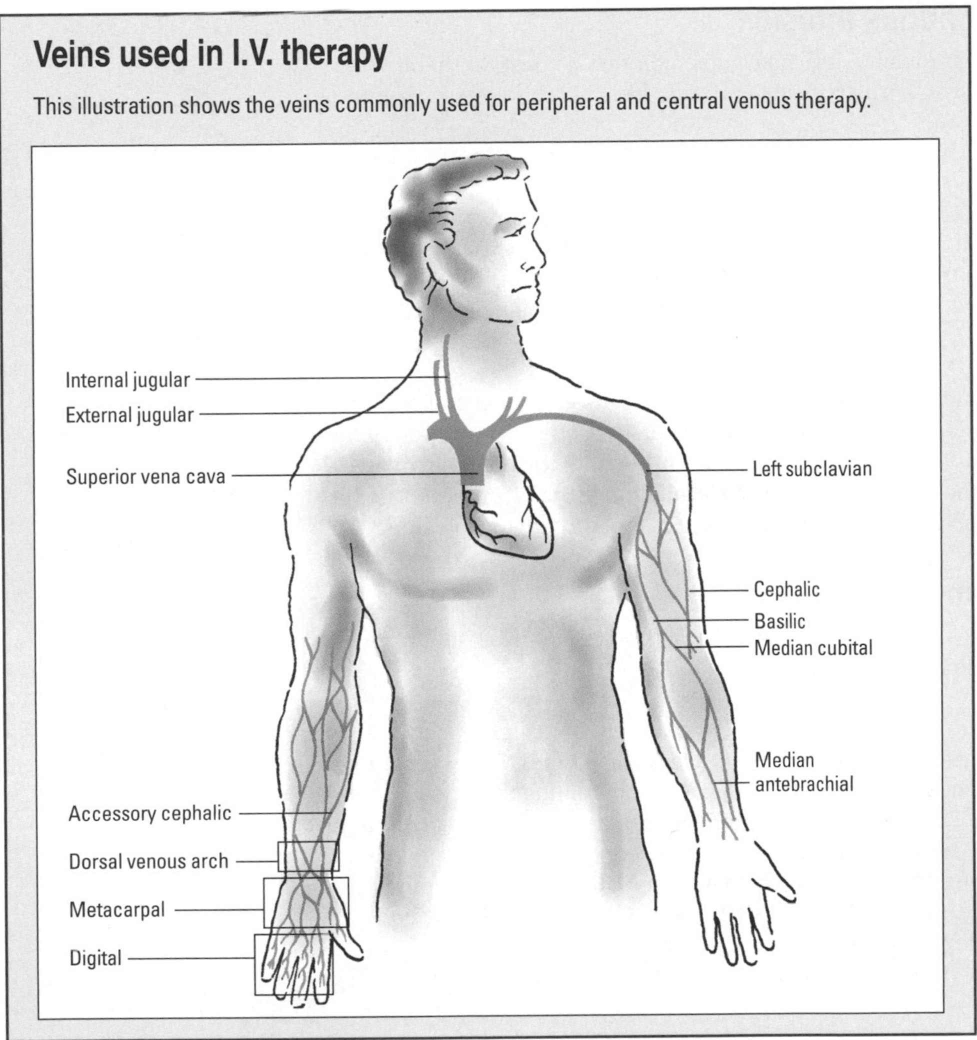

Making the right choice

The choice of I.V. delivery method depends on the purpose and duration of therapy as well as the patient's condition, age, and health history.

At times, a patient may receive I.V. therapy by more than one delivery method. Also, variations of each delivery method may be used. Some therapies require extra equipment. For example, in some long-term chemotherapy, an implanted central venous access device is needed.

Continuous infusion

A continuous I.V. infusion helps maintain a constant therapeutic drug level. It's also used to provide I.V. fluid therapy or parenteral nutrition.

Upside...

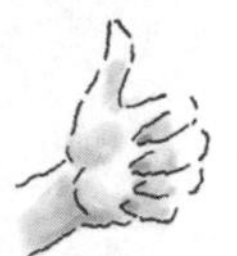

Continuous I.V. infusion has its advantages. For example, less time is spent mixing solutions and hanging containers than with the intermittent method. You'll also handle less tubing and access the patient's I.V. device less often, decreasing the risk of infection.

...and downside

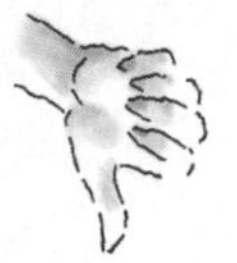

Continuous administration has some disadvantages, too. For example, the patient may become distressed if the equipment hinders mobility and interferes with other activities of daily living. Also, the drip rate must be carefully monitored to ensure that the I.V. fluid and medication don't infuse too rapidly or too slowly.

I can be flexible. Use intermittent infusion to administer drugs over short periods at varying intervals.

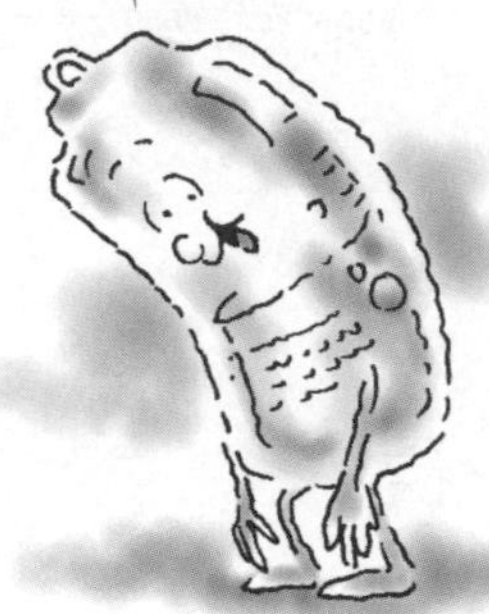

Intermittent infusion

The most common and flexible method of administering I.V. medications is by intermittent infusion.

On again, off again

In intermittent infusion, drugs are administered over a specified period at varying intervals, thereby maintaining therapeutic blood levels. The volume may be delivered over several minutes or a few hours, depending on the infusion prescription. You can deliver an intermittent infusion through a primary line (the most common method) or secondary line. The secondary line is usually connected or piggybacked into the primary line by way of a Y-site (a Y-shaped section of tubing with a self-sealing access port).

Direct injection

You might say that I.V. therapy by direct injection gets right to the point. You give a direct injection through an intermittent infusion device (called a heparin or saline lock) that's already in place. A direct injection may also be administered using a Y-port on I.V. tubing and injecting the drug into the solution.

Administration sets

You need to choose the correct administration set for the patient's infusion. Your choice depends on the type of infusion to be provided, the infusion container, and whether you're using a volume-control device.

Vented and unvented

I.V. administration sets come in two forms: vented and unvented. The vented set is for containers that have no venting system (I.V. plastic bags and some bottles). The unvented set is for compatible bottles that have their own venting system.

Other features and options

I.V. administration sets come with other features as well, including ports for infusing secondary medications and filters for blocking microbes, irritants, or large particles. The tubing also varies. Some types are designed to enhance the proper functioning of devices that help regulate the flow rate. Other tubing is used specifically for continuous or intermittent infusion or for infusing parenteral nutrition and blood.

Some I.V. administration sets come equipped with special tubing to facilitate specific types of infusions.

Infusion flow rates

A key aspect of administering I.V. therapy is maintaining accurate flow rates for the solutions. If an infusion runs too fast or too slow, your patient may suffer complications, such as phlebitis, infiltration, circulatory overload (possibly leading to heart failure and pulmonary edema), and adverse drug reactions.

Volume-control devices and the correct administration set help prevent such complications. You can help as well by being familiar with all of the information in doctors' orders and being able to recognize incomplete or incorrectly written orders for I.V. therapy. (See *Reading an I.V. order.*)

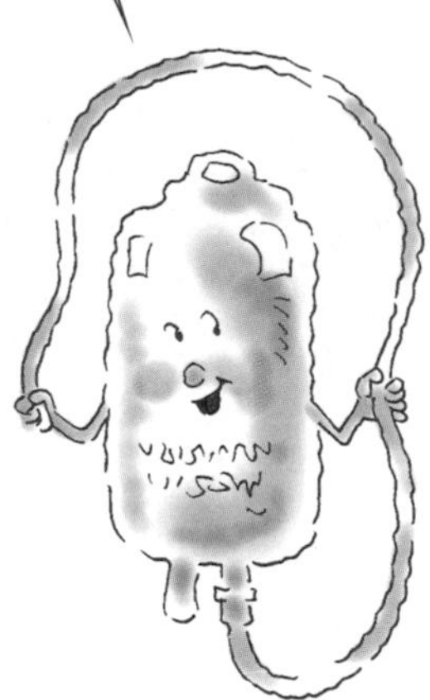

Calculating flow rates

There are two basic types of flow rates available with I.V. administration sets: macrodrip and microdrip. Each set delivers a specific number of drops per milliliter (gtt/ml). Macrodrip delivers 10, 15, or 20 gtt/ml; microdrip delivers 60 gtt/ml. Regardless of the type of set you use, the formula for calculating flow rates is the same. (See *Calculating flow rates*, page 21.)

Regulating flow rates

When a patient's condition requires you to maintain precise I.V. flow rates, use an infusion control device such as:

- clamps
- volumetric pumps
- rate minders.

ml/hour or gtt/minute?

When you regulate I.V. flow rate with a clamp, the rate is usually measured in drops per minute (gtt/minute). If you use a pump, the flow rate is measured in milliliters per hour (ml/hour).

I.V. clamps

You can regulate the flow rate with two types of clamps: slide and roller. The roller clamp is used for standard fluid therapy and is easy to manipulate. The slide clamp can stop or start the flow but can't regulate the rate. (See *Using I.V. clamps*, page 22.)

Pumps

New pumps are being developed all the time; be sure to attend instruction sessions to learn how to use them. On your unit, keep a file of instruction manuals (provided by the manufacturers) for each piece of equipment used.

(Text continues on page 21.)

Reading an I.V. order

Orders for I.V. therapy may be standardized for different illnesses and therapies (such as burn treatment) or individualized for a particular patient. Some facility policies dictate an automatic stop order for I.V. fluids. For example, I.V. orders are good for 24 hours from the time they're written, unless otherwise specified.

It's complete

A complete order for I.V. therapy should specify:

- type and amount of solution
- any additives and their concentrations (such as 10 mEq potassium chloride in 500 ml dextrose 5% in water)
- rate and volume of infusion
- duration of infusion.

When it isn't complete

If you find that an order isn't complete or if you think an I.V. order is inappropriate because of the patient's condition, consult with the practitioner.

Calculating flow rates

When calculating the flow rate (drops per minute) of I.V. solutions, remember that the number of drops required to deliver 1 ml varies with the type of administration set used and its manufacturer:

- Administration sets are of two types—macrodrip (the standard type) and microdrip. Macrodrip delivers 10, 15, or 20 gtt/ml; microdrip usually delivers 60 gtt/ml (see illustrations).
- Manufacturers calibrate their devices differently, so be sure to look for the "drop factor"—expressed in drops per milliliter, or gtt/ml—in the packaging that accompanies the set you're using. (This packaging also has crucial information about such things as special infusions and blood transfusions.)

When you know your device's drop factor, use the following formula to calculate specific flow rates:

$$\frac{\text{volume of infusion (in milliliters)}}{\text{time of infusion (in minutes)}} \times \text{drop factor (in drops per milliliter)} = \text{flow rate (in drops per minute)}$$

After you calculate the flow rate for the set you're using, remove your watch or position your wrist so you can look at your watch and the drops at the same time. Next, adjust the clamp to achieve the ordered flow rate and count the drops for 1 full minute. Readjust the clamp as necessary and count the drops for another minute. Keep adjusting the clamp and counting the drops until you have the correct rate.

Macrodrip

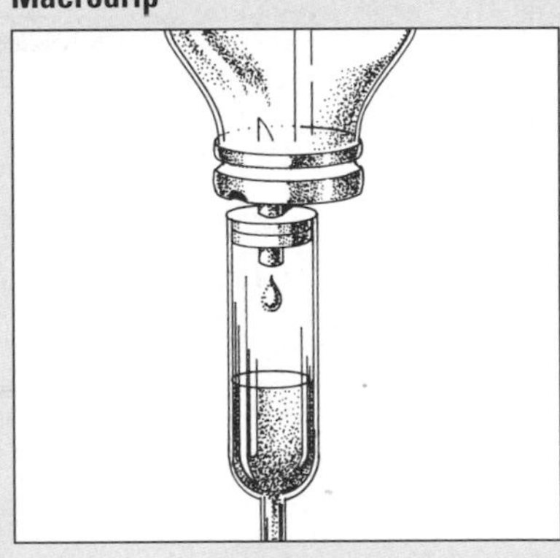

Microdrip

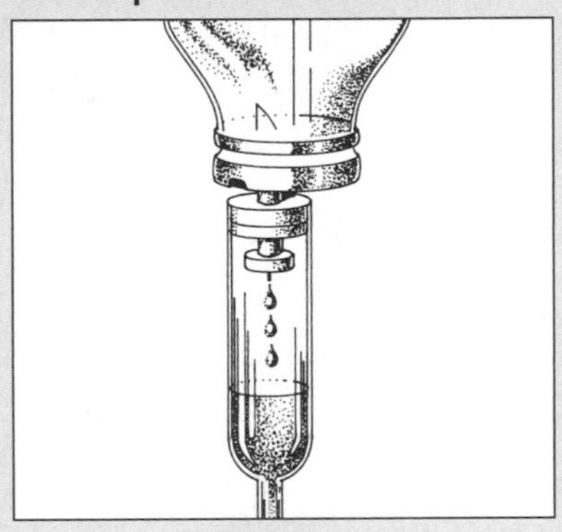

Rate minder

Another type of flow control device is the rate minder, which resembles a roller clamp. This device is added to the I.V. tubing. By setting the rate minder to the desired flow rate, you adjust the clamp to deliver that rate. Be sure to label the infusion bag with the rate in milliliters per hour.

Mind these limitations

Rate minders have some limitations. Because the flow rate may vary by as much as 5%, the infusion must be checked frequently to prevent too-rapid infusion or nonflow situations. The other drawback is that the rate minders usually don't deliver infusions at rates lower than 5 to 10 ml/hour. For this reason, they're used mainly for adult patients and only with noncritical infusions.

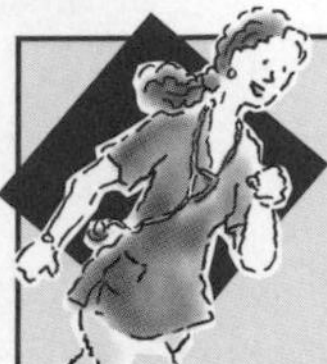

Running smoothly

Using I.V. clamps

You may use a roller clamp to regulate the flow of a solution. With this type of clamp, a wheel increases or decreases the flow rate through the administration site. A slide clamp moves horizontally to open and close the I.V. line. It can stop and start the flow but doesn't allow fine adjustments to regulate the flow. The illustrations below show both types of clamps, with arrows to indicate the direction you turn or push to open the clamp.

Roller clamp

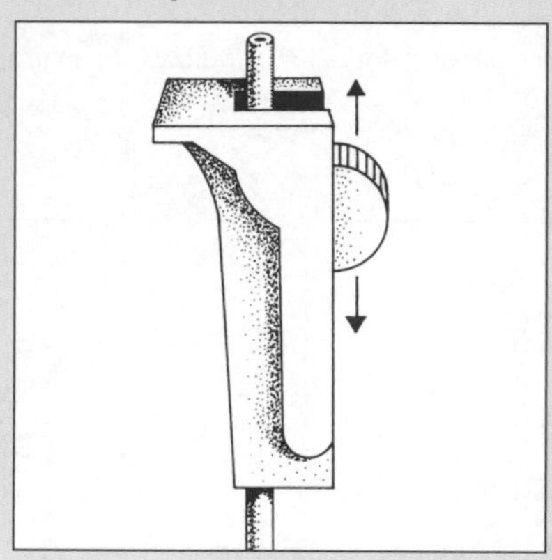

Slide clamp

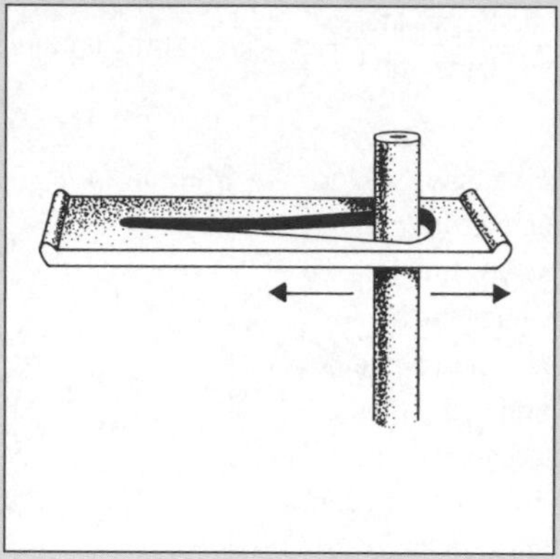

Factor these in

When you're using a clamp for flow regulation, you must monitor the flow rate closely and adjust it as needed. Such factors as vein spasm, vein pressure changes, patient movement, manipulations of the clamp, and bent or kinked tubing can cause the rate to vary markedly. For easy monitoring, use a time tape, which marks the prescribed solution level at hourly intervals. (See *Using a time tape*, page 23.)

Other factors that affect flow rate include the type of I.V. fluid and its viscosity, the height of the infusion container, the type of administration set, and the size and position of the venous access device.

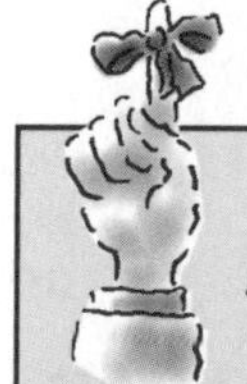

Memory jogger

To remind yourself of the need to check and adjust flow rates, remember the following tongue twister:

Fight fickle flow with frequent follow-up.

Checking flow rates

Flow rates can be fickle; they should be checked and adjusted regularly. The frequency of flow rate checks depends on the patient's condition and age and the solution or medication being administered.

How isotonic solutions affect cells

An isotonic solution has the same solute concentration (or osmolarity) as serum and other body fluids. Infusing the solution doesn't alter the concentration of serum; therefore, osmosis doesn't occur. (For osmosis to occur, there must be a difference in solute concentration between serum and the interstitial fluid.)

The isotonic solution stays where it's infused, inside the blood vessel, and doesn't affect the size of cells.

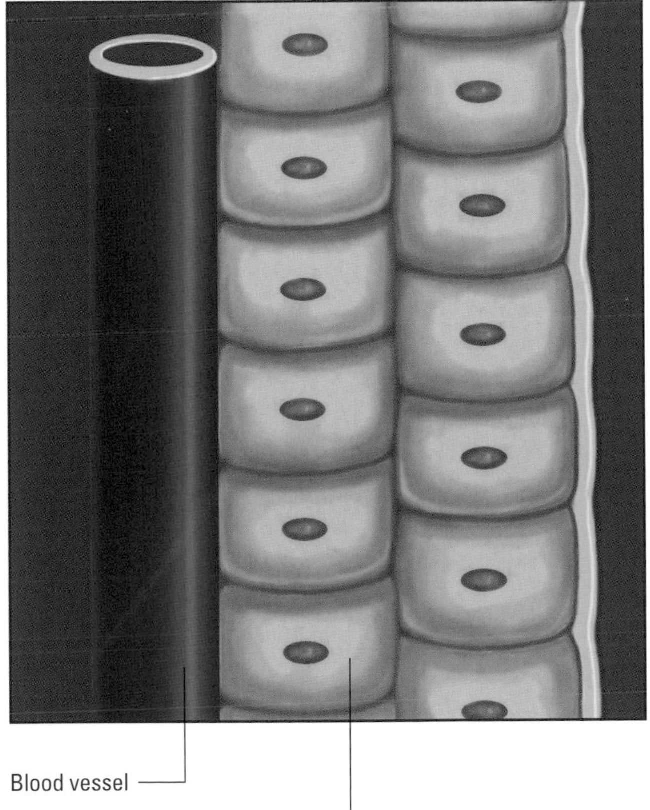

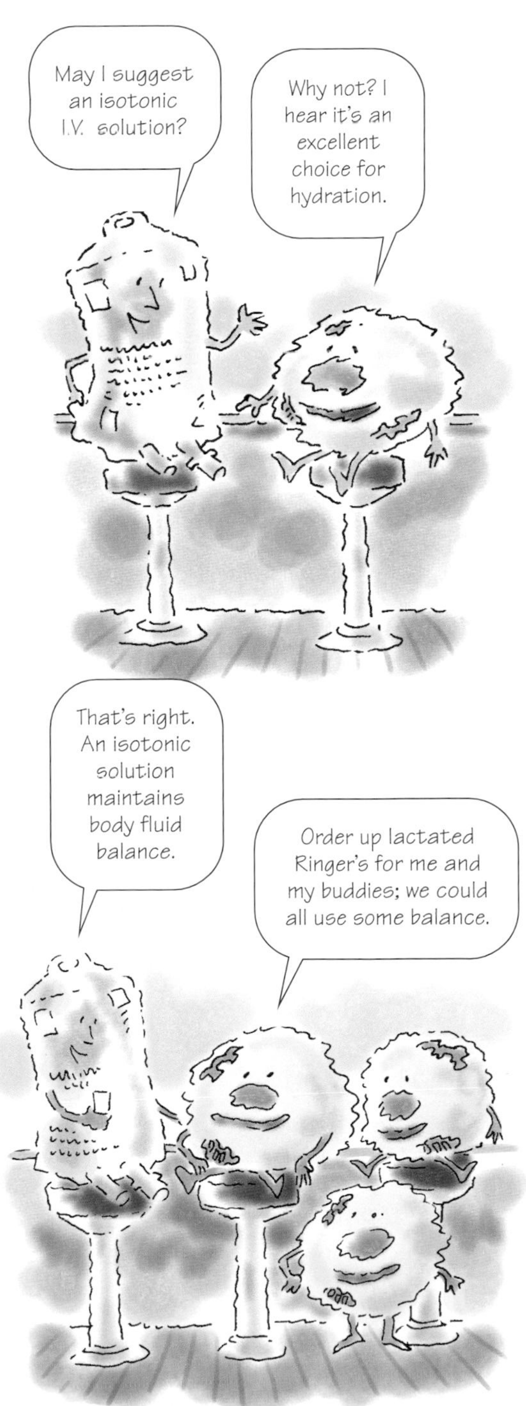

How hypertonic solutions affect cells

A hypertonic I.V. solution has a solute concentration higher than the solute concentration of serum. Infusing a hypertonic solution increases the solute concentration of serum. Because the solute concentration of serum is now different from the interstitial fluid, osmosis occurs. Fluid is pulled from the cells and the interstitial compartment into the blood vessels.

Many patients receive hypertonic fluids postoperatively. The shift of fluid into the blood vessels reduces the risk of edema, stabilizes blood pressure, and regulates urine output.

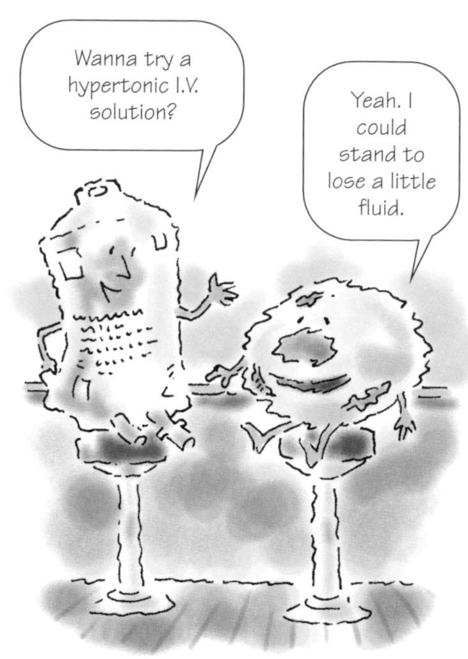

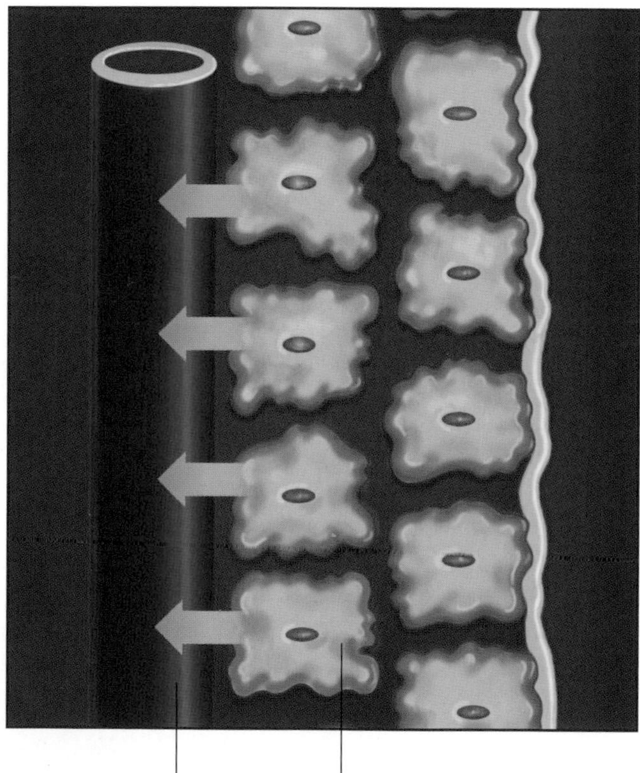

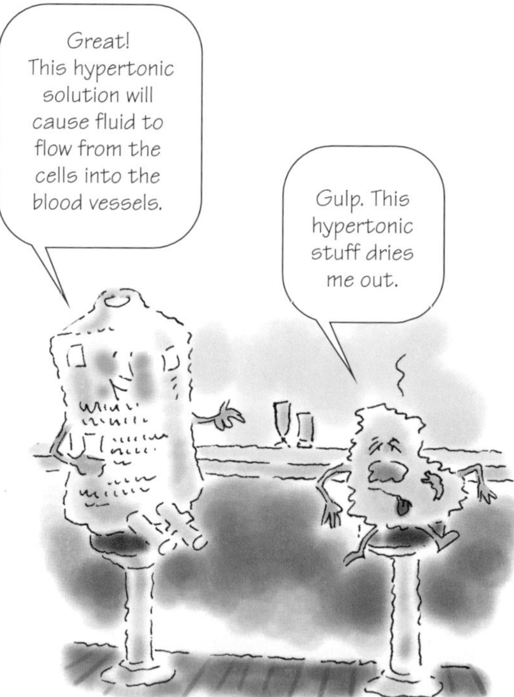

How hypotonic solutions affect cells

A hypotonic I.V. solution is the opposite of a hypertonic solution. It has a lower solute concentration than serum. Infusion of a hypotonic solution causes the solute concentration of serum to decrease. Because the solute concentration of serum is now different from the interstitial fluid, osmosis occurs.

This time, the fluid shift is in the opposite direction than that of a hypertonic fluid. Fluid shifts out of the blood vessels and into the cells and interstitial spaces, where the solute concentration is higher.

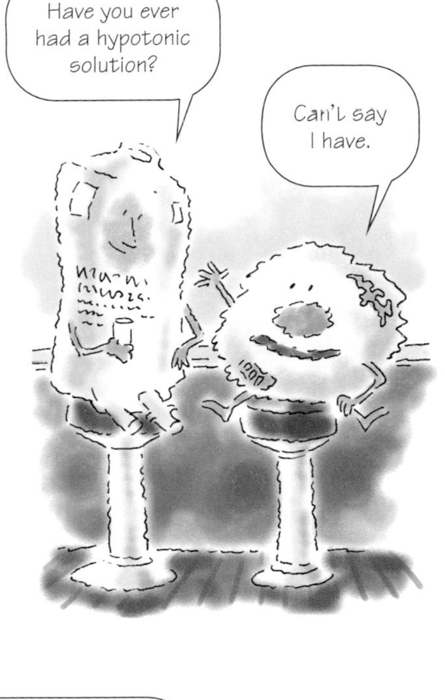

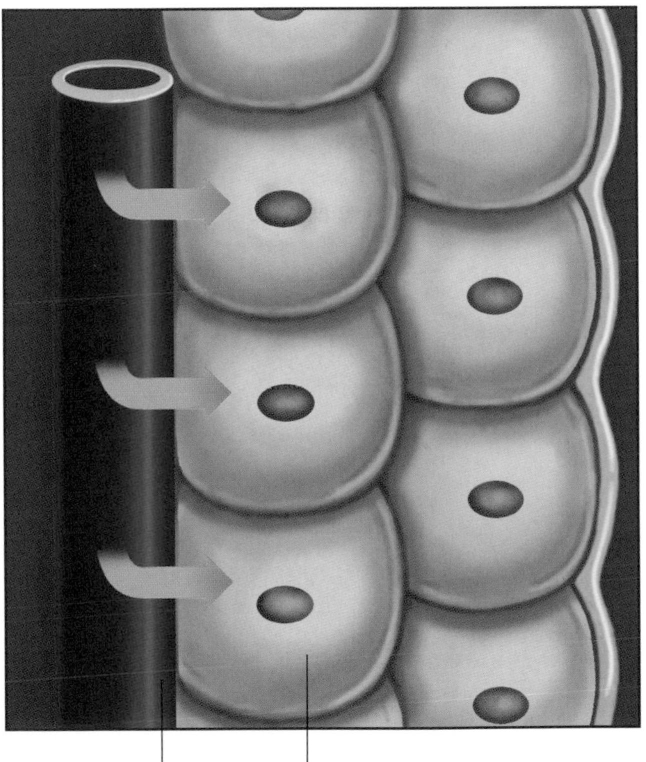

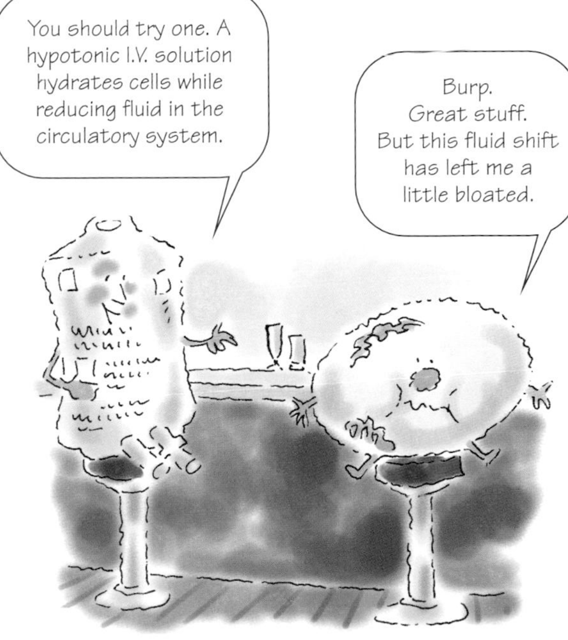

Common catheter insertion sites

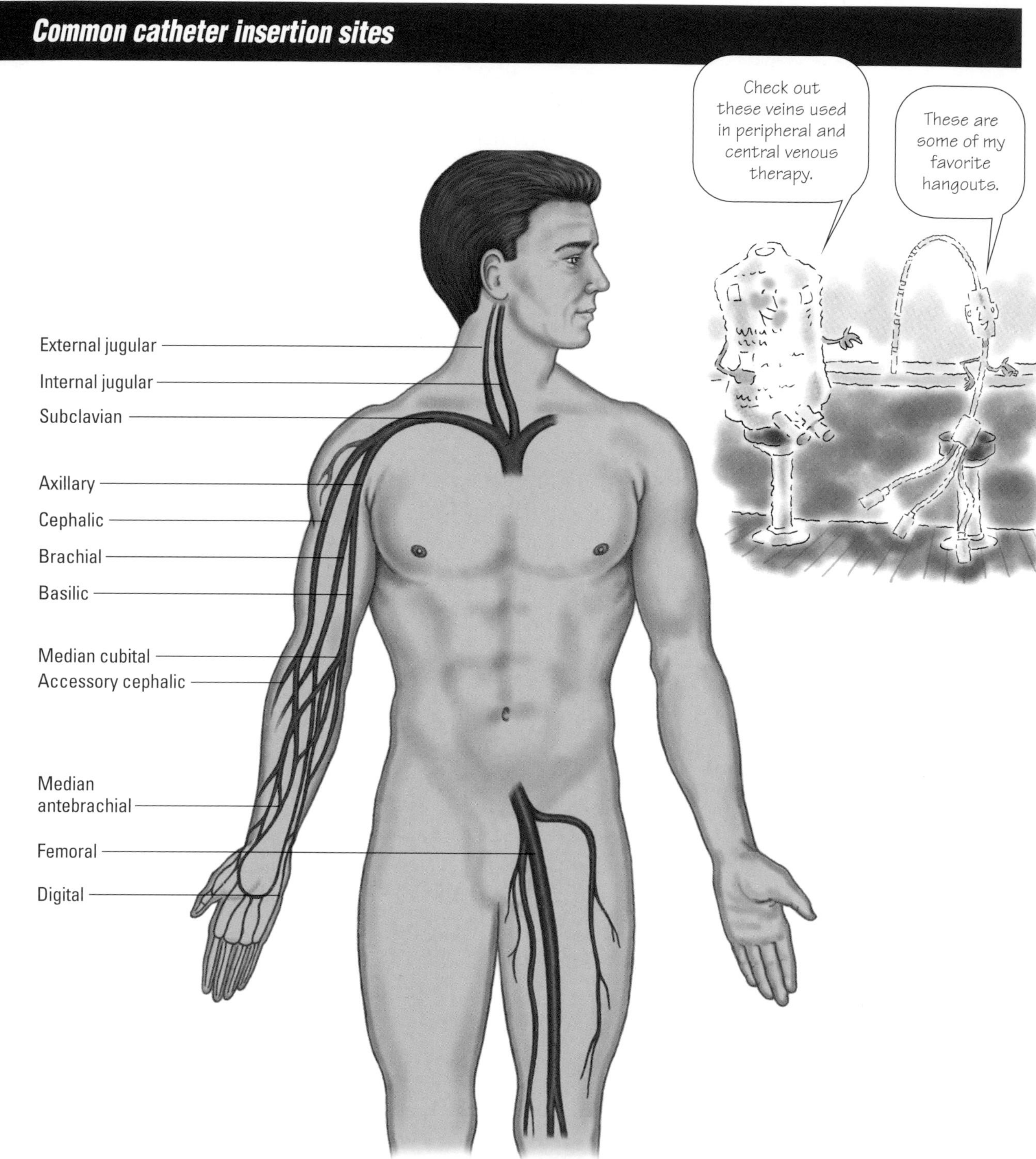

I'll be back soon!

Many nurses check the I.V. flow rate every time they're in a patient's room and after each position change. Flow rate should be assessed more frequently for:

- critically ill patients
- patients with conditions that might be exacerbated by fluid overload
- pediatric patients
- elderly patients
- patients receiving a drug that can cause tissue damage if infiltration occurs.

While you're there

When checking the flow rate, inspect and palpate the I.V. insertion site, and ask the patient how it feels.

Minor (not major) adjustments

If the infusion rate slows significantly, you can usually get it back on schedule by adjusting the rate slightly. Don't make a major adjustment, though. If the rate must be increased by more than 30%, check with the practitioner.

You should also time an infusion control device or rate minder for 1 to 2 hours per shift. (These devices have an error rate ranging from 2% to 10%.) Before using any infusion control device, become thoroughly familiar with its features. Attend instruction sessions and perform return demonstrations until you learn the system.

Using a time tape

Here's a simple way to monitor I.V. flow rate: Attach a piece of tape or a preprinted strip to the I.V. container; then write hourly times on the tape or strip beginning with the time you hung the solution.

By comparing the actual time with the label time, you can quickly see if the rate needs to be adjusted. Remember that you should never increase I.V. rates by more than 30% unless you first check with the practitioner.

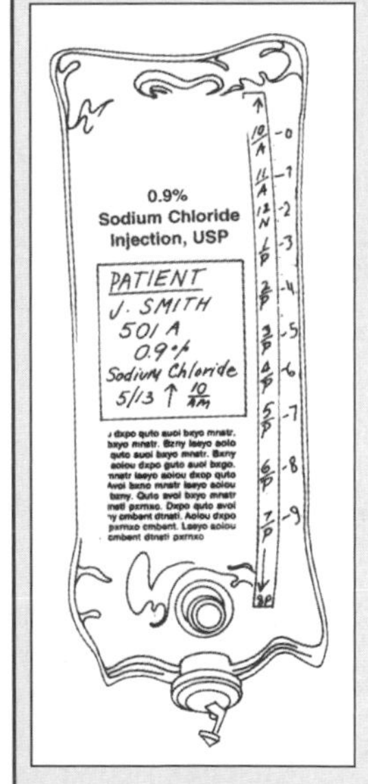

Professional and legal standards

Administering drugs and solutions to patients is one of the most legally significant tasks nurses perform. Unfortunately, the number of lawsuits directed against nurses who are involved in I.V. therapy is increasing. For example, one study reported a high incidence of errors involving I.V. solution administration, in which wrong solutions were used or solutions were administered by an incorrect route. Many lawsuits have centered on errors in infusion pump use.

Lawsuits may also result from administration of the wrong medication dosage, inappropriate placement of an I.V. catheter, and failure to monitor for adverse reactions, infiltration, dislodgment of I.V. equipment, or other mishaps.

Court cases

Mistakes
can be fatal to
your patient
and costly
to your facility.
Be alert!

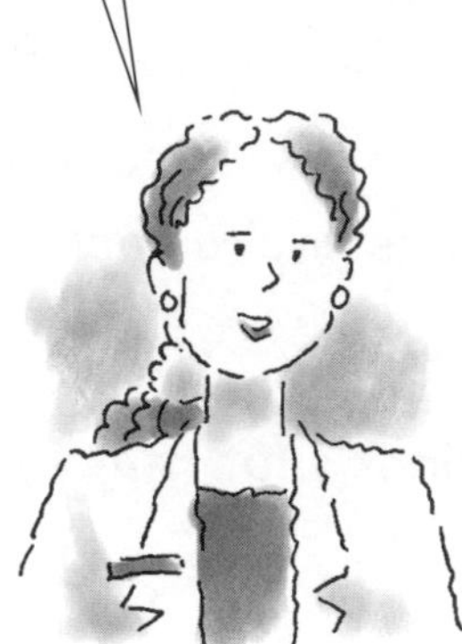

The following are examples of lawsuits involving I.V. therapy.

Midazolam mistake

In Los Angeles, a nurse administered midazolam through a port in an I.V. line to an infant, leading to the infant's death. This nurse had never administered I.V. midazolam to an infant or child before. A facility protocol prohibited the use of midazolam on the pediatric floor. The manufacturer recommended a dosage of 0.1 mg/kg, and the infant weighed 9 kg. The hospital record indicated that 5 mg had been administered. A settlement awarded the plaintiff $225,000.

Still accountable

In another Los Angeles case, continuous infusion of 145 mg of morphine over 18 hours led to a patient's death. The doctor failed to limit the amount to be infused. Nevertheless, the charge nurse and staff nurse were held accountable for failing to recognize a "gross overdose." The patient's widow and children were awarded more than $2 million for lost wages and general damages.

Syringe confusion

In Illinois, a nurse administered the wrong dose of lidocaine (Xylocaine). The order was for 100 mg; the nurse injected 2 g. The packaging caused confusion: the lidocaine was provided in a 2-g syringe for mixing into an I.V. solution and in a 100-mg syringe for direct injection. The nurse accidentally used the 2-g syringe. However, information about previous overdose incidents from the Food and Drug Administration and medical literature had been available to the hospital.

Clamp error

In Ohio, a nurse failed to clamp a pump regulating the flow of an antibiotic through a central venous access device to a child. This resulted in delivery of nearly seven times the prescribed dosage of gentamicin, causing the child to become totally deaf.

Infiltration injury

In Pennsylvania, an emergency department nurse placed an I.V. catheter that infiltrated in the patient's hand, resulting in reflex sympathetic dystrophy. The patient couldn't return to work and won a $702,000 award.

Striking a nerve

Several recent lawsuits have involved allegations that a nurse struck a patient's radial nerve during insertion of an I.V. catheter.

Such injuries can cause compartment syndrome; uncorrected, compartment syndrome can progress to gangrene and amputation of fingers. One New York case involving finger amputation resulted in a $40 million jury verdict, which was later reduced to $5 million.

Don't give all your attention to me — listen to the patient as well!

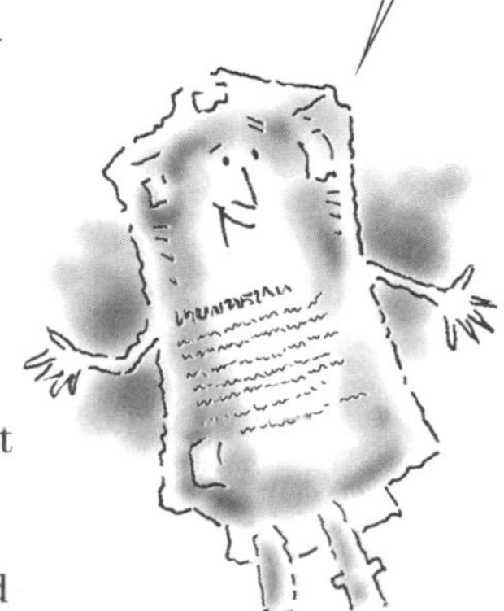

Listen up

When monitoring I.V. therapy, listening to the patient is as important as monitoring the site, pump, and tubing. In the Tampa, Florida, case of *Frank v. Hillsborough County Hospital*, a patient's frequent complaints of pain were ignored. The patient suffered permanent nerve damage and later obtained an award of almost $60,000.

Know your responsibility

As a nurse, you have a legal and ethical responsibility to your patients. The good news is that if you honor these duties and meet the appropriate standards of care, you'll be able to hold your own in court.

By becoming aware of professional standards and laws related to administering I.V. therapy, you can provide the best care for your patients and protect yourself legally. Professional and legal standards are defined by state nurse practice acts, federal regulations, and facility policies.

State nurse practice acts

Each state has a nurse practice act that broadly defines the legal scope of nursing practice. Your state's nurse practice act is the most important law affecting your nursing practice.

Know your limits

Every nurse is expected to care for patients within defined limits. If a nurse gives care beyond those limits, she becomes vulnerable to charges of violating her state nurse practice act. For a copy of your state nurse practice act, contact your state nurse's association or your state board of nursing or access its Web site.

Many states' nurse practice acts don't specifically address scope of practice issues regarding I.V. therapy by registered nurses (RNs). However, many states' nurse practice acts do address whether licensed practical nurses (LPNs) or licensed vocational nurses (LVNs) can administer I.V. therapy. It's important for LPNs and LVNs as well as for the RNs who are supervising or training them to be familiar with this information.

Federal regulations

Don't take chances when it comes to complying with regulatory standards!

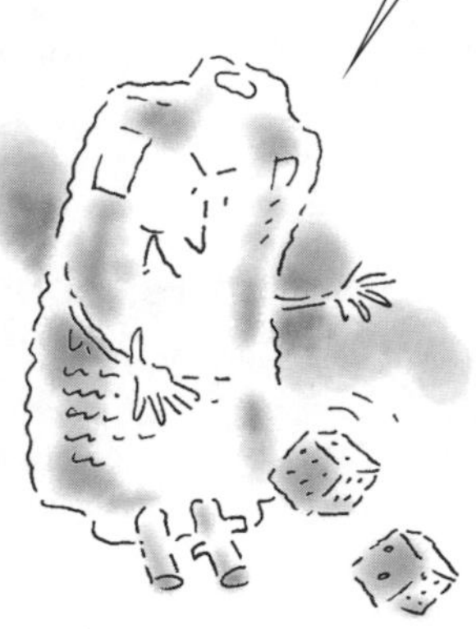

The federal government issues regulations and establishes policies related to I.V. therapy administration. For example, it mandates adherence to standards of I.V. therapy practice for health care facilities so that they can be eligible to receive reimbursement under Medicare, Medicaid, and other programs.

Millions served

Medicare and Medicaid, the two major federal health care programs, serve millions of Americans. They're run by the Centers for Medicare and Medicaid Services (CMS), which is part of the U.S. Department of Health and Human Services. CMS formulates national Medicare policy, including policies related to I.V. therapy, but contracts with private insurance companies to oversee claims and make payment for services and supplies provided under Medicare. These agencies, in turn, enforce CMS policy by accepting or denying claims for reimbursement. When reviewing claims, agencies may evaluate practices and quality of care — an important factor underlying the emphasis on proper documentation in health care.

Medicaid, which serves certain low-income people, is a state-federal partnership administered by a state agency. There are broad federal requirements for Medicaid, but states have a wide degree of flexibility to design their own programs.

One patient, many regulators

To be eligible for reimbursement, health care agencies must comply with the standards of a complex network of regulators. Consider, for example, a patient receiving I.V. medications at home with a reusable pump. This patient is primarily covered by Medicare with secondary Medicaid coverage. Various carriers, fiscal intermediaries, and agencies share responsibility for reimbursement and regulatory oversight of the patient's care:

- An insurance carrier contracts with Medicare to cover such services as refilling the pump.
- A separate insurance carrier (a durable medical equipment carrier designated by CMS) covers administered drugs, the pump, and pump supplies.
- Another insurance carrier (called a *fiscal intermediary*) contracts with Medicare to cover preliminary in-hospital training of the patient in I.V. therapy techniques.
- A Medicaid agency also covers a portion of the patient's care.

Nursing documentation must be complete to meet the requirements of all of these different agencies. The underlying (although unstated) philosophy of these agencies is: "If it isn't documented, it isn't done." The regulatory network is becoming more complicated as many Medicare and Medicaid patients are being covered by managed care organizations that have their own rules and procedures.

Facility policy

Every health care facility has I.V. therapy policies for nurses. Such policies are required to obtain accreditation from The Joint Commission and other accrediting bodies. These policies can't go beyond what a state's nurse practice act permits, but they more specifically define your duties and responsibilities.

Awareness of facility policy is important in all areas of practice because the intensity of service and patient needs is increasing dramatically. For example, home health nurses need to be acutely aware of patient and family education policies because infusion systems are being used in the home 24 hours per day without the presence of full-time nursing staff.

INS — not just about immigration

The Infusion Nurses Society (INS) has developed a set of standards, the *Infusion Nursing Standards of Practice*, that are commonly used by committees developing facility policy. According to the INS, the goals of these standards are to "protect and preserve the patient's right to safe, quality care and protect the nurse who administers infusion therapy." These standards address all aspects of I.V. nursing. For more information, contact the INS at (781) 440-9408 or at *www.ins1.org*.

Documentation

You must document I.V. therapy for several reasons. Proper documentation provides:

- accurate description of care that can serve as legal protection (for example, as evidence that a prescribed treatment was administered)
- mechanism for recording and retrieving information
- record for health care insurers of equipment and supplies used.

Forms, forms, forms

I.V. therapy may be documented on progress notes, a computerized chart, a special I.V. therapy sheet or flow sheet, a nursing care plan on the patient's chart, or an intake and output sheet. I.V. therapy is also commonly recorded on the patient's medication sheet, which provides specifics about the medications used.

Document your I.V. care on the proper forms, such as progress notes, I.V. flow sheets, and the patient's medication sheet.

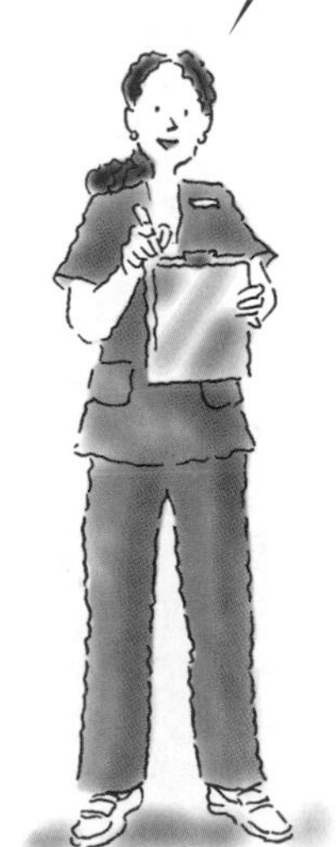

Documenting initiation of I.V. therapy

When documenting the insertion of a venous access device or the beginning of therapy, specify:

- size, length, and type of the device
- name of the person who inserted the device
- date and time
- site location (anatomical vein name preferred)
- type of dressing used
- condition of the site
- type of solution
- any additives
- flow rate
- use of an electronic infusion device or other type of flow controller
- complications, patient response, and nursing interventions
- patient teaching and evidence of patient understanding (for example, ability to explain instructions or perform a return demonstration)
- number of attempts (both successful and unsuccessful).

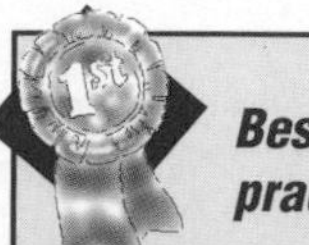

Best practice

How to label a dressing

To label a new dressing over an I.V. site, include:

- date of insertion
- gauge and length of venipuncture device
- date and time of the dressing change
- your initials.

Label that dressing!

In addition to documentation in the patient's chart, you need to label the dressing on the catheter insertion site. Whenever you change the dressing, label the new one. (See *How to label a dressing.*)

You should also label the fluid container and place a time tape on it. With a child, you may need to label the volume-control set as well. In labeling the container and the set, follow your facility's policy and procedures. (See *How to label an I.V. bag.*)

Remember to label your patient's dressing on the catheter insertion site and the I.V. bag of the solution you're infusing.

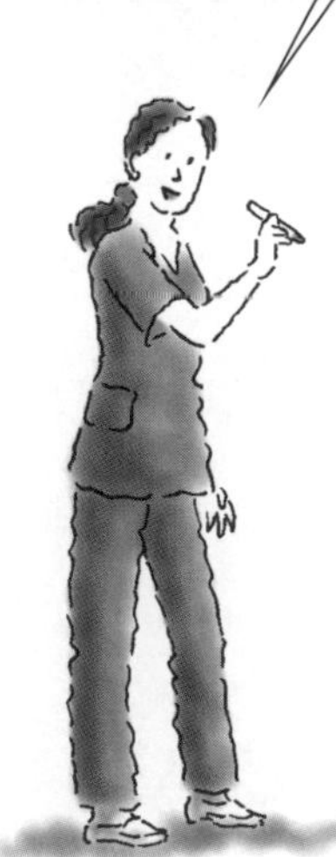

Documenting I.V. therapy maintenance

When documenting I.V. therapy maintenance, specify:

- condition of the site
- site care provided
- dressing changes
- tubing and solution changes
- your teaching and evidence of patient understanding.

Sequential system

One way to document I.V. solutions throughout therapy is to number each container sequentially. For example, if a patient is to receive normal saline solution at 125 ml/hour (3,000 ml/day) on day 1, number the 1,000-ml containers as 1, 2, and 3. If another 3,000 ml is ordered on day 2, number those containers as 4, 5, and 6. This system can help reduce administration errors. Also, check your facility's policy and procedures; some facilities require beginning the count again if the type of fluid changes, whereas others keep the count sequential regardless of the type of fluid.

Flow sheets

Flow sheets highlight specific patient information according to preestablished parameters of nursing care. They have spaces for recording dates, times, and specific interventions. When you use an I.V. flow sheet, record:

- date
- flow rate
- use of an electronic flow device or flow controller
- type of solution
- sequential solution container
- date and time of dressing and tubing changes.

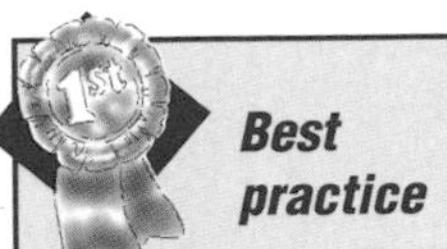

Best practice

How to label an I.V. bag

To properly label an I.V. solution container, include (in addition to the time tape):

- patient's name, identification number, and room number
- date and time the container was hung
- any additives and their amounts
- rate at which the solution is to run
- sequential container number
- expiration date and time of infusion
- your name.

When you place the label on the bag, be sure not to cover the name of the I.V. solution.

Intake and output sheets

When you're documenting I.V. therapy on an intake and output sheet, follow these guidelines:

- If the patient is a child, note fluid levels on the I.V. containers hourly. If the patient is an adult, note these levels at least twice per shift.
- With children and critical care patients, record intake of all I.V. infusions, including fluids, medications, flush solutions, blood and blood products, and other infusates, every 1 to 2 hours.
- Document the total amount of each infusate and totals of all infusions at least every shift so you can monitor fluid balance. Make sure that the math is correct.
- Note output hourly or less often (but at least once per shift), depending on the patient's condition. Output includes urine, stool, vomitus, and gastric drainage. For an acutely ill or unstable patient, you may need to assess urine output every 15 minutes.
- Read fluid levels from the infusate containers or electronic volume-control device to estimate the amounts infused and the amounts remaining to be infused.

Documenting discontinuation of I.V. therapy

All things come to an end; when that time comes in infusion therapy, make sure you have a record of it. When you document the discontinuation of I.V. therapy, be sure to specify:

- time and date
- reason for discontinuing therapy
- assessment of venipuncture site before and after the venous access device is removed
- complications, patient reactions, and nursing interventions

- integrity of the venous access device on removal
- follow-up actions (for example, restarting the I.V. infusion in another extremity)
- amount of I.V. fluid infused before discontinuing therapy.

Patient teaching

Although you may be accustomed to I.V. therapy, many patients aren't. Your patient may be apprehensive about the procedure and concerned that his condition has worsened. A child may be even more afraid. He may imagine he's about to be poisoned or that the needle will never be removed.

Teaching the patient and, when appropriate, members of his family will help him relax and take the mystery out of I.V. therapy.

Good teaching will help I.V. therapy appear less mysterious to the patient.

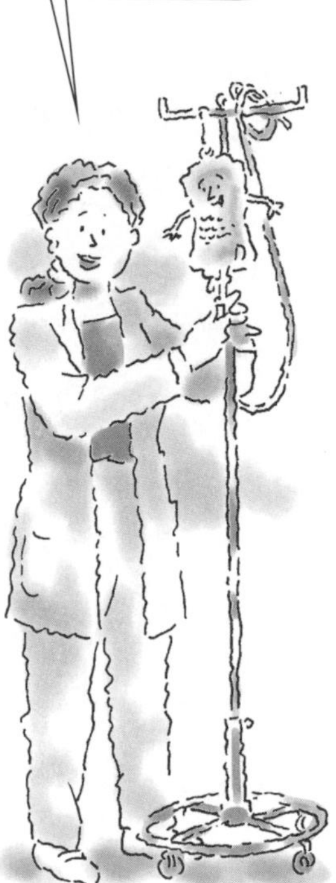

Based on past experience

Begin by assessing the patient's previous infusion experience, his expectations, and his knowledge of venipuncture and I.V. therapy. Then base your teaching on your assessment.

Your teaching should include these steps:

- Describe the procedure. Tell the patient that *I.V.* means "inside the vein" and that a plastic catheter will be placed in his vein.
- Explain that fluids containing certain nutrients or medications will flow from a bag or bottle through a length of tubing, and then through the catheter (the plastic tube) into his vein.
- Tell the patient how long the catheter might stay in place, and explain that his practitioner will decide how much and what type of fluid and medication he needs.

The whole story

Give the patient as much information as possible. Consider providing pamphlets, sample catheters and I.V. equipment, slides, videotapes, and other appropriate information. Some practice areas, such as home care, use patient-teaching checklists that must be signed by the patient or his caregiver. Be sure to tell the whole story:

- Tell the patient that, although he may feel transient pain as the needle goes in, the discomfort will stop when the catheter is in place.
- Explain why I.V. therapy is needed and how the patient can help by holding still and not withdrawing if he feels pain when the needle is inserted.
- Explain that the I.V. fluids may feel cold at first, but the sensation should last only a few minutes.

- Instruct the patient to report any discomfort he feels after therapy begins.
- Explain activity restrictions such as those regarding bathing and ambulating.

Easing anxiety

Give the patient time to express his concerns and fears, and take the time to provide reassurance. Also, encourage the patient to use stress-reduction techniques such as deep, slow breathing. Allow the patient and his family to participate in his care as much as possible.

But did they get it?

Be sure to evaluate how well the patient and his family understand your instruction. Evaluate their understanding while you're teaching and when you're done. You can do so by asking frequent questions and having them explain or demonstrate what you've taught.

Don't forget the paperwork

Document all your teaching in the patient's records. Note what you taught and how well the patient understood it.

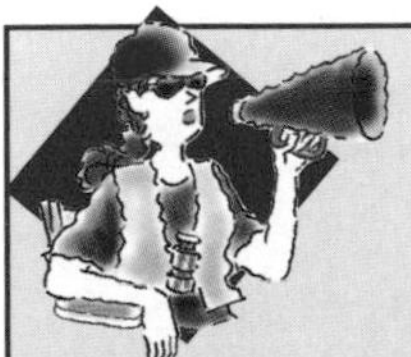

That's a wrap!

Introduction to I.V. therapy review

Objectives of I.V. therapy

- To restore and maintain fluid and electrolyte balance
- To provide medications and chemotherapeutic agents
- To transfuse blood and blood products
- To deliver parenteral nutrients and nutritional supplements

Benefits

- Administers fluids, drugs, nutrients, and other solutions when a patient can't take oral substances
- Allows for more accurate dosing
- Allows medication to reach the bloodstream immediately

Risks

- Blood vessel damage
- Infiltration
- Infection
- Overdose
- Incompatibility of drugs and solutions when mixed
- Adverse or allergic reactions
- May limit patient activity
- Expensive

Fluids, electrolytes, and I.V. therapy

Fluid functions

- Helps regulate body temperature
- Transports nutrients and gases throughout the body
- Carries cellular waste products to excretion sites

(continued)

Introduction to I.V. therapy review *(continued)*

• Includes intracellular fluid (fluid existing inside cells) and extracellular fluid, which is composed of interstitial fluid (fluid that surrounds each cell of the body) and intravascular fluid (blood plasma)

Electrolyte functions

• Conducts current that's necessary for cell function

• Includes sodium and chloride (major extracellular electrolytes), potassium and phosphorus (major intracellular electrolytes), calcium, and magnesium

Fluid and electrolyte balance

• Fluid balance involves the kidneys, heart, liver, adrenal glands, pituitary glands, and nervous system.

• Fluid volume and concentration are regulated by the interaction of antidiuretic hormone (regulates water retention) and aldosterone (retains sodium and water).

• The thirst mechanism helps regulate water volume.

• Fluid movement is influenced by membrane permeability and colloid osmotic and hydrostatic pressures.

• Water and solutes move across capillary walls by capillary filtration and reabsorption.

Types of I.V. solutions

Isotonic solutions

• Have the same osmolarity or tonicity as serum and other body fluids

• Include lactated Ringer's and normal saline

• Indicated for hypovolemia

Hypertonic solutions

• Have a higher osmolarity than serum and cause fluid to be pulled from the interstitial and intracellular compartments into the blood vessels

• Include dextrose 5% in half-normal saline and dextrose 5% in lactated Ringer's

• Used to reduce risk of edema, stabilize blood pressure, and regulate urine output

Hypotonic solutions

• Have a lower serum osmolarity and cause fluid to shift out of the blood vessels into the cells and interstitial spaces

• Include half-normal saline, 0.33% sodium chloride, and dextrose 2.5%

• Used when diuretic therapy dehydrates cells or for hyperglycemic conditions

I.V. delivery methods

• *Continuous infusion* provides constant therapeutic drug level, fluid therapy, or parenteral nutrition.

• *Intermittent infusion* administers drugs over a specified time.

• *Direct injection* is used for a single-dose drug or solution.

Administration sets

• Selection depends on the type of infusion, infusion container, and need for volume-control device

• May be vented for those containers that have no venting system or unvented for those that do

Infusion flow rates

• Macrodrip delivers 10, 15, or 20 gtt/ml.

• Microdrip delivers 60 gtt/ml.

Calculating flow rates

• Divide the volume of the infusion (in ml) by the time of infusion (in minutes), and then multiply this value by the drop factor (in drops per ml).

Regulating flow rates

• Use clamps, volumetric pumps, or rate minders.

• Factors affecting flow rate include vein spasm, vein pressure changes, patient movement, manipulations of the clamp, bent or kinked tubing, I.V. fluid and viscosity, height of the infusion container, type of administration set, and size and position of the venous access device.

Checking flow rates

• Assess flow rates more frequently in patients who are critically ill, those with conditions that might be exacerbated by fluid overload, pediatric patients, elderly patients, and those receiving a drug that can cause tissue damage if infiltration occurs.

Professional and legal standards

• Events that may result in lawsuits include administration of the wrong dosage or solution, use of an incorrect route of administration, inappropriate placement of an I.V. line, and failure to monitor for such problems as adverse reactions, infiltration, and dislodgment of I.V. equipment.

• Professional and legal standards are defined by state nurse practice acts, federal regulations, and facility policy.

• To be eligible for reimbursement, compliance with standards of regulators is necessary.

Introduction to I.V. therapy review *(continued)*

Documentation of I.V therapy
When therapy is initiated, label the dressing on the catheter insertion site and the fluid container according to facility policy and procedures, and document:
- size, length, and type of device
- name of person inserting the device
- date and time
- site location
- type of dressing
- condition of site
- type of solution and any additives used
- flow rate
- use of an electronic infusion device or other type of flow controller
- complications
- patient response
- nursing interventions
- patient teaching and evidence of patient understanding
- number of attempts.

Maintenance
Documentation for I.V. therapy maintenance includes:
- condition of the site
- site care provided
- dressing changes
- tubing and solution changes
- teaching and evidence of patient understanding.

Discontinued
Documentation for discontinuing I.V. therapy includes:
- time and date
- reason for discontinuing therapy
- assessment of site before and after venous access device is removed
- complications
- patient reactions
- nursing interventions
- integrity of the venous access device on removal
- follow-up actions.

Patient teaching
- Describe the procedure and why it's needed.
- State the solution to be infused and the estimated infusion time.
- Discuss activity restrictions.
- Consider using pamphlets, sample catheters, I.V. equipment, slides, or videotapes.
- Be honest about potential discomfort.
- Document the teaching and evaluate the patient's understanding.

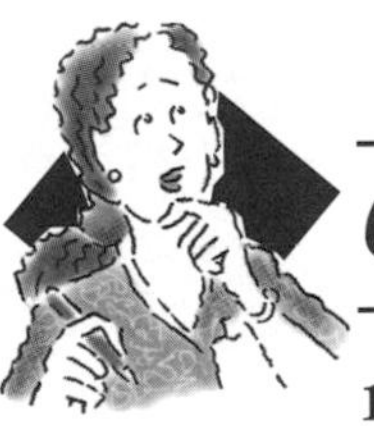

Quick quiz

1. What percentage of body weight is attributed to ECF?
A. 5%
B. 10%
C. 20%
D. 40%

Answer: C. ECF makes up about 20% of body weight.

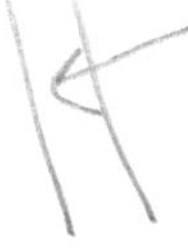

2. Which type of solution raises serum osmolarity and pulls fluid and electrolytes from the intracellular and interstitial compartments into the intravascular compartment?
A. Isotonic
B. Solvent
C. Hypotonic
D. Hypertonic

Answer: D. The higher osmolarity of hypertonic solutions draws fluid into the intravascular compartment.

3. Which electrolyte participates in neurotransmitter release at synapses?

A. Calcium
B. Magnesium
C. Phosphorus
D. Chloride

Answer: A. Calcium participates in neurotransmitter release at synapses.

4. Intravascular infections can be prevented by which of the following precautions?

A. Securing the venous access device with gauze
B. Changing insertion sites according to facility policy
C. Applying the tourniquet 6″ to 8″ (15 to 20 cm) above the insertion site
D. Washing your hands after inserting the device

Answer: B. Intravascular infection can be prevented by alternating insertion sites.

5. When capillary blood pressure exceeds colloid osmotic pressure:

A. water and diffusible solutes leave the capillaries and circulate into the ISF.
B. water and diffusible solutes return to the capillaries.
C. there's no change.
D. intake and output are affected.

Answer: A. When capillary blood pressure exceeds colloid osmotic pressure, water and diffusible solutes leave the capillaries and circulate into the ISF. When capillary blood pressure falls below colloid osmotic pressure, water and diffusible solutes return to the capillaries.

Scoring

☆☆☆ If you answered all five questions correctly, congratulations! Clearly, reading this chapter has infused you with a great deal of knowledge.

☆☆ If you answered three or four questions correctly, good job! Whether hypertonic, hypotonic, or isotonic, you have most of the correct solutions.

☆ If you answered fewer than three questions correctly, don't fret! Put this book under your pillow at night and see if you can absorb the material by osmosis.

2

Peripheral I.V. therapy

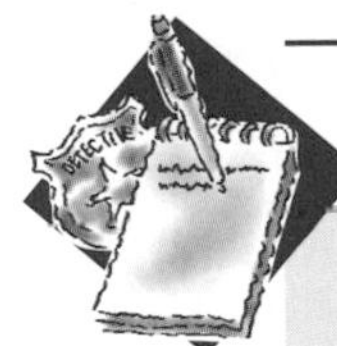

Just the facts

In this chapter, you'll learn:

- the purpose of peripheral I.V. therapy
- proper preparation of a peripheral I.V. venipuncture
- the proper way to perform a peripheral I.V. venipuncture
- peripheral infusion maintenance
- the signs of complications of peripheral I.V. therapy and how to respond to them
- the proper way to discontinue a peripheral infusion.

Understanding peripheral I.V. therapy

Few nursing responsibilities require more time, knowledge, and skill than administering peripheral I.V. therapy. At the bedside, you need to assemble the equipment, prepare the patient, insert the venous access device, regulate the I.V. flow rate, and monitor the patient for possible adverse effects. You also have behind-the-scenes responsibilities, such as checking the practitioner's orders, ordering or preparing supplies and equipment, labeling solutions and tubing, and documenting your nursing interventions.

Practice, practice, practice

Perhaps the most challenging aspect of peripheral I.V. therapy is performing the venipuncture itself. You need steady hands and a sharp eye, plus lots of practice — it's worth the effort, both in terms of positive outcome and patient satisfaction. As you gain experience, you'll learn to perform even difficult venipunctures confidently and successfully.

Peripheral I.V. therapy requires time, knowledge, and skill — at the bedside and behind the scenes.

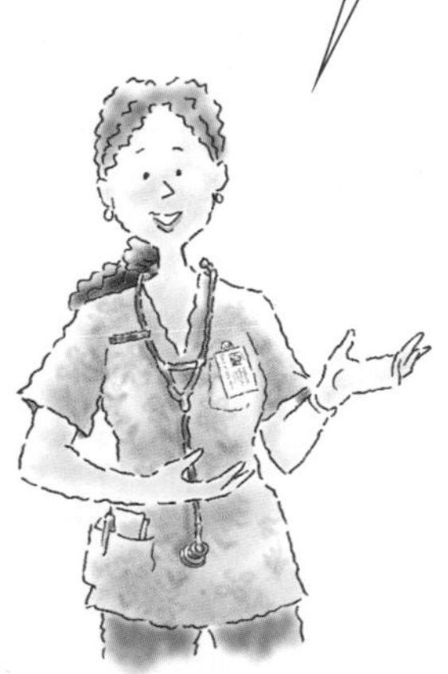

Basics of peripheral I.V. therapy

Peripheral I.V. therapy is ordered whenever venous access is needed; for example, when a patient requires surgery, transfusion therapy, or emergency care. You may also use peripheral I.V. therapy to maintain hydration, restore fluid and electrolyte balance, provide fluids for resuscitation, or administer I.V. drugs, blood and blood components, and nutrients for metabolic support.

Quick and easy

Peripheral I.V. therapy offers easy access to veins and rapid administration of solutions, blood, and drugs. It allows continuous administration of drugs to produce rapid systemic changes. It's also easy to monitor.

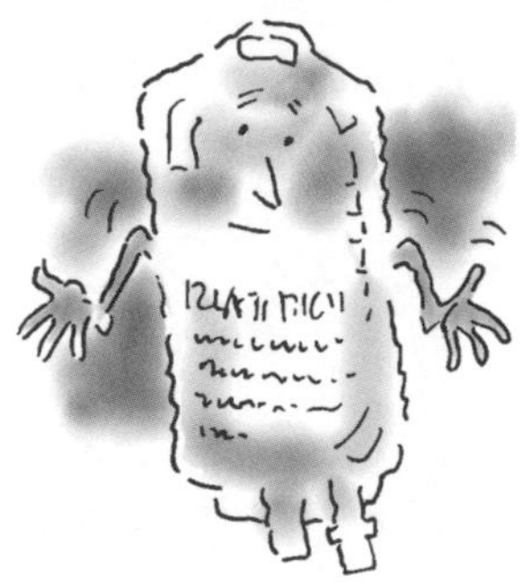

Peripheral concerns — and cost

Peripheral I.V. therapy is an invasive vascular procedure that carries such associated risks as bleeding, infiltration, and infection. Rapid infusion of some drugs can produce hearing loss, bone marrow depression, kidney or heart damage, and other irreversible adverse effects. Finally, peripheral I.V. therapy can't be used indefinitely and costs more than oral, subcutaneous, or I.M. drug therapy.

A mainstay and crucial contributor

Despite its risks, peripheral I.V. therapy remains a mainstay of modern medicine and a crucial contribution that nurses make to their patients' well being. The key is to do it well, and that starts with preparation.

Preparing for venipuncture and infusion

Before performing a venipuncture, talk with the patient, select and prepare the proper equipment, and choose the best access site and venous access device.

Preparing the patient

Before approaching the patient, check his medical record for allergies, his medical history, and his current diagnosis and care plan. Review the practitioner's orders, noting pertinent laboratory studies that might affect the administration or outcome of the prescribed therapy.

Care + confidence = a relaxed, cooperative patient

Keep in mind that the patient may be apprehensive. Among other things, this anxiety may cause vasoconstriction, making the venipuncture more difficult for you and more painful for the patient. Careful patient teaching and a confident, understanding attitude will help the patient relax and cooperate during the procedure. (See *Teaching a patient about peripheral I.V. therapy.*)

Teaching a patient about peripheral I.V. therapy

Many patients feel apprehensive about peripheral I.V. therapy. So, before you begin therapy, teach your patient what to expect before, during, and after the procedure. Thorough patient teaching can reduce his anxiety, making therapy easier. Follow the guidelines below.

Describe the procedure

- Tell the patient that "intravenous" means inside the vein and that a plastic catheter (plastic tube) will be placed in his vein. Explain that fluids containing certain nutrients or medications will flow from an I.V. bag or bottle through a length of tubing, and then through the plastic catheter into his vein.
- Tell the patient approximately how long the I.V. catheter will stay in place (if known). Explain that the practitioner will decide how much and what type of fluid he needs.
- Mention that he may feel some pain during insertion but that the discomfort will stop once the catheter is in place.
- Tell him that the I.V. fluid may feel cold at first, but this sensation should last only a few minutes.

Do's and Don'ts

- Tell the patient to report any discomfort after the catheter has been inserted and the fluid has begun to flow.
- Explain any restrictions, as ordered. If appropriate, tell the patient that he can walk while receiving I.V. therapy. Depending on the insertion site and the device, he may also be able to shower or take a tub bath during therapy.
- Teach the patient how to assist in the care of the I.V. system. Tell him not to pull at the insertion site or tubing and not to remove the container from the I.V. pole. Also, tell him not to kink the tubing or lie on it. Explain that he should call a nurse if the flow rate suddenly slows down or speeds up.

The worst (and it wasn't that bad) is over

- Explain that removing a peripheral I.V. line is a simple procedure. Tell the patient that pressure will be applied to the site until the bleeding stops. Reassure him that, once the device is out and the bleeding stops, he'll be able to use his arm as usual.

What goes on behind drawn curtains

After you complete your teaching, ensure the patient's privacy by asking visitors to leave and drawing the curtains around the bed if another patient is present. However, if the patient requests that his family stay during the procedure, respect his wishes. Have him put on a gown if he isn't already wearing one, and remove any jewelry from the arm where the I.V. catheter will be inserted. When the patient is ready, position him comfortably in the bed, preferably on his back. Make sure that the area is well lit and that the bed is in a position that allows you to maneuver easily when inserting the device.

Selecting the equipment

Besides the venous access device, peripheral I.V. therapy requires a solution container, an administration set (sometimes with an in-line filtration system) and, if needed, an infusion pump.

Solution containers

Some health care facilities use glass I.V. solution containers; however, most use plastic bags for the routine administration of I.V. fluids. Glass must be used to deliver medications that are absorbed by plastic (such as nitroglycerin) and for albumin and immune globulin preparations.

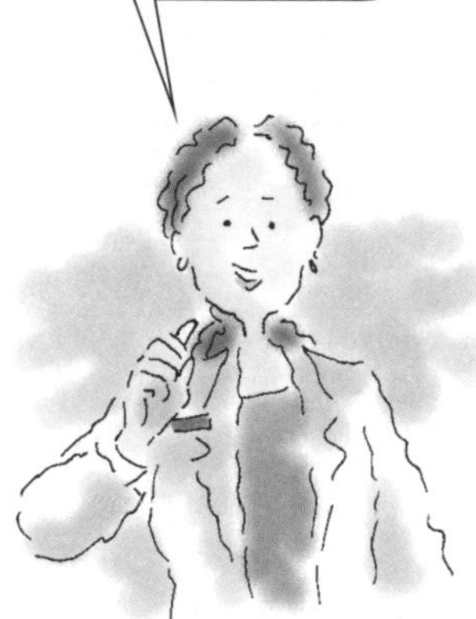

Plastic or glass?

Because they're available in soft, flexible bags or semi-rigid rectangular containers, plastic solution containers allow easy storage, transportation, and disposal. Unlike glass bottles, they collapse as fluid flows out and don't require air venting, thus reducing the risk of air embolism or airborne contamination. In addition, plastic containers aren't likely to break.

In contrast, glass containers don't collapse as fluid flows out and require vented tubing. A vented I.V. administration set has an extra filtered port near the spike that allows air to enter and displace fluid. This helps the solution flow correctly.

Administration sets

There are three major types of I.V. administration sets:

- basic, or *primary*
- add-a-line, or *secondary line*
- volume-control.

Comparing I.V. administration sets

I.V. administration sets come in three major types: basic (also called *primary*), add-a-line (also called *secondary*), and volume-control. The basic set is used to administer most I.V. solutions. An add-a-line set delivers an intermittent secondary infusion through one or more additional Y-sites, or Y-ports. A volume-control set delivers small, precise amounts of solution. All three types come with vented or nonvented drip chambers.

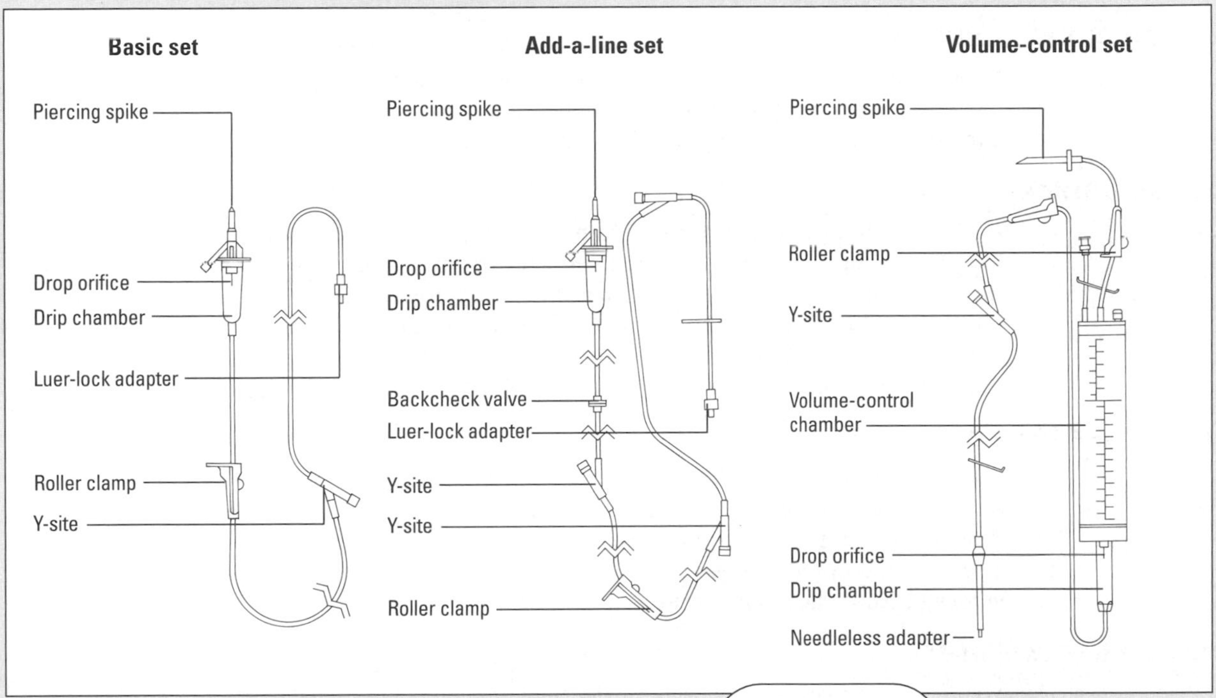

Basic set

Piercing spike
Drop orifice
Drip chamber
Luer-lock adapter
Roller clamp
Y-site

Add-a-line set

Piercing spike
Drop orifice
Drip chamber
Backcheck valve
Luer-lock adapter
Y-site
Y-site
Roller clamp

Volume-control set

Piercing spike
Roller clamp
Y-site
Volume-control chamber
Drop orifice
Drip chamber
Needleless adapter

A macrodrip system delivers a solution in large quantities at rapid rates.

All three have drip chambers that may be vented or nonvented (Glass containers require venting, plastic ones don't.) and two drip systems: macrodrip and microdrip. (See *Comparing I.V. administration sets.*)

A microdrip system delivers a smaller amount of solution with each drop.

Drip, drip, drip…

A macrodrip system delivers a solution in large quantities at rapid rates. A microdrip system delivers a smaller amount of solution with each drop and is used for pediatric patients and adults who need small or closely regulated amounts of I.V. solution.

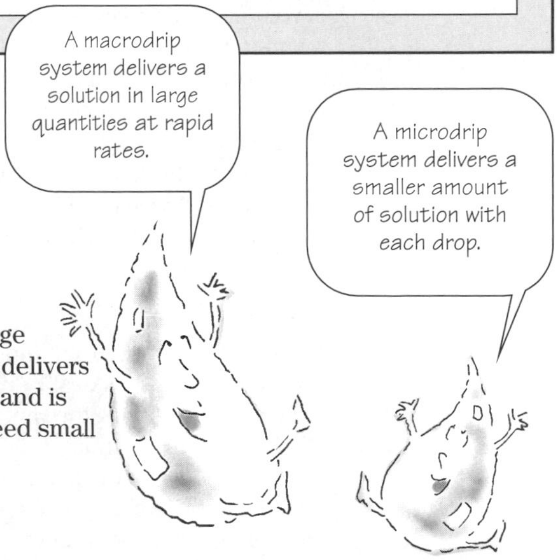

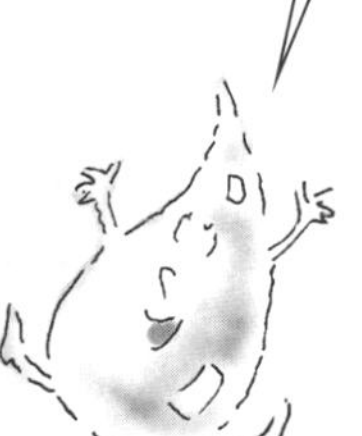

Sizing up the situation

Selecting the correct set requires knowing the type of solution container and comparing the set's flow rate with the nature of the I.V. solution — the more viscous the solution, the larger the drops and, thus, the fewer drops per milliliter. Also, make sure that the intended solution can be infused using a filtration system; otherwise, you'll need an infusion set without the filtration component.

Supplemental supplies

Depending on the type of therapy ordered, you may need to supplement the administration set with other equipment, such as stopcocks, extension loops, and needleless systems.

Back to basics

Basic I.V. administration sets range from 70″ to 110″ (178 to 279 cm) long. They're used to deliver an I.V. solution or to infuse solutions through an intermittent infusion device. The Y-site provides a secondary injection port for a separate or simultaneous infusion of two compatible solutions. A macrodrip set generally delivers 10, 15, or 20 gtt/ml. A microdrip set always delivers 60 gtt/ml.

Add-a-line? Here's Y...

Add-a-line sets can deliver intermittent secondary infusions through one or more additional Y-sites. A backcheck valve prevents backflow of the secondary solution into the primary solution. After the secondary solution has been infused, the set automatically resumes infusing the primary one.

Down to the milliliter

Volume-control sets — used primarily for pediatric patients — deliver small, precise amounts of fluid and medication from a volume-control chamber that's calibrated in milliliters. This chamber is placed at the top of the I.V. tubing, just above the drip chamber. Also called *burette sets* or *Buretrols*, volume-control sets are available with or without an in-line filter. They may be attached directly to the venous access device or connected to the Y-site of a primary I.V. administration set. Macrodrip and microdrip systems are available.

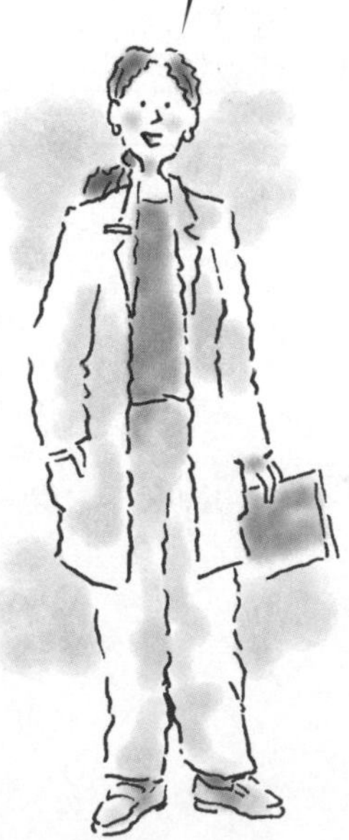

In-line filters

In-line filters are located in a segment of the I.V. tubing through which the fluid passes. In-line filters remove pathogens and particles, thus reducing the risk of infection and phlebitis. Filters also help prevent air from entering the patient's vein by venting it through the filter housing. Filters range in size from 0.2 micron (the most common) to 170 microns. Some are built into the line; others need to be added.

Keeping in line with in-line filters

Most facilities have guidelines for using in-line filters; these guidelines usually include the following instructions:

- When using a filter with an infusion pump, make sure that it can withstand the pump's infusion pressure. Some filters are made for use only with gravity flow and may crack if the pressure exceeds a certain level.
- The filter should be distal in the tubing and located close to the patient.
- Carefully prime the in-line filter to eliminate all the air from it, following the manufacturer's directions.
- Be sure to change the filter according to the manufacturer's recommendation to prevent bacteria from accumulating and releasing endotoxins and pyrogens small enough to pass through the filter into the bloodstream.

I don't like pathogens and particles. That's why I hooked up with an in-line filter.

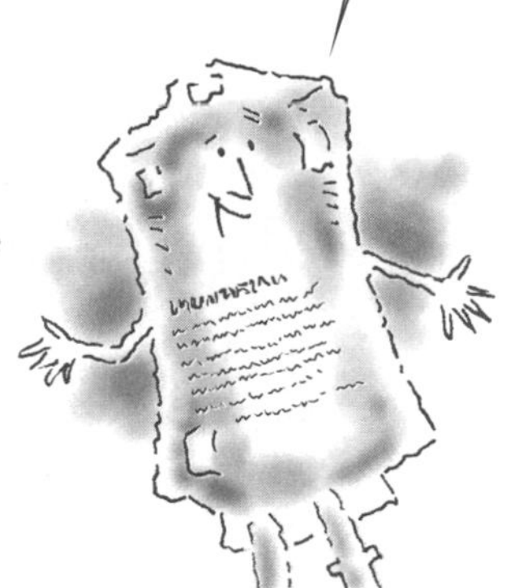

Is there a filter in your future?

Routine use of filters increases costs. Therefore, filters may not be indicated in all situations. When can you expect to use an in-line filter? Usually in situations when:

- treating an immunosuppressed patient
- administering total parenteral nutrition
- using additives composed of many separate particles (such as antibiotics that require reconstitution) or when administering several additives
- the risk of phlebitis is high.

Don't expect to use a 0.2-micron filter if you're administering blood, blood components, or lipid emulsions; the larger particles in these solutions could clog the filter. The same is true of low-dose (less than 5 mcg/ml), low-volume medications because the filter membrane may absorb them.

Preparing the equipment

After you select and gather the infusion equipment, you'll need to prepare it for use. Preparation involves inspecting the I.V. container and solution, preparing the solution, attaching and priming the administration set, and setting up the controller or infusion pump.

Inspecting the container and solution

Check that the container size is appropriate for the volume to be infused and that the type of I.V. solution is correct. Note the expiration date; discard an outdated solution.

When in doubt, throw it out

Make sure that the solution container is intact. Examine a glass container for cracks or chips and a plastic container for tears or leaks. (Plastic bags commonly come with an outer wrapper, which you must remove before inspecting the container.) Discard a damaged container, even if the solution appears clear. If the solution isn't clear, discard the container and notify the pharmacy or dispensing department. Solutions may vary in color, but they should never appear cloudy, turbid, or separated.

Discard a damaged or suspicious looking I.V. container, and always use sterile technique when preparing to attach the container to the administration set. Better safe than sorry!

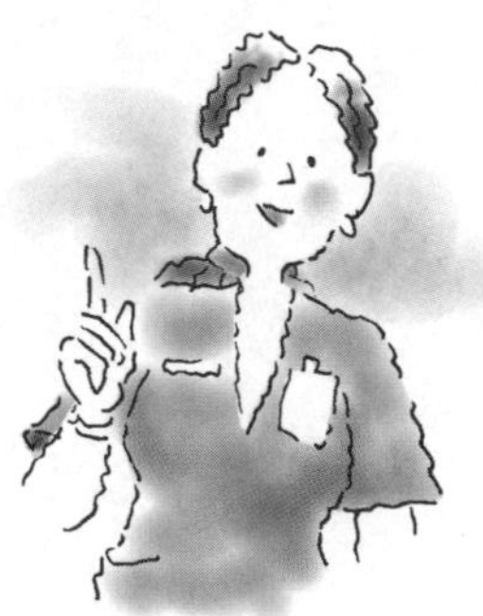

Preparing the solution

Make sure that the container is labeled with the following information: your name; the patient's name, identification number, and room number; the date and time the container was hung; any additives; and the container number (if such information is required by your facility). For a pediatric patient, you may label the volume-control set instead of the container.

After the container is labeled, use sterile technique to remove the cap or pull tab. Be careful not to contaminate the port or the spike from the administration set.

Attaching the administration set

Make sure that the administration set is correct for the patient and the type of I.V. container and solution you're using. Also make sure that the set has no cracks, holes, or missing clamps. If the solution container is glass, check whether it's vented or nonvented to determine how to prepare it before attaching it to the administration set. (Plastic containers are prepared differently.)

Nonvented bottle

When attaching a nonvented bottle to an administration set, take the following steps:

1. Remove the metal cap and inner disk, if necessary.
2. Place the bottle on a stable surface, and wipe the rubber stopper with an alcohol swab.
3. Close the flow clamp on the administration set.
4. Remove the protective cap from the spike.
5. Push the spike through the center of the rubber stopper. Avoid twisting or angling the spike to prevent pieces of the stopper from breaking off and falling into the solution.

Invert the bottle. Hang the bottle on the I.V. pole, about 36″ (91 cm) above the venipuncture site.

Vented bottle

When attaching a vented bottle to an administration set, take the following steps:

Remove the metal cap and latex diaphragm to release the vacuum. If the vacuum isn't intact, discard the bottle (unless a medication has been added).

Place the bottle on a stable surface, and wipe the rubber stopper with an alcohol swab.

Close the flow clamp on the administration set.

Remove the protective cap from the spike.

Push the spike through the insertion port, which is located next to the air vent.

Hang the bottle on the I.V. pole about 36″ above the venipuncture site.

Plastic bag

When attaching a plastic bag to an administration set, take the following steps:

Place the bag on a flat, stable surface or hang it on an I.V. pole.

Remove the protective cap or tear the tab from the tubing insertion port.

Slide the flow clamp up close to the drip chamber, and close the clamp.

Remove the protective cap from the spike.

Hold the port carefully and firmly with one hand, and then quickly insert the spike with your other hand.

Hang the bag about 36″ above the venipuncture site.

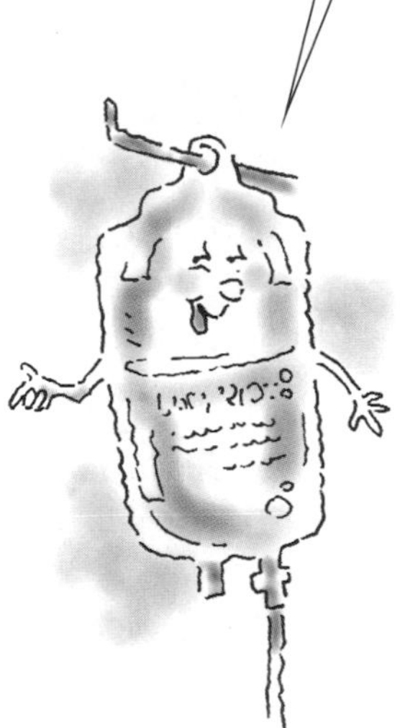

Priming the administration set

Before you prime an administration set, label it with the date and time you opened it. Make sure that you have also labeled the container. When priming a set with an electronic infusion device, the procedure is similar to priming other infusion sets. (See *Electronic infusion devices.*)

Basic training

When priming a basic set, take the following steps:

1. Close the roller clamp below the drip chamber.
2. Squeeze the drip chamber until it's half full.
3. Aim the distal end of the tubing at a receptacle.
4. Open the roller clamp, and allow the solution to flow through the tubing to remove the air. (Most distal tube coverings allow the solution to flow without having to remove the protective end.)
5. Close the clamp after the solution has run through the line and all the air has been purged from the system.

My sweet add-a-line

Follow the same steps you would use to prime a basic set, along with these additional steps:

1. As the solution flows through the tubing, invert the backcheck valves so that the solution can flow into them. Tap the backcheck valve to release any trapped air bubbles.
2. Straighten the tubing and continue purging air in the usual manner.

Taking control

To prime a volume-control set, take the following steps:

1. Attach the set to the solution container, and close the lower clamp on the I.V. tubing below the drip chamber.
2. Open the clamp between the solution container and the fluid chamber, and allow about 50 ml of the solution to flow into the chamber.
3. Close the upper clamp.
4. Open the lower clamp, and allow the solution in the chamber to flow through the remainder of the tubing. Make sure that some fluid remains in the chamber so that air won't fill the tubing below it.

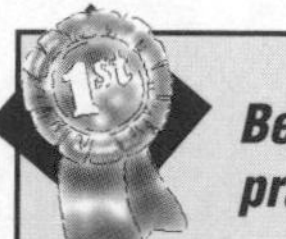

Best practice

Electronic infusion devices

An electronic infusion device, such as a pump, helps regulate the rate and volume of infusions, improving the safety and accuracy of drug and fluid administration.

Priming the set

Follow the steps below to prime an infusion set with an electronic infusion device:

1. Fill the drip chamber to the halfway mark.
2. Slowly open the roller clamp.
3. As gravity assists the flow, invert the chambered sections of the tubing to expel the air and fill them with the I.V. fluid or infusate. The chambered sections fit into the pump of the electronic infusion device; they must be filled exactly so they won't activate the air-in-line alarm during use.
4. Reinvert the pump chamber, continuing to purge the air along the fluid path and out of the tubing.

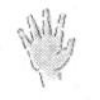 Close the lower clamp.

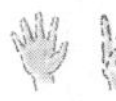 Fill the chamber with the desired amount of solution.

What about a filter?

If you're using a filter on any of these sets and it isn't an integral part of the infusion path, attach it to the primed distal end of the I.V. tubing and follow the manufacturer's instructions for filling and priming it. Most filters are positioned with the distal end of the tubing facing upward so the solution will wet the filter membrane completely and the line will be purged of all air bubbles.

Setting up and monitoring an infusion pump

Infusion pumps help maintain a steady flow of liquid at a set rate over a specified period. After gathering your equipment, follow these steps:

Attach the pump to the I.V. pole. Insert the administration spike into the I.V. container.

Fill the drip chamber completely to prevent air bubbles from entering the tubing. To avoid fluid overload, clamp the tubing whenever the pump door is open.

Follow the manufacturer's instructions for priming and placing the I.V. tubing.

Be sure to flush all of the air out of the tubing before connecting it to the patient to lower the risk of an air embolism.

Place the infusion pump on the same side of the bed as the I.V. setup and the venipuncture site.

Set the appropriate controls to the desired infusion rate or volume.

Connect the tubing to the venous access site, watch for infiltration, and monitor the accuracy of the infusion rate.

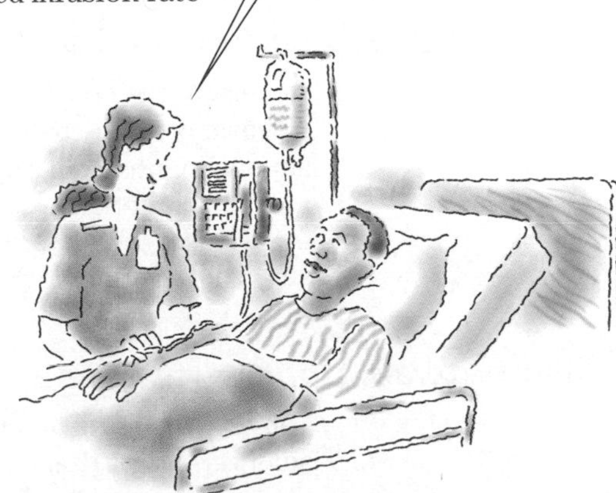

Don't alarm the patient

Be sure to explain the alarm system to the patient so he isn't frightened when a change in the infusion rate triggers the alarm. Also, be prepared to disengage the device if infiltration occurs, otherwise the pump may continue to infuse medication in the infiltrated area.

Frequently check the infusion pump to make sure that it's working properly — specifically, note the flow rate. Monitor the patient for signs of infiltration and other complications such as infection.

Change the tubing

After the equipment is up and running, you'll also need to change the tubing according to the manufacturer's instructions and your facility's policy.

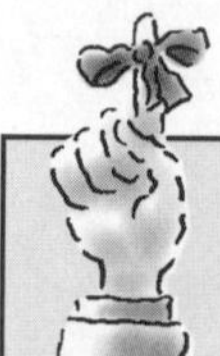

Memory jogger

In selecting the best site for a venipuncture, remember the abbreviation **VIP:**

Vein

Infusion

Patient.

For the vein, consider its location, condition, and physical path along the extremity.

For the infusion, consider its purpose and duration.

For the patient, consider his degree of cooperation and compliance, along with his preference.

Selecting the insertion site

Here are general suggestions for selecting the vein:

- Keep in mind that the most prominent veins aren't necessarily the best veins — they're frequently sclerotic from previous use.
- Never select a vein in an edematous or impaired arm.
- Never select a vein in the arm closest to an area that's surgically compromised — for example, veins compromised by a mastectomy or placement of dialysis access.
- Never select a vein in the affected arm of a patient following a stroke.
- Select a vein in the nondominant arm or hand when possible.
- For subsequent venipunctures, select sites above the previously used or injured vein.
- Make sure that you rotate access sites.
- Try to avoid areas of flexion.

Commonly used veins

The veins commonly used for placement of venipuncture devices include the metacarpal, cephalic, and basilic veins, along with the branches or accessory branches that merge with them. (See *Comparing peripheral venipuncture sites.*)

Superficial advice: Try the hand and forearm

Generally, the superficial veins in the dorsum of the hand and forearm offer the best choices. The dorsum of the hand is well supplied with small, superficial veins that can be dilated easily and accommodate a catheter. The dorsum of the forearm has long, straight veins with fairly large diameters, making them convenient sites for introducing the large-bore long catheters used in prolonged I.V. therapy.

Alternatives: Upper arms, legs, feet, and more

Veins of the hand and forearm are suitable for most drugs and solutions. For irritating drugs and solutions with a high osmolarity, the cephalic and basilic veins in the upper arm are more suitable.

Comparing peripheral venipuncture sites

Venipuncture sites located in the hand, forearm, foot, and leg offer various advantages and disadvantages. This chart includes some of the major benefits and drawbacks of common venipuncture sites.

Site	Advantages	Disadvantages
Digital veins Along lateral and dorsal portions of fingers	• May be used for short-term therapy • May be used when other means aren't available	• Requires splinting fingers with a tongue blade, which decreases ability to use hand • Uncomfortable for patient • Significant risk of infiltration • Not used if veins in dorsum of hand already used • Won't accommodate large volumes or fast I.V. rates
Metacarpal veins On dorsum of hand; formed by union of digital veins between knuckles	• Easily accessible • Lie flat on back of hand; more difficult to dislodge • In adult or large child, bones of hand act as splint	• Wrist movement limited unless short catheter is used • Painful insertion likely because of large number of nerve endings in hands • Phlebitis likely at site
Accessory cephalic vein Along radial bone as a continuation of metacarpal veins of thumb	• Large vein excellent for venipuncture • Readily accepts large-gauge catheters • Doesn't impair mobility • Doesn't require an arm board in an older child or adult	• Some difficulty positioning catheter flush with skin • Discomfort during movement due to location of device at bend of wrist • Danger of radial nerve injury
Cephalic vein Along radial side of forearm and upper arm	• Large vein excellent for venipuncture • Readily accepts large-gauge catheters • Doesn't impair mobility	• Decreased joint movement due to proximity of device to elbow • Possible difficulty stabilizing vein
Median antebrachial vein Rising from palm and along ulnar side of forearm	• Holds winged catheters well • A last resort when no other means are available	• Painful insertion or infiltration damage possible due to large number of nerve endings in area • High risk of infiltration in this area
Basilic vein Along ulnar side of forearm and upper arm	• Straight, strong vein suitable for venipuncture • Takes large-gauge catheter easily	• Inconvenient position for patient during insertion • Painful insertion due to penetration of dermal layer of skin where nerve endings are located • Possible difficulty stabilizing vein

(continued)

Comparing peripheral venipuncture sites *(continued)*

Site	Advantages	Disadvantages
Antecubital veins In antecubital fossa (median cephalic, on radial side; median basilic, on ulnar side; median cubital, which rises in front of elbow joint)	• Large vein; facilitates drawing blood • Commonly visible or palpable in children when other veins won't dilate • May be used in an emergency or as a last resort	• Difficult to splint elbow area with arm board • Veins may be small and scarred if blood has been drawn frequently from this site
Dorsal venous network On dorsal portion of foot	• Suitable for infants and toddlers	• Difficult to see or find vein if edema is present • Difficult to walk with device in place • Increased risk of deep vein thrombosis
Scalp veins	• Suitable for infants • Commonly visible and palpable in infants • May be used as a last resort	• Difficult to stabilize • May require clipping hair at site • Increased infiltration risk due to vein fragility

When leg or foot veins must be used, the saphenous vein of the inner aspect of the ankle and the veins of the dorsal foot network are best—but only as an absolute last resort. Venous access in the lower extremities can cause thrombophlebitis. In infants younger than age 6 months, scalp veins are commonly used. Veins in the feet are commonly used in nonambulatory children and infants. In neonates, the umbilical veins may be accessed; for example, in an emergency situation.

The lowdown on the upper arm

An upper arm vein may seem like an excellent site for a venous access device— it's comfortable for the patient and reasonably safe from accidental dislodging. Even so, it has a serious drawback. When an upper arm vein has a venous access device in place, the use of sites distal to the upper arm is compromised. Moreover, upper arm veins can be difficult to locate in obese patients and in those with shorter arms such as pediatric patients.

You aren't an artery, are you?

Before choosing a vein as an I.V. site, make sure that it's actually a vein—not an artery. Arteries are located deep in soft tissue and muscles; veins are superficial. Arteries contain bright red blood that flows away from the heart; veins contain dark red blood that flows toward the heart.

A single artery supplies a large area; many veins supply and remove blood from the same area. If you puncture an artery (which is difficult to do because of the artery's depth), the blood pulsates from the site; if you puncture a vein, the blood flows slowly. (See *Reviewing skin and vein anatomy,* page 50.)

Avoid valves

All veins have valves, but they're usually apparent only in long, straight arm veins or in large, well-developed veins that have good tone. If the tip of the venous access device terminates near a valve, the flow rate may be affected. Look for a vein that's straight and smooth for about 1″ (2.5 cm). Sclerosed valves appear as painless knots within veins. Insert the venous access device above the knot.

Selection guidelines

When selecting an I.V. site, choose distal veins first, unless the solution is very irritating (for example, potassium chloride). Generally, your best choice is a peripheral vein that's full and pliable and appears long enough to accommodate the length of the intended catheter (about 1″). It should be large enough to allow blood flow around the catheter to minimize venous lumen irritation. If the patient has an area that's bruised, tender, or phlebitic, choose a vein proximal to it. Avoid flexion areas, such as the wrist and antecubital fossa.

Refrain from these veins

Some veins are best to avoid, including those in:

- legs (Circulation may be easily compromised.)
- inner wrist and arm (They're small and uncomfortable for the patient.)
- affected arm of a mastectomy patient
- arm with an arteriovenous shunt or fistula
- arm being treated for thrombosis or cellulitis
- arm that has experienced trauma (such as burns or scarring from surgery).

How long?

The size and health (tone) of the vein help determine how long the venous access device can remain in place before irritation develops. However, the key to determining how long the venous access device will remain functional is the effect of the fluid or drug on the vein. Drugs and solutions with high osmolarity and high or low pH will cause vein irritation sooner. Concentrated solutions of drugs and rapid infusion rates can also affect how long the I.V. site remains symptom-free.

Reviewing skin and vein anatomy

Understanding the anatomy of skin and veins can help you locate appropriate venipuncture sites and perform venipunctures with minimal patient discomfort.

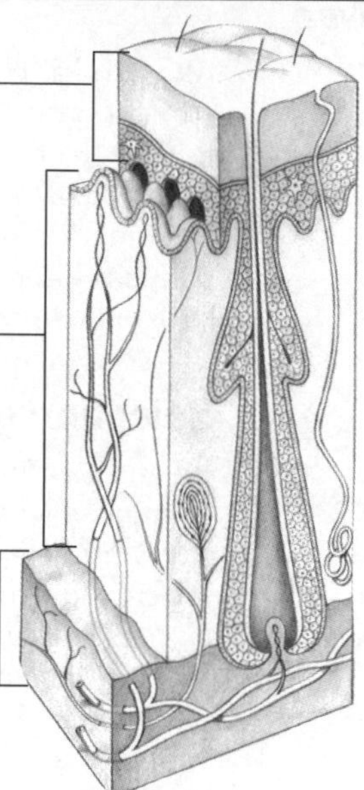

Layers of the skin

Epidermis

- Top layer that forms a protective covering for the dermis
- Varied thickness in different parts of the body—usually thickest on palms of hands and soles of feet, thinnest on inner surface of limbs
- Varied thickness depending on age; possibly thin in elderly people
- Contains about 25 layers of cells with bacteria located in the top 5 layers

Dermis

- Highly sensitive and vascular because it contains many capillaries
- Location of thousands of nerves, which react to temperature, touch, pressure, and pain
- Varied number of nerve fibers throughout the body; some I.V. sites more painful than others (for example, the inner aspect of the wrist is more painful than the dorsum of the hand or the forearm)

Subcutaneous tissue

- Located below the two layers of skin
- Site of superficial veins
- Varied thickness that loosely covers muscles and tendons
- Potential site of cellulitis if strict aseptic technique isn't observed during venipuncture and care of I.V. site

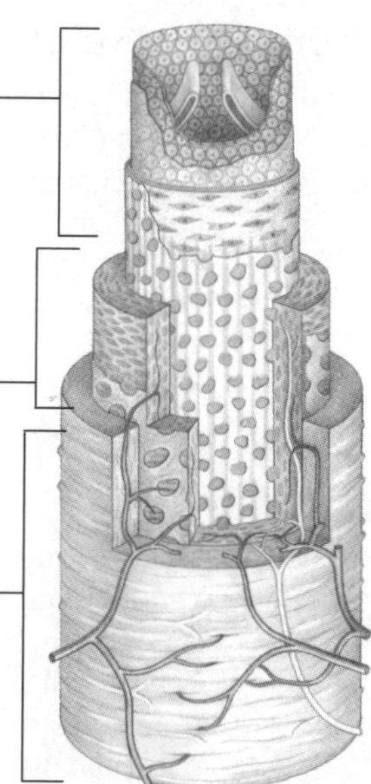

Layers of veins

Tunica intima (inner layer)

- Inner elastic endothelial lining made up of layers of smooth, flat cells, which allow blood cells and platelets to flow smoothly through the blood vessels (unnecessary movement of the venous access device may scratch or roughen this inner surface, causing thrombus formation)
- Valves in this layer located in the semilunar folds of the endothelium (valves prevent backflow and ensure that blood flows toward the heart)

Tunica media (middle layer)

- Muscular and elastic tissue
- Location of vasoconstrictor and vasodilator nerve fibers that stimulate the veins to contract and relax (these fibers are responsible for venous spasm that can occur as the result of anxiety or infusion of I.V. fluids that are too cold)

Tunica adventitia (outer layer)

- Connective tissue that surrounds and supports the vessel and holds it together
- Reduced thickness and amount of connective tissue with age, resulting in fragile veins

Selecting the venous access device

Basically, you should select the device with the shortest length and the smallest diameter that allows for proper administration of the therapy. Other considerations include:

- length of therapy or time the device will stay in place
- type of therapy
- type of procedure or surgery to be performed
- patient's age and activity level
- type of solution used (blood, for instance, will require a larger-gauge device)
- condition of veins.

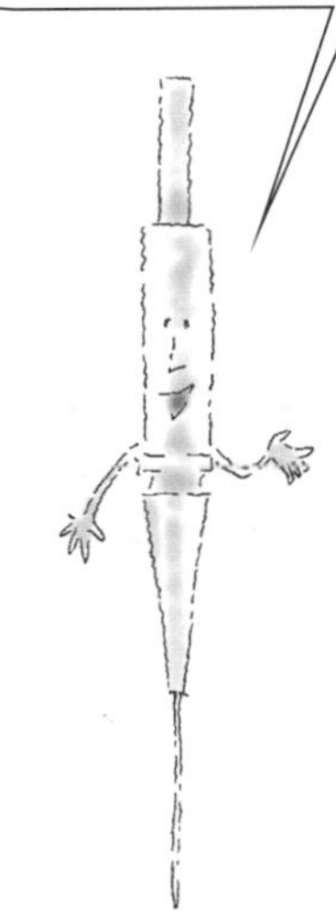

Venous access devices

The two most commonly used devices are plastic catheter sets and winged-set type infusion sets. As a rule, plastic catheters allow more patient movement and activity and are less prone to infiltration than winged-set type infusion sets. However, they're more difficult to insert. (See *Comparing basic venous access devices*, page 52.)

Let's go over this needle

An over-the-needle catheter is the most commonly used device for peripheral I.V. therapy. It consists of a plastic outer tube and an inner needle that extends just beyond the catheter. It's available in lengths of ¾″ to 3″, with gauges ranging from 14 to 26. Longer-length models, used mainly in the operating room, are for insertion into a deep vein. (See *Guide to needle and catheter gauges*, page 53.)

The needle is removed after insertion, leaving the catheter in place. Typically, you should change an over-the-needle catheter every 2 to 3 days, depending on your facility's policy and procedures. If a patient has poor venous access and therapy is to be continued indefinitely, consult with the practitioner about line placement alternatives.

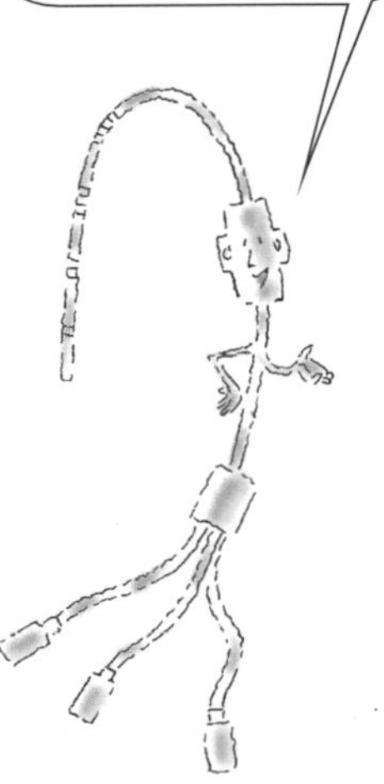

Taking wing

Winged-set type infusion sets have flexible wings you can grasp when inserting the device. When the device is in place, the wings lie flat and can be taped to the surrounding skin.

Winged-set type infusion sets have short, small-bore tubing between the catheter and hub. The catheter stays in place after the needle is removed. This type of catheter is available in a ¾″ length for wider gauges. It's especially useful for hard veins and for insertion in an elderly patient or child.

Comparing basic venous access devices

Use the chart below to compare the two major types of venous access devices. To improve I.V. therapy and guard against accidental needlesticks, you should use a needle-free system and a shielded or retracting peripheral I.V. catheter.

Over-the-needle catheter

Purpose

- Long-term therapy for the active or agitated patient

Advantages

- Inadvertent puncture of vein less likely than with a winged-set type infusion set
- More comfortable for the patient
- Radiopaque thread for easy location
- Safety needles that prevent accidental needlesticks
- Activity-restricting device, such as arm board, rarely required

Disadvantages

- Difficult to insert
- Extra care required to ensure that needle and catheter are inserted into vein

Winged-set type

Purpose

- Short-term therapy for cooperative adult patient
- Therapy of any duration for an infant or child or for an elderly patient with fragile or sclerotic veins

Advantages

- Easiest intravascular device to insert because needle is thin-walled and extremely sharp
- Ideal for nonirritating I.V. push drugs

Disadvantage

- Infiltration easily caused if rigid needle winged infusion device is used

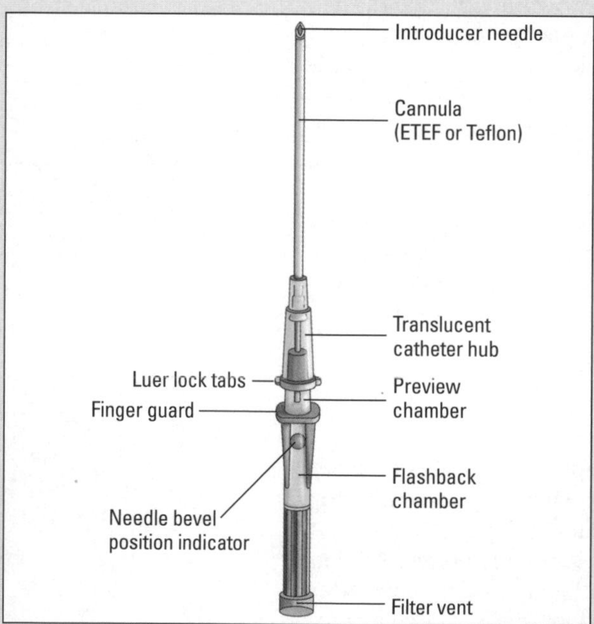

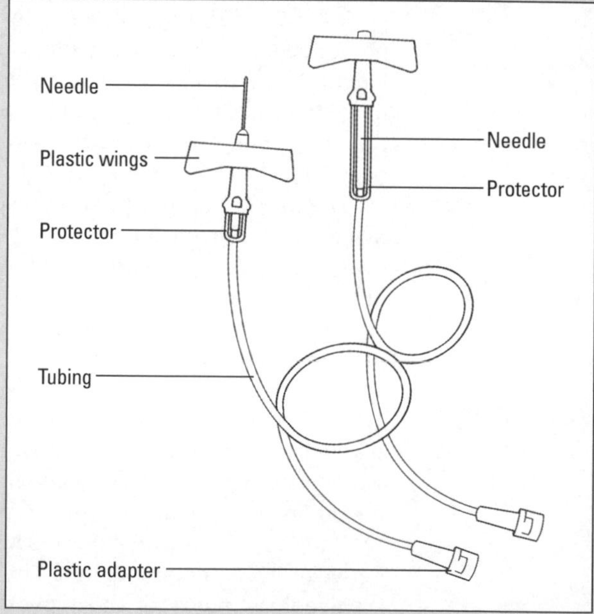

Guide to needle and catheter gauges

How do you know which gauge needle and catheter to use for your patient? The answer depends on the patient's age, his condition, and the type of infusion he's receiving. This chart lists the uses and nursing considerations for various gauges.

Gauge	Uses	Nursing considerations
16	• Adolescents and adults • Major surgery • Trauma • Whenever large amounts of fluids must be infused rapidly	• Painful insertion • Requires large vein
18	• Older children, adolescents, and adults • Administration of blood and blood components and other viscous infusions • Routinely used preoperatively	• Painful insertion • Requires large vein
20	• Children, adolescents, and adults • Suitable for most I.V. infusions, blood, blood components, and other viscous infusions	• Commonly used
22	• Toddlers, children, adolescents, and adults (especially elderly) • Suitable for most I.V. infusions	• Easier to insert into small veins • Commonly used for most infusions
24, 26	• Neonates, infants, toddlers, school-age children, adolescents, and adults (especially elderly) • Suitable for most infusions, but flow rates are slower	• For extremely small veins—for example, small veins of fingers or veins of inner arms in elderly patients • Possible difficulty inserting into tough skin

An intermittent adaptation

Any venous access device that includes a catheter can be made into an intermittent infusion device by placing an access cap over the catheter's adapter end. These caps are commonly called "locks," and a saline solution is flushed into them to keep the device patent. The cap is a luer-locking attachment or add-on. Intermittent venous access devices should be flushed with saline solution before and after each use, at least once per day, or according to the facility's policy and procedures.

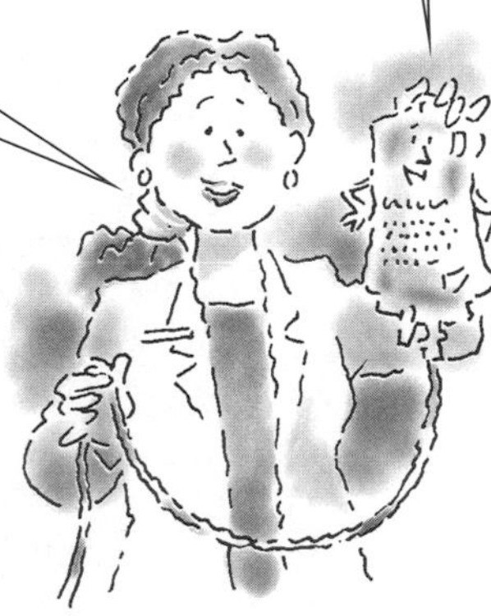

Performing venipuncture

To perform a venipuncture, you need to dilate the vein, prepare the access site, and insert the device. After the infusion starts, you can complete the I.V. placement by securing the device with tape or a transparent semipermeable dressing.

Dilating the vein

To dilate or distend a vein effectively, you may need to use a tourniquet, which traps blood in the veins by applying enough pressure to impede venous flow. A properly distended vein should appear and feel round, firm, and fully filled with blood as well as rebound when gently compressed. Because the amount of trapped blood depends on circulation, a patient who's hypotensive, very cold, or experiencing vasomotor changes (such as septic shock) may have inadequate filling of the peripheral blood vessels.

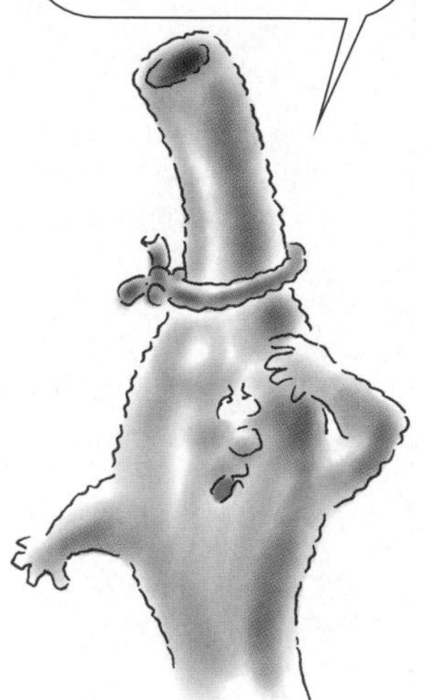

Pretourniquet prep

Before applying the tourniquet, place the patient's arm in a dependent position to increase capillary flow to the lower arm and hand. If his skin is cold, warm it by rubbing and stroking his arm or by covering the entire arm with warm moist towels for 5 to 10 minutes. As soon as you remove the warm towels, apply the tourniquet and continue to perform the insertion procedure.

Applying a tourniquet

The ideal tourniquet is one that can be secured easily, doesn't roll into a thin band, stays relatively flat, and releases easily. The most common type is a soft rubber band about 2″ (5 cm) wide. (To tie a tourniquet, follow the steps outlined in *Applying a tourniquet*, page 55.)

Intend to distend

After you have applied the tourniquet about 6″ to 8″ (15 to 20 cm) above the intended site, have the patient open and close his fist tightly four to six times to distend the vein. If necessary, gently flick the skin over the vein with one or two short taps of your forefinger. This is less traumatic than slapping the skin, but it achieves the same result. If the vein still feels small and uniform, release the tourniquet, reapply it, and reassess the intended access site. If the vein still isn't well distended, remove the tourniquet; apply a warm, moist towel for 5 minutes; then reapply the tourniquet. This step is especially helpful if the patient's skin feels cool.

Best practice

Applying a tourniquet

To safely apply a tourniquet, follow these steps:

1. Place the tourniquet under the patient's arm, about 6″ (15 cm) above the venipuncture site. Position the arm on the middle of the tourniquet.
2. Bring the ends of the tourniquet together, placing one on top of the other.
3. Holding one end on top of the other, lift and stretch the tourniquet and tuck the top tail under the bottom tail. Don't allow the tourniquet to loosen.
4. Tie the tourniquet smoothly and snugly; be careful not to pinch the patient's skin or pull his arm hair.

No more than 2 minutes

Leave the tourniquet in place for no more than 2 minutes. If you can't find a suitable vein and prepare the venipuncture site in this amount of time, release the tourniquet for a few minutes. Then reapply it and continue the procedure. You may need to apply the tourniquet, find the vein, remove the tourniquet, prepare the site, and then reapply the tourniquet for the venipuncture.

As flat as possible

Keep the tourniquet as flat as possible. It should be snug but not uncomfortably tight. If it's too tight, it will impede arterial as well as venous blood flow. Check the patient's radial pulse. If you can't feel it, the tourniquet is too tight and must be loosened. Also loosen and reapply the tourniquet if the patient complains of severe tightness.

Following these guidelines will ensure safety and promote blood flow, making venipuncture easier.

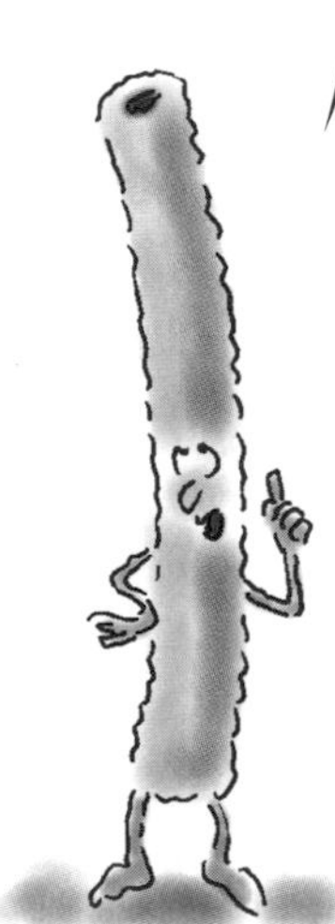

Top tourniquet technique

A tourniquet that's kept in place too long or is applied too tightly may cause increased bruising, especially in elderly patients whose veins are fragile. Release the tourniquet as soon as you have placed the venous access device in the vein. You'll know the device is in the vein when you see blood in the flashback chamber.

Infection control

For infection control reasons, tourniquets should be discarded after use on one patient. When available, use latex-free tourniquets to reduce the chance of an allergic reaction.

Preparing the access site

Before performing the venipuncture, you'll need to clean the site and stabilize the vein; you may also need to administer a local anesthetic.

Cleaning the venipuncture site

Wash your hands and then put on gloves. If necessary, clip the hair over the insertion site to make the veins and the site easier to see and reduce pain when the tape is removed. Avoid shaving the patient because it can cause microabrasion of the skin, which increases the risk of infection.

Clean the skin with 2% chlorhexidine. Using a swab, start at the center of the insertion site and move outward in a back-and-forth motion. Be careful not to go over an area you have already cleaned. Allow the solution to dry thoroughly.

Have a hairy patient? Clip hair at the insertion site. Shaving may cause microabrasion of the skin.

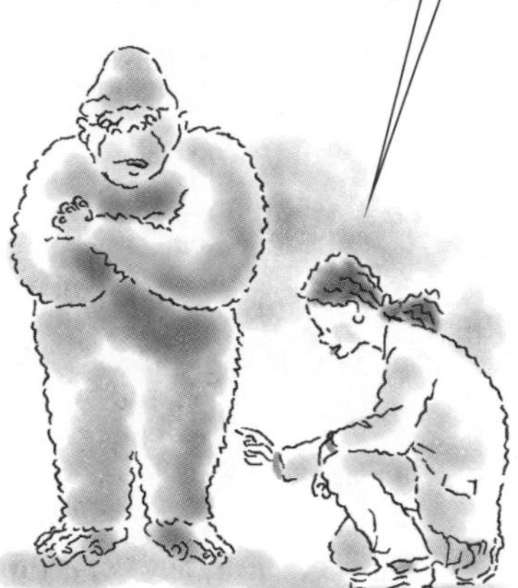

Using a local anesthetic

If an anesthetic is ordered, first check with the patient and review his record for an allergy to lidocaine, iodine, or other drugs. Then describe the procedure to him and explain that it will reduce the discomfort of the venipuncture.

Next, administer the local anesthetic as ordered. The anesthetic will begin to work in 2 to 3 seconds. Lidocaine anesthetizes the site to pain but allows the patient to feel touch and pressure. Also, normal saline solution has proven effective. (See *Administering a local anesthetic*, page 57.)

Creaming the pain

Transdermal analgesic cream may also be used before accessing a peripheral vein. Like injectable anesthetics, transdermal analgesic cream reduces pain, but the patient still feels pressure and touch. To be effective, a transdermal analgesic cream should be applied at least 30 minutes before insertion of the venous access device. The cream form is a good choice for anesthetizing I.V. sites in children.

It's electric

Another option is to use iontophoresis, a technique that delivers dermal analgesia in 10 to 20 minutes with minimal discomfort and without distorting the tissue. A handheld device with two electrodes uses a mild electric current to deliver charged ions of lidocaine 2% and epinephrine 1:100,000 solution into the skin. Because iontophoresis acts quickly, it's an excellent choice for numbing an I.V. injection site in a child.

Administering a local anesthetic

A local anesthetic may be prescribed when starting peripheral I.V. therapy. If a local anesthetic is ordered, follow the steps below.

Using a U-100 insulin syringe with a 27G needle, draw 0.1 ml of lidocaine 1% without epinephrine.

Clean the venipuncture site.

Insert the needle next to the vein, introducing about one-third of it into the skin at a 30-degree angle. The side approach carries less risk of accidental vein puncture (indicated by blood appearing in the syringe). If the vein is deep, however, inject the lidocaine over the top of it. To make sure that you don't inject lidocaine into the vein—thus allowing it to circulate systemically—aspirate to check for a blood return. If this occurs, withdraw the needle and begin the procedure again.

Hold your thumb on the plunger of the syringe during insertion to avoid unnecessary movement when the needle is under the skin.

Without aspirating, quickly inject the lidocaine until a small wheal appears (as shown). You may not have to administer the entire amount in the syringe.

Quickly withdraw the syringe and massage the wheal with an alcohol swab. This will make the wheal disappear so the vein won't be hidden—although you'll see a small pinprick of blood. The skin numbness will last about 30 minutes.

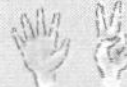 Insert the venous access device into the vein.

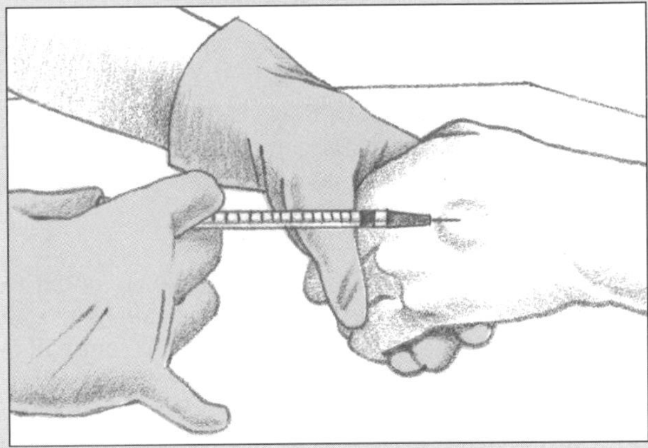

Stabilizing the vein

Stabilizing the vein helps ensure a successful venipuncture the first time and decreases the chance of bruising. If the tip of the venous access device repeatedly probes a moving vein wall, it can nick the vein and cause it to leak blood. When a vein gets nicked, it can't be reused immediately and a new venipuncture site must be found. Thus, the patient will experience the discomfort of another needle puncture.

Hold still, vein

To stabilize the vein, stretch the skin and hold it taut, and then lightly press it with your fingertips about 1½″ (3.5 cm) from the insertion site. (Never touch the prepared site or you'll recontaminate it.) The vein should feel round, firm, fully engorged, and resilient. Remove your fingertips. If the vein returns to its original position and appears larger than it did before you applied the tourniquet, it's adequately distended.

To help prevent the vein from "rolling," apply adequate traction with your nondominant hand to hold the skin and vein in place. This traction is particularly helpful in those with poor skin turgor or loosely anchored veins. (See *How to stabilize veins*, page 59.)

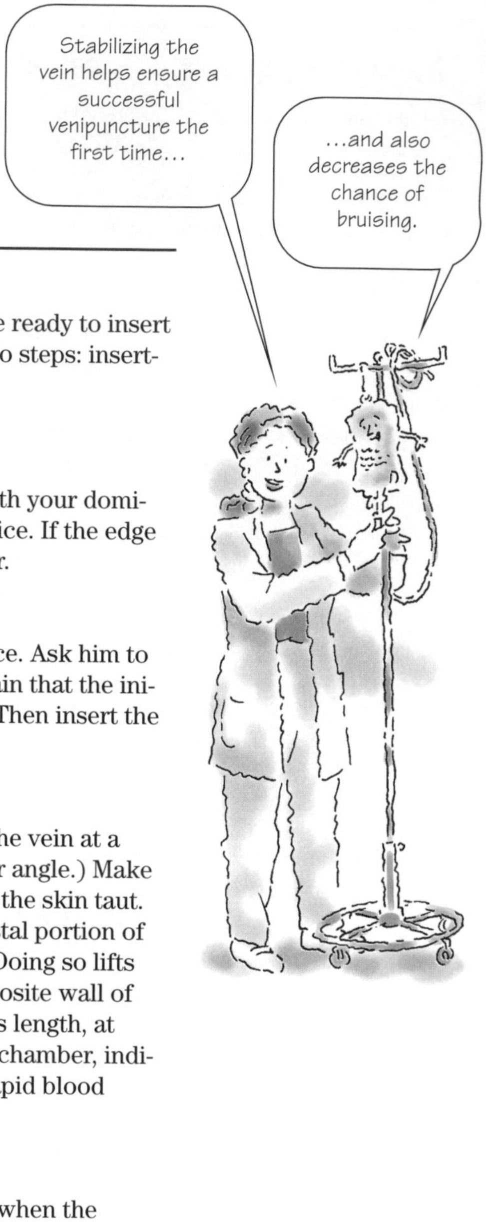

Stabilizing the vein helps ensure a successful venipuncture the first time...

...and also decreases the chance of bruising.

Insertion

Once you've prepared the venipuncture site, you're ready to insert the venous access device. The process involves two steps: inserting and advancing.

Inserting the venous access device

While still wearing gloves, grasp the plastic hub with your dominant hand, remove the cover, and examine the device. If the edge isn't smooth, discard the device and obtain another.

You need-le to know this

Tell the patient that you're about to insert the device. Ask him to remain still and to refrain from pulling away. Explain that the initial needle stick will hurt but will quickly subside. Then insert the device, using the direct approach.

Steady and direct

Keeping the bevel up, enter the skin directly over the vein at a 5- to 15-degree angle. (Deeper veins require a wider angle.) Make sure to use a steady, smooth motion while keeping the skin taut. As soon as the device enters the vein, lower the distal portion of the adapter until it's almost parallel with the skin. Doing so lifts the tip of the needle so it doesn't penetrate the opposite wall of the vein. Then advance the device to at least half its length, at which point you should see blood in the flashback chamber, indicating that you're in the vein. (You may not see a rapid blood return with a small vein.)

We're in!

Sometimes you'll feel a "pop" or a sense of release when the device enters the vein. However, this usually occurs only when a venous access device enters a large, thick-walled vein or when the patient has good tissue tone. You'll know for sure that the device is in the vein when you see a blood return in the flashback chamber.

How to stabilize veins

To help ensure successful venipuncture, you need to stabilize the patient's vein by stretching the skin and holding it taut. The stretching technique you'll use varies with the venipuncture site. This chart lists the various venipuncture sites along with a description of the stretching technique used for each.

Vein	Stretching technique
Metacarpal (hand) veins	Stretch the patient's hand and wrist downward, and hold the skin taut with your thumb.
Cephalic vein above wrist	Stretch the patient's fist laterally downward, and immobilize the skin with the thumb of your other hand.
Basilic vein at outer arm	Have the patient flex his elbow. While standing behind the flexed arm, retract the skin away from the site, and anchor the vein with your thumb. As an alternative, rotate the patient's extended lower arm inward, and approach the vein from behind the arm. (This position may be difficult for the patient to maintain.)
Inner aspect of wrist	Extend the patient's open hand backward from the wrist. Anchor the vein with your thumb below the insertion site.
Inner arm	Anchor the vein with your thumb above the wrist.
Antecubital fossa	Have the patient extend his arm completely. Anchor the skin with your thumb, about 2″ to 3″ (5 to 7.5 cm) below the antecubital fossa.
Saphenous vein of ankle	Extend the patient's foot downward and inward. Anchor the vein with your thumb, about 2″ to 3″ below the ankle.
Dorsum of foot	Pull the patient's foot downward. Anchor the vein with your thumb, about 2″ to 3″ below the vein (usually near the toes).
Scalp	Hold the skin taut with your thumb and forefinger.

Don't wing it, follow these steps. . .

If you're using a winged-set type infusion set, hold the edges of the wings between your thumb and forefinger, with the bevel facing upward. Then squeeze the wings together. Remove the protective cover from the needle, being careful not to contaminate the needle or the catheter. Then insert the device in the same manner as a standard I.V. catheter.

Advancing the venous access device

To advance the catheter before starting the infusion, first release the tourniquet. While stabilizing the vein with one hand, use the other to advance the catheter up to the hub. Be sure to advance only the catheter to avoid puncturing the vein with the needle. Next, remove the inner needle. Apply digital pressure to the catheter (to minimize blood exposure) and, using aseptic technique, attach the primed I.V. tubing or flush the inserted device with saline solution. The advantage of this method is that it usually results in less blood being spilled.

In the midst of infusion

To advance the catheter while infusing the I.V. solution, release the tourniquet and remove the inner needle. Using aseptic technique, attach the I.V. tubing and begin the infusion. While stabilizing the vein with one hand, use the other to advance the catheter into the vein. When the catheter is advanced, slow the I.V. flow rate. The advantage of using this method for advancing the catheter is that it reduces the risk of puncturing the vein wall because the catheter is advanced without the needle and the rapid flow dilates the vein. However, this method increases the risk of infection. A winged-set type infusion set is advanced using the same method.

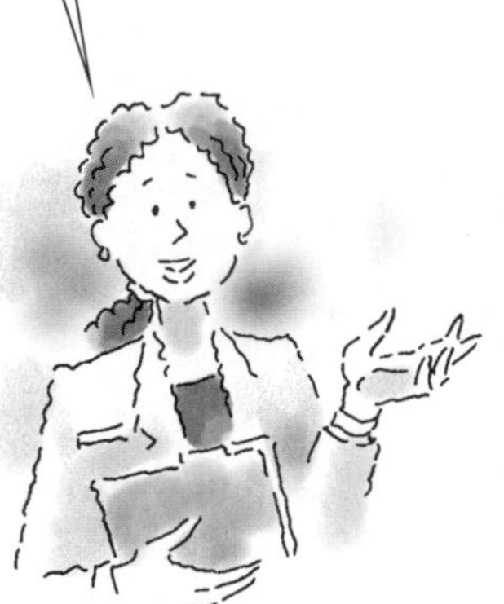

Wrapping it up

After the venous access device has been successfully inserted, secure the device using a commercial catheter securement device or sterile tape or sterile surgical strips. Dispose of the inner needle in a nonpermeable receptacle. Finally, regulate the flow rate, and then remove your gloves and wash your hands.

Intermittent infusion device

Also called a *saline lock*, an intermittent infusion device may be used when venous access must be maintained for intermittent use and a continuous infusion isn't necessary. This device keeps the access device sterile and prevents blood and other fluids from leaking from an open end. Much like the administration set injection port, the intermittent injection cap is self-sealing after the needle or needleless injector is removed. The ends of these devices are universal in size and fit the female end of any catheter or tubing designed for infusion therapy. Caps should have a luer-lock design to prevent disconnections.

Continuous infusion not required

The intermittent infusion device can be flushed with diluted saline solution to expel air from the equipment. Doing so makes it possible to maintain venous access in patients who must receive I.V. medications regularly or intermittently but don't require continuous infusion.

Less means more

The intermittent infusion device has many benefits. It minimizes the risks of fluid overload and electrolyte imbalance that may be associated with a keep-vein-open infusion. By eliminating the continuous use of I.V. solution containers and administration sets, it reduces the risk of contamination and lowers costs. Finally, it allows for patient mobility, which helps reduce anxiety.

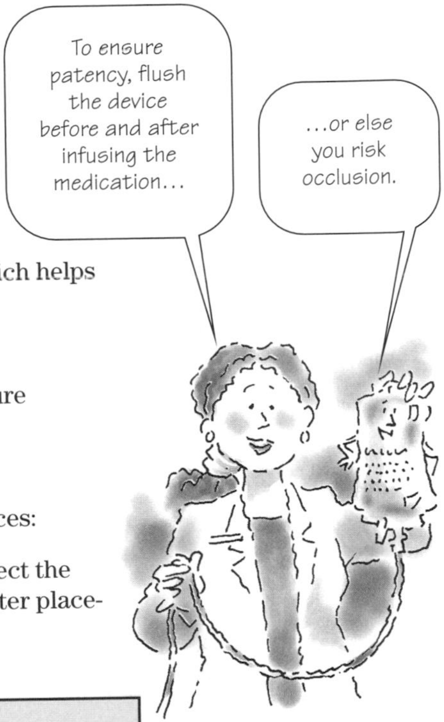

To ensure patency, flush the device before and after infusing the medication…

…or else you risk occlusion.

Flush before and after

Occlusion is possible if the device isn't flushed to ensure patency before and after medication is infused.

Two tips

Here are two tips related to intermittent infusion devices:

- If the patient feels a burning sensation as you inject the saline solution, stop the injection and check the catheter place-

From continuous to intermittent

The male adapter plug shown below allows you to convert an existing I.V. line into an intermittent infusion device.

To make the conversion:

1. Prime the male adapter plug with saline solution.
2. Clamp the I.V. tubing and remove the administration set from the catheter or needle hub.
3. Insert a male adapter plug.
4. Flush the access with the remaining solution to prevent occlusion.

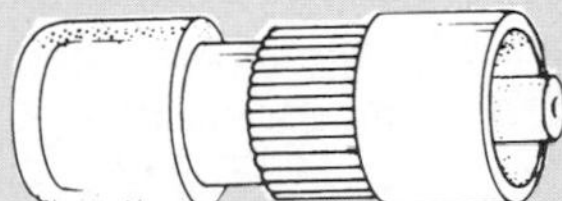

The male luer-lock adapter plug twists into place.

ment. If it's in the vein, inject the solution at a slower rate to minimize irritation.

If the practitioner orders discontinuation of an I.V. infusion, you can convert the existing line from a continuous to an intermittent venous access device. Just disconnect the I.V. tubing and insert an adapter plug into the device that's already in place. (See *From continuous to intermittent*, page 61.)

Insertion into deep veins

If a superficial vein isn't available, you may have to insert the venous access device into a deep vein that isn't visible. Here's how. First, put on gloves. Then palpate the area with your fingertips until you feel the vein. Next, clean the skin over the vein with chlorhexidine, using a back-and-forth motion. Then aim the device directly over the intended vein, stretch the skin with your gloved fingertips, and insert the venous access device at a 15-degree angle to the skin.

Making sure

Expect to insert the device one-half to two-thirds its length; that way you'll make sure that the needle and the catheter are in the vein lumen. When you see blood in the flashback chamber, remove the tourniquet and inner needle and advance the catheter with or without infusing fluid.

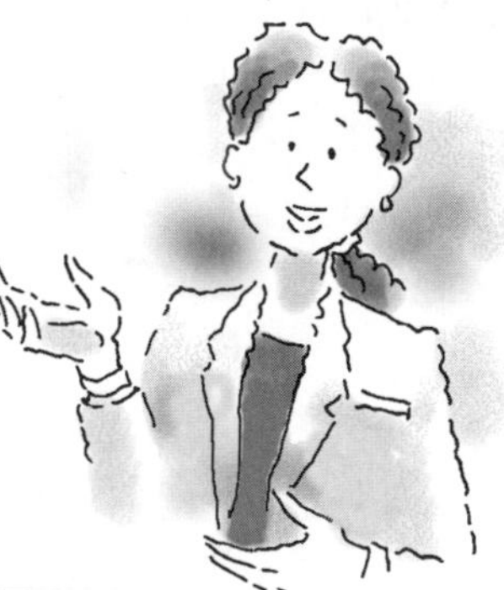

Take this sample

To smoothly and safely collect a blood sample, follow these step-by-step techniques after assembling your equipment and making the venipuncture:

- Place a pad underneath the site to protect the bed linens.
- When the venous access device is correctly placed, remove the inner needle.
- Leave the tourniquet tied.
- Attach the syringe to the venous access device's hub, and withdraw the appropriate amount of blood.
- Release the tourniquet and disconnect the syringe.
- Quickly attach the saline lock or I.V. tubing, regulate the flow rate, and stabilize the device.
- Attach a needleless device to the syringe, and transfer the blood into the laboratory tubes.
- Properly dispose of the equipment, and then complete I.V. catheter placement.

Collecting a blood sample

If a blood sample is ordered, you can collect it while performing the venipuncture. First, gather the necessary equipment: one or more laboratory tubes, an appropriate-size syringe without a needle, a needleless device, and a protective pad. Then follow the steps outlined in *Take this sample.* The Infusion Nurses Society and the Centers for Disease Control and Prevention recommend only drawing a blood sample from an I.V. catheter when it's inserted, not at any other time.

Securing the venous access device

After the infusion begins, secure the venous access device at the insertion site using a catheter securement device, sterile tape or sterile surgical strips, or a transparent semipermeable dressing. A stretch net or an arm board may also be used.

Applying a catheter securement device

A catheter securement device decreases the risk of infiltration, phlebitis, and I.V. line dislodgment. After inserting the venous access device, use an alcohol pad to wipe the skin near the insertion site. Place an adhesive strip, which usually comes with the device, over the catheter hub. Then apply a skin preparation solution and let it dry. Place the device under the luer lock of the venous access device and press it into place. A catheter securement device should be changed as often as the I.V. site, or every 7 days.

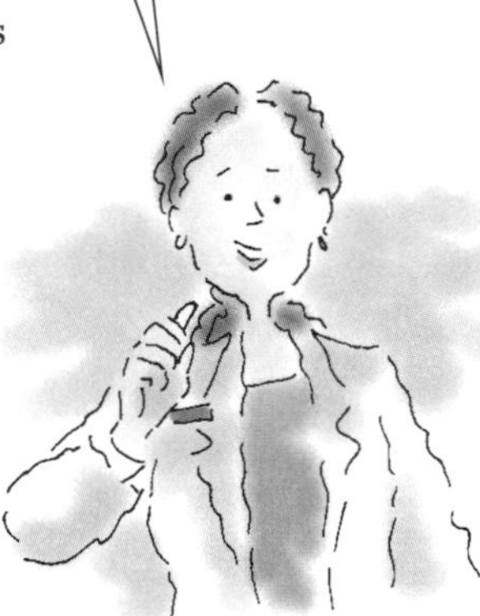

Applying tape

Stabilize the device and keep the hub from moving by using a standard taping method, such as the chevron, U, or H method. (See *Taping techniques*.)

Taping technique

Use as little tape as possible, and don't let the tape ends meet. Doing so reduces the risk of a tourniquet effect if infiltration occurs. Clip any hair from around the access area. Besides improving visibility and reducing pain when the tape is removed, clipping hair helps decrease colonization by bacteria present on the hair. Don't let the tape cover the patient's skin too far beyond the infusion device's entry site because it could obscure swelling and redness, signs of impending complications.

Taping techniques

If you use sterile tape to secure the venous access device to the insertion site, use one of these methods.

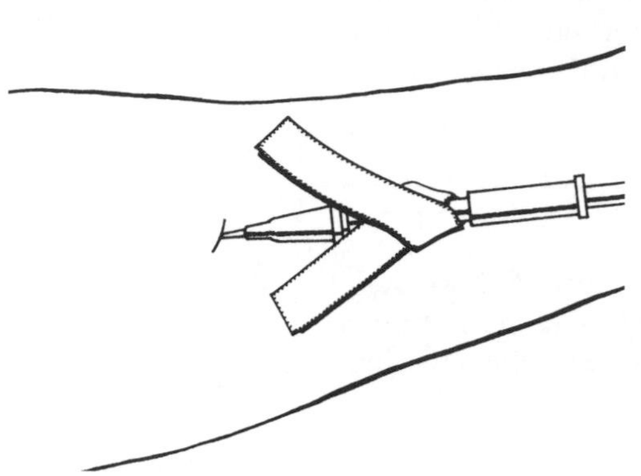

Chevron method

1. Cut a long strip of ½″ tape. Place it sticky side up under the hub.
2. Cross the ends of the tape over the hub, and secure the tape to the patient's skin on the opposite sides of the hub, as shown at left.
3. Apply a piece of 1″ tape across the two wings of the chevron. Loop the tubing and secure it with another piece of 1″ tape. Once a dressing is secured, apply a label. On the label, write the date and time of insertion, type and gauge of the needle, and your initials.

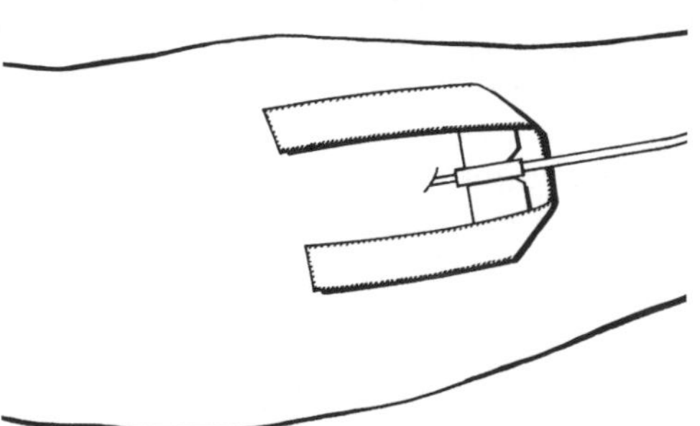

U method

1. Cut a strip of ½″ tape. With the sticky side up, place it under the hub of the catheter.
2. Bring each side of the tape up, folding it over the wings of the catheter, as shown at left. Press it down, parallel to the hub.
3. Next, apply tape to stabilize the catheter. After a dressing is secured, apply a label. On the label, write the date and time of insertion, type and gauge of the catheter, and your initials.

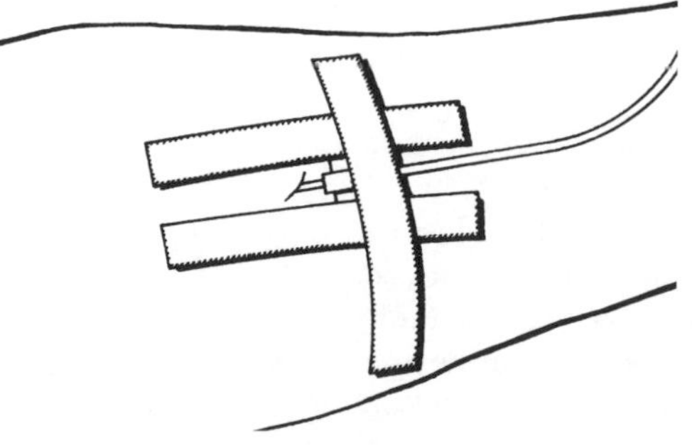

H method

1. Cut three strips of ½″ tape.
2. Place one strip of tape over each wing, keeping the tape parallel to the catheter.
3. Place the third strip of tape perpendicular to the first two, as shown at left. Put the tape directly on top of the wings. Make sure that the catheter is secure, and then apply a dressing and label. On the label, write the date and time of insertion, type and gauge of the catheter, and your initials.

Tale of the tape

If the patient has had a previous sensitivity reaction to tape, use a nonallergenic tape, preferably one that's lightweight and easy to remove. Paper tape usually isn't satisfactory for I.V. sites because it shreds and is difficult to remove after prolonged contact with skin and body heat.

It isn't fair!
Air can get through transparent dressings but I can't!

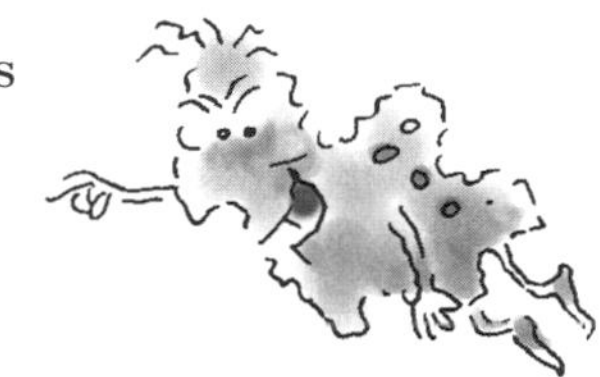

Applying a transparent dressing

To prevent infection, nurses in many health care facilities cover the insertion site with a transparent, semipermeable dressing. This dressing allows air to pass through but is impervious to microorganisms. (For instructions, see *How to apply a transparent semipermeable dressing.*)

The benefits are transparent

If this dressing remains intact, daily changes aren't necessary. Other advantages include fewer skin reactions and a clearly visible insertion site (especially helpful in detecting early signs of phlebitis and infiltration). The dressing is waterproof, so it protects the site

1st

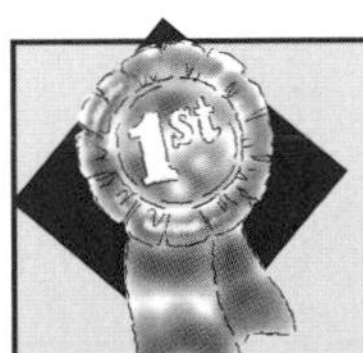

Best practice

How to apply a transparent semipermeable dressing

Here's how to apply a transparent semipermeable dressing, which allows for visual assessment of the catheter insertion site:

- Make sure the insertion site is clean and dry.
- Remove the dressing from the package and, using aseptic technique, remove the protective seal. Avoid touching the sterile surface.
- Place the dressing directly over the insertion site and the hub, as shown. Don't cover the tubing. Also, don't stretch the dressing; doing so may cause itching.
- Tuck the dressing around and under the catheter hub to make the site occlusive to microorganisms.

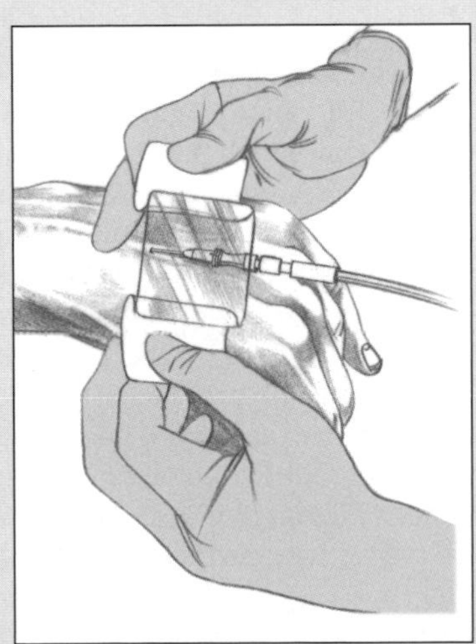

Grasp, lift, stretch

To remove the dressing, grasp one corner, stabilize the catheter, and then lift and stretch.

from contamination if it gets wet. In addition, because the dressing adheres well to the skin, the venous access device is less likely to accidentally dislodge.

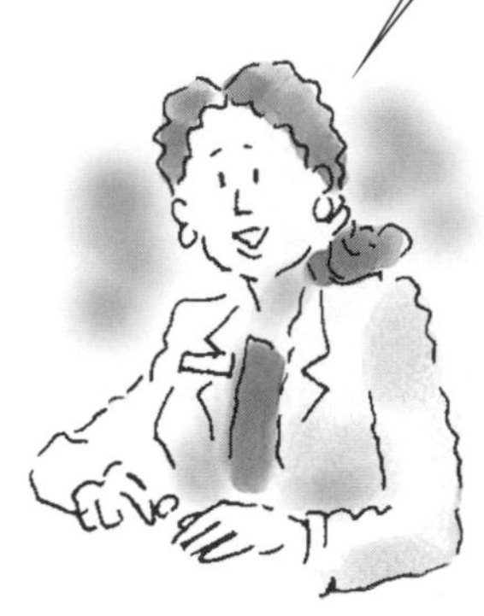

Using a stretch net

You can make the venous access device more secure by applying a stretch net to the affected limb. (If you'll be using the net on the patient's hand, cut a hole in the net sleeve for his thumb.) The net reduces the risk of accidental dislodgment, especially with patients who are confused or very active, and cuts down on the amount of tape needed to prevent dislodgment, which works particularly well for children.

Using an arm board

An arm board is an immobilization device that helps secure correct venous access device positioning and prevent unnecessary motion that could cause infiltration or inflammation. This immobilization device is sometimes necessary when the insertion site is near a joint or in the dorsum of the hand. An arm board may be used with a restraint in certain situations (for example, if the patient is confused or disoriented).

Arms restrictions

Because it's an immobilization device, the use of an arm board may be restricted by state or facility policies — so check first. Better yet, don't place the tip of the infusion device in a flexion area. Then you won't need an arm board.

The range-of-motion test

To determine whether an arm board is called for, move the patient's arm through its full range of motion (ROM) while watching the I.V. flow rate. If the flow stops during movement, you may need to use the arm board to prevent flexion of the extremity. Choose one that's long enough to prevent flexion and extension at the tip of the device. If necessary, cover it with a soft material before you secure it to the patient's arm. Make sure that you can still observe the insertion site.

Keep in mind that an arm board applied too tightly can cause nerve and tendon damage. If you need to use an arm board, remove it periodically according to facility policy so the patient can perform ROM activities and you can better observe for complications from restricted activity and infusion therapy.

Documenting the venipuncture

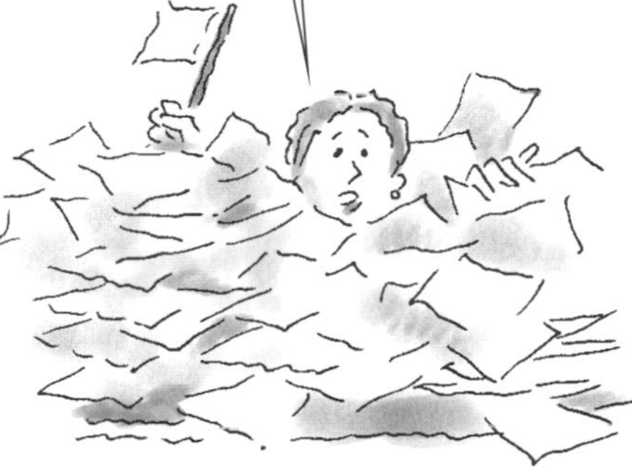

When you start an I.V. line, be sure to document:
- date and time of the venipuncture
- number of the solution container (if required by facility policy and procedures)
- type and amount of solution
- name and dosage of additives in the solution
- type of venipuncture device used, including length and gauge
- venipuncture site
- number of insertion attempts, if more than one
- flow rate
- adverse reactions and the actions taken to correct them
- patient teaching and evidence of patient understanding
- name of the person initiating the infusion.

Remember to document this information in all areas required by your facility's policy, such as the progress notes, intake and output flow sheets, the patient's chart, and medication sheets.

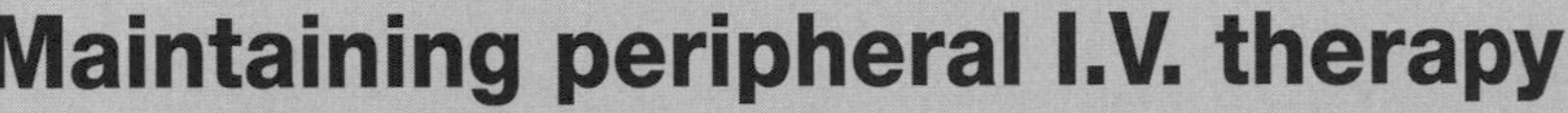

Maintaining peripheral I.V. therapy

After the I.V. infusion starts, focus on maintaining therapy and preventing complications. Doing so involves routine and special care measures as well as discontinuing the infusion when therapy is completed. Also, you should be prepared to meet the special needs of pediatric, elderly, and home care patients who require I.V. therapy.

Routine care

Routine care measures help prevent complications. They also give you an opportunity to observe the I.V. site for signs of inflammation or infection — two of the most common complications. Perform these measures according to your facility's policy and procedures. Wash your hands and wear gloves whenever you work near the venipuncture site.

Changing the dressing

The insertion site should be inspected and palpated for tenderness daily, through the intact dressing.

Time to change

Depending on your facility's policy, gauze dressings should be changed routinely every 48 hours. A transparent semipermeable dressing should be changed whenever its integrity is compromised because it has become soiled, wet, or loose or every 7 days.

Getting ready

Before performing a dressing change, gather this equipment:
- alcohol swab or other approved solution
- catheter securement device, sterile tape, or sterile surgical strips
- transparent semipermeable dressing
- sterile gloves.

To change a dressing, follow the steps outlined in *Changing a peripheral I.V. dressing.* Of course, use aseptic technique.

Changing the I.V. solution

To avoid microbial growth, don't allow an I.V. container to hang for more than 24 hours. Before changing the I.V. container, check the new one for cracks, leaks, and other damage. Also check the solution for discoloration, turbidity, and particulates. Note the date and time the solution was mixed and the expiration date.

I can't stand those microbes so please don't leave me hanging for more than 24 hours.

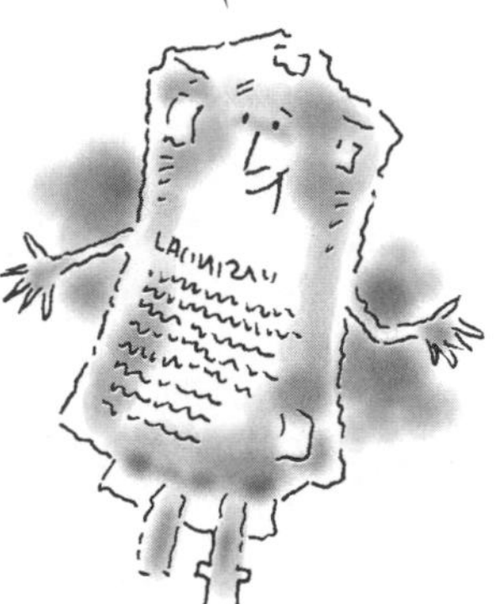

Changing a peripheral I.V. dressing

To change a peripheral I.V. dressing, follow these steps:

1. Wash your hands and put on sterile gloves.
2. Hold the catheter in place with your nondominant hand to prevent movement or dislodgment that could lead to infiltration; then gently remove the tape and the dressing.
3. Assess the venipuncture site for signs of infection (redness and tenderness), infiltration (coolness, blanching, edema), and thrombophlebitis (redness, firmness, pain along the path of the vein, edema).
4. If you detect these signs, apply pressure to the area with a sterile gauze pad and remove the catheter. Maintain pressure on the area until the bleeding stops, and then apply an adhesive bandage. Using new equipment, insert the I.V. access device at another site.
5. If you don't detect complications, hold the catheter at the hub and carefully clean around the site with an alcohol swab or other approved solution. Work in a swiping motion to avoid introducing pathogens into the cleaned area. Allow the area to dry completely.
6. Resecure the device and apply a transparent semipermeable dressing.

Cleanliness is key

After washing your hands, clamp the line, remove the spike from the old container, and quickly insert the spike into the new one. Then hang the new container and adjust the flow rate as prescribed.

Changing the administration set

Change the administration set according to your facility's policy (usually every 72 hours if it's a primary infusion line) and whenever you note or suspect contamination. If possible, change the set when you start a new venous access device during routine site rotation.

Getting equipped again

Before changing the set, gather:

- I.V. administration set
- sterile 2″ × 2″ gauze pad
- adhesive tape for labeling or appropriate labeling tapes supplied by your facility
- gloves.

Then follow the guidelines set out in *A change in administration*.

A change in administration

To quickly change the administration set for a peripheral infusion, follow these steps:

1. Wash your hands and put on gloves.
2. Reduce the I.V. flow rate. Then remove the old spike from the container, and place the cover of the new spike over it loosely.
3. Keeping the old spike upright and above the patient's heart level, insert the new spike into the I.V. container and prime the system.
4. Place a sterile gauze pad under the hub of the plastic catheter to create a sterile field.
5. Disconnect the old tubing from the venous access device, being careful not to dislodge or move the device. If you have trouble disconnecting the old tubing, try one of these techniques: Use a pair of hemostats to hold the hub securely while twisting and removing the end of the tubing, or grasp the venous access device with one pair of hemostats and the hard plastic of the luer-lock end of the administration set with another pair and pull the hemostats in opposite directions. *Don't clamp the hemostats shut; this may crack the tubing adapter or the venous access device.*
6. Using aseptic technique, quickly attach the new primed tubing to the device.
7. Adjust the flow to the prescribed rate.
8. Label the new tubing with the date and time of the change.

Changing the I.V. site

As a standard of care, rotate the I.V. site every 72 hours, according to facility policy. Sometimes, limited venous access will prevent you from changing sites this often. If that's the case, notify the practitioner of the situation and discuss alternatives for long-term insertion.

A complete change may be in order

Be prepared to change the entire system, including the venous access device, if you detect signs of thrombophlebitis, cellulitis, or I.V. therapy-related bacteremia.

Documentation

Record dressing, tubing, and solution changes, and note the condition of the venipuncture site. If you obtain a blood sample for culture and sensitivity testing, record the date and time and the practitioner's name.

Special care procedures

In addition to your routine care procedures, be prepared to handle special situations such as administering additive infusions. Also, when peripheral venous access is no longer possible, you may need to assist the practitioner with other venous access interventions such as insertion of a central line.

Additive infusions

To piggyback an I.V. drug into a primary line, use an add-a-line administration set. To infuse two compatible solutions simultaneously, connect an administration set with an attached needleless access catheter to the secondary solution container and prime the tubing. Hang the container at the same level as the primary solution.

"Y" marks the site

Next, clean a Y-site in the lower part of the primary tubing using an alcohol swab. Attach the secondary infusion set to the Y-site and secure it. Adjust each infusion rate independently. Remember that, with this setup, you may not have a backcheck valve above the Y-site, so one solution may flow back into the other.

Complications of therapy

Complications of peripheral I.V. therapy can arise from the venous access device, the infusion, or the medication being administered and can be local or systemic.

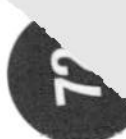

Local trouble? It may become systemwide...

Local complications include:
- infiltration
- phlebitis
- cellulitis
- catheter dislodgment (extravasation)
- occlusion
- vein irritation or pain at the I.V. site
- severed or fractured catheter
- hematoma
- venous spasm
- vasovagal reaction
- thrombosis
- thrombophlebitis
- nerve, tendon, or ligament damage.

Systemic complications include air embolism and allergic reactions. A complication may begin locally and become systemic — as when an infection at the venipuncture site progresses to septicemia. (For a complete description of local and systemic complications, see *Risks of peripheral I.V. therapy*, pages 73 to 77.)

Infiltrated!

Perhaps the greatest threat to a patient receiving I.V. therapy is infiltration (infused fluid leaking into the surrounding tissues). Infiltration occurs when the venous access device punctures the vein wall or migrates out of the vein. Infiltration is more likely to occur one or more days later, usually because the flexible tip of the catheter has penetrated the vein wall.

A joint risk

The risk of infiltration increases whenever you insert it near a joint. If the tip of the venous access device isn't inserted far enough into the vein lumen, part of the tip remains outside the vein and infiltration develops quickly.

More complications

Infiltration of a drug or solution can result in extravasation or breakdown of tissue (necrosis) because of the drug or solution's vesicant properties.

The fluid factor

The type of fluid being infused determines how much discomfort the patient feels during infiltration. Isotonic fluids usually don't cause much discomfort. Fluids with an acidic or alkaline pH, or those that are more than slightly hypertonic, are usually more irritating. Don't depend on the patient to complain of discomfort;

large amounts of I.V. fluid — as much as 1 L — can escape into the surrounding tissues without the patient knowing it.

Proper technique and careful monitoring are a winning team!

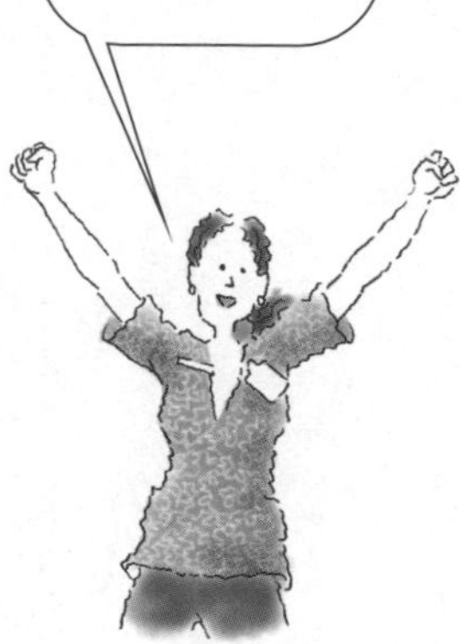

It's in your hands

Fortunately, you can minimize or prevent most complications by using proper insertion techniques and carefully monitoring the patient. I.V. sites should be checked by a nurse every 2 to 4 hours, or according to facility policy.

Always document — thoroughly document!

If complications do occur, document the signs and symptoms, patient complaints, name of the practitioner notified, and treatment. If the patient develops a severe infusion-related problem — for instance, vesicant infiltration (extravasation), circulatory compromise, a skin tear, fluid overload, or a severe allergic reaction — fill out an incident report according to your facility's policy and procedures. For legal purposes, document the details of the complication as well as any medical and nursing interventions provided.

Discontinuing the infusion

To discontinue the infusion, first clamp the infusion line and then remove the venous access device using aseptic technique. Here's how to proceed:

- After putting on gloves, lift the tape from the skin to expose the insertion site. You don't need to remove the tape or dressing as long as you can peel it back to expose the venous access device and skin.
- Be careful to avoid manipulating the device in the skin to prevent skin organisms from entering the bloodstream. Moving the device may also cause discomfort, especially if the insertion site has become phlebitic.
- Apply a sterile 2″ × 2″ dressing directly over the insertion site, and then quickly remove the device. (Never use an alcohol pad to clean the site when discontinuing an infusion; this may cause bleeding and a burning sensation.)
- Maintain direct pressure on the I.V. site for several minutes, and then tape a dressing over it, being careful not to encircle the limb. If possible, hold the limb upright for about 5 minutes to decrease venous pressure.
- Tell the patient to restrict his activity for about 10 minutes and to leave the site dressing in place for at least 8 hours. If he feels lingering tenderness at the I.V. site, apply warm, moist packs.
- Dispose of the used venipuncture equipment, tubing, and solution containers in a receptacle designated by your facility.

I need a break. Follow these steps to finish up the infusion.

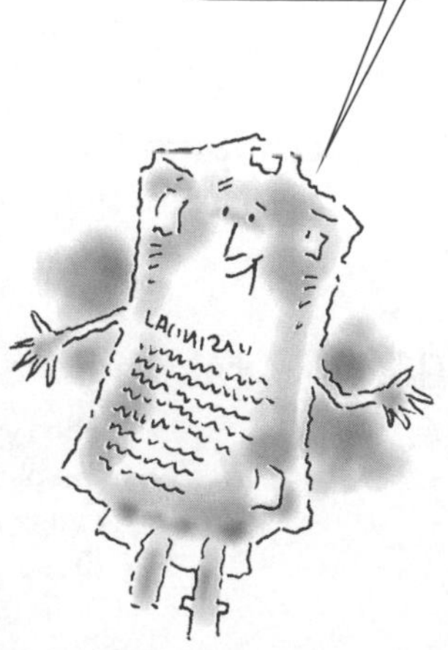

(Text continues on page 79.)

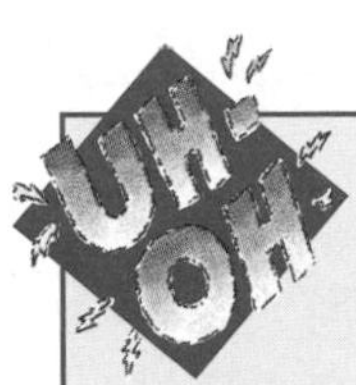

Warning!

Risks of peripheral I.V. therapy

Complications of peripheral I.V. therapy may be local or systemic. This chart lists some common complications along with their signs and symptoms, possible causes, and nursing interventions, including preventive measures.

Signs and symptoms	Possible causes	Nursing interventions
Local complications		
Phlebitis • Tenderness at tip of device and above • Redness at tip of catheter and along vein • Puffy area over vein • Vein hard on palpation • Elevated temperature	• Poor blood flow around device • Friction from catheter movement in vein • Device left in vein too long • Clotting at catheter tip (thrombophlebitis) • Solution with high or low pH or high osmolarity	• Remove the device. • Apply a warm pack. • Notify the practitioner. • Document the patient's condition and your interventions. *Prevention:* • Restart the infusion in a different vein using a larger vein for irritating infusate, or restart with a smaller-gauge device to ensure adequate blood flow. • Tape device securely to prevent motion.
Infiltration • Swelling at and around I.V. site (may extend along entire limb) • Discomfort, burning, or pain at site • Feeling of tightness at site • Decreased skin temperature around site • Blanching at site • Continuing fluid infusion even when vein is occluded, although rate may decrease • Absent backflow of blood • Slower flow rate	• Device dislodged from vein • Perforated vein	• Remove the device. • Apply warm soaks to aid absorption. • Elevate the limb. • Notify the practitioner if severe. • Periodically assess circulation by checking for pulse, capillary refill, and numbness or tingling. • Restart the infusion, preferably in another limb or above the infiltration site. • Document the patient's condition and your interventions. *Prevention:* • Check the I.V. site frequently, especially when using an I.V. pump. • Don't obscure area above site with tape. • Teach the patient to report discomfort, pain, or swelling.
Catheter dislodgment • Catheter partly backed out of vein • Infusate infiltrating	• Loosened tape or tubing snagged in bedclothes, resulting in partial retraction of catheter	• If no infiltration occurs, retape without pushing catheter back into vein. *Prevention:* • Tape the device securely on insertion.

(continued)

Risks of peripheral I.V. therapy *(continued)*

Signs and symptoms	Possible causes	Nursing interventions
Local complications *(continued)*		
Occlusion • No increase in flow rate when I.V. container is raised • Blood backup in line • Discomfort at insertion site	• I.V. flow interrupted • Intermittent device not flushed • Blood backup in line when patient walks • Hypercoagulable patient • Line clamped too long	• Use a low flush pressure syringe during injection. Don't use force. If resistance is met, stop immediately. If unsuccessful, reinsert the I.V. device. *Prevention:* • Maintain the I.V. flow rate. • Flush promptly after intermittent piggyback administration. • Have the patient walk with his arm below heart level to reduce the risk of blood backup.
Vein irritation or pain at I.V. site • Pain during infusion • Possible blanching if vasospasm occurs • Red skin over vein during infusion • Rapidly developing signs of phlebitis	• Solution with high or low pH or high osmolarity, such as potassium chloride, phenytoin, and some antibiotics (vancomycin and nafcillin)	• Slow the flow rate. • Try using an electronic flow device to achieve a steady regulated flow. *Prevention:* • Dilute solutions before administration. For example, give antibiotics in 250-ml rather than 100-ml solution. • If long-term therapy is planned, ask the practitioner to use central access device.
Severed catheter • Leakage from catheter shaft	• Catheter inadvertently cut by scissors • Reinsertion of needle into catheter	• If the broken part is visible, attempt to retrieve it. If unsuccessful, notify the practitioner. • If a portion of the catheter enters the bloodstream, place a tourniquet above the I.V. site to prevent progression. • Notify the practitioner and radiology. • Document the patient's condition and your interventions. *Prevention:* • Don't use scissors around the I.V. site. • Never reinsert a needle into catheter. • Remove the unsuccessfully inserted catheter and needle together.

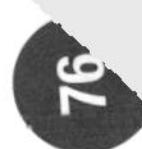

Risks of peripheral I.V. therapy *(continued)*

Signs and symptoms	Possible causes	Nursing interventions
Local complications *(continued)*		
Hematoma • Tenderness at venipuncture site • Bruising around site • Inability to advance or flush I.V. line	• Vein punctured through ventral wall at time of venipuncture • Leakage of blood from needle displacement	• Remove the venous access device. • Apply pressure and warm soaks to the affected area. • Recheck for bleeding. • Document the patient's condition and your interventions. *Prevention:* • Choose a vein that can accommodate the size of the intended device. • Release the tourniquet as soon as successful insertion is achieved.
Venous spasm • Pain along vein • Sluggish flow rate when clamp is completely open • Blanched skin over vein	• Severe vein irritation from irritating drugs or fluids • Administration of cold fluids or blood • Very rapid flow rate (with fluids at room temperature)	• Apply warm soaks over the vein and surrounding area. • Slow the flow rate. *Prevention:* • Use blood warmer for blood or packed red blood cells when appropriate.
Thrombosis • Painful, reddened, and swollen vein • Sluggish or stopped I.V. flow	• Injury to endothelial cells of vein wall, allowing platelets to adhere and thrombus to form	• Remove the device; restart the infusion in the opposite limb if possible. • Apply warm soaks. • Watch for I.V. therapy-related infection. (Thrombi provide an excellent environment for bacterial growth.) *Prevention:* • Use proper venipuncture techniques to reduce injury to the vein.
Thrombophlebitis • Severe discomfort • Reddened, swollen, and hardened vein	• Thrombosis and inflammation	• Remove the device; restart the infusion in the opposite limb if possible. • Apply warm soaks. • Notify the practitioner. • Watch for I.V. therapy-related infection. (Thrombi provide an excellent environment for bacterial growth.) *Prevention:* • Check the site frequently. Remove the device at the first sign of redness and tenderness.

(continued)

Risks of peripheral I.V. therapy *(continued)*

Signs and symptoms	Possible causes	Nursing interventions
Local complications *(continued)*		
Nerve, tendon, or ligament damage • Extreme pain (similar to electric shock when nerve is contracted) • Numbness and muscle contraction • Delayed effects, including paralysis, numbness, and deformity	• Improper venipuncture technique, resulting in injury to surrounding nerves, tendons, or ligaments • Tight taping or improper splinting with arm board	• Stop procedure and remove the device. *Prevention:* • Don't repeatedly penetrate tissues with the venous access device. • Don't apply excessive pressure when taping or encircle the limb with tape. • Pad the arm board and, if possible, pad the tape securing the arm board.
Systemic complications		
Circulatory overload • Discomfort • Neck vein engorgement • Respiratory distress • Increased blood pressure • Crackles • Large positive fluid balance (intake is greater than output)	• Roller clamp loosened to allow run-on infusion • Flow rate too rapid • Miscalculation of fluid requirements	• Raise the head of the bed. • Slow the infusion rate (but don't remove the venous access device). • Administer oxygen as needed. • Notify the practitioner. • Administer medications (probably furosemide) as ordered. *Prevention:* • Use a pump, volume-control set, or rate minder for elderly or compromised patients. • Recheck calculations of fluid requirements. • Monitor the infusion frequently.
Systemic infection (septicemia or bacteremia) • Fever, chills, and malaise for no apparent reason • Contaminated I.V. site, usually with no visible signs of infection at site	• Failure to maintain aseptic technique during insertion or site care • Severe phlebitis, which can set up ideal conditions for organism growth • Poor taping that permits venous access device to move, which can introduce organisms into bloodstream • Prolonged indwelling time of device • Immunocompromised patient	• Notify the practitioner. • Administer medications as prescribed. • Culture the site and the device. • Monitor the patent's vital signs. *Prevention:* • Use scrupulous aseptic technique when handling solutions and tubings, inserting the venous access device, and discontinuing the infusion. • Secure all connections. • Change I.V. solutions, tubing, and venous access device at recommended times.

Risks of peripheral I.V. therapy *(continued)*

Signs and symptoms	Possible causes	Nursing interventions
Systemic complications *(continued)*		
Air embolism • Respiratory distress • Unequal breath sounds • Weak pulse • Increased central venous pressure • Decreased blood pressure • Confusion, disorientation, loss of consciousness	• Empty solution container • Solution container empties; next container pushes air down line • Tubing disconnected from venous access device or I.V. bag	• Discontinue the infusion. • Place the patient in Trendelenburg's position on his left side to allow air to enter the right atrium and disperse through the pulmonary artery. • Administer oxygen. • Notify the practitioner. • Document the patient's condition and your interventions. *Prevention:* • Purge the tubing of air completely before the infusion. • Use an air-detection device on the pump or an air-eliminating filter proximal to the I.V. site. • Secure all connections.
Allergic reaction • Itching • Tearing eyes and runny nose • Bronchospasm • Wheezing • Urticarial rash • Edema at I.V. site • Anaphylactic reaction (within minutes or up to 1 hour after exposure), including flushing, chills, anxiety, agitation, generalized itching, palpitations, paresthesia, throbbing in ears, wheezing, coughing, seizures, and cardiac arrest	• Allergens such as medications	• If a reaction occurs, stop the infusion immediately and infuse normal saline solution. • Maintain a patent airway. • Notify the practitioner. • Administer an antihistaminic steroid, an anti-inflammatory, and antipyretic drugs, as ordered. • Give 0.2 to 0.5 ml of 1:1,000 aqueous epinephrine subcutaneously. Repeat at 3-minute intervals and as needed, as ordered. • Administer cortisone if ordered. *Prevention:* • Obtain the patient's allergy history. Be aware of cross-allergies. • Assist with test dosing. • Monitor the patient carefully during the first 15 minutes of administration of a new drug.

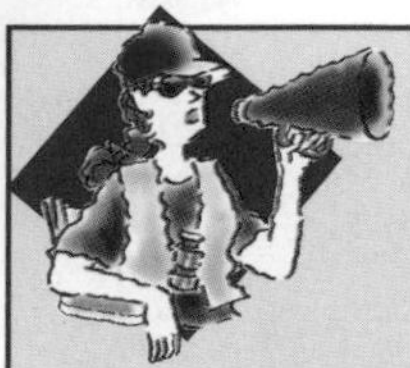

That's a wrap!

Peripheral I.V. therapy review

Basics of peripheral I.V. therapy

Peripheral I.V. therapy involves:

- checking the practitioner's orders
- ordering supplies and equipment
- labeling solutions and tubing
- documenting nursing interventions.

Peripheral I.V. therapy is ordered when venous access is needed for:

- surgery
- transfusions
- emergency care
- maintaining hydration
- restoring fluid and electrolyte balance
- providing fluids for resuscitation
- administering I.V. medications or nutrients.

Preparing for venipuncture and infusion

- Check the patient's medical record for allergies, disease history, and his current diagnosis and care plan.
- Review the practitioner's orders and the patient's laboratory studies.
- Describe the procedure to the patient and provide patient teaching.
- Provide privacy, and then have the patient put on a gown and remove all jewelry.
- Position the patient comfortably.
- Select the appropriate insertion site, venous access device, solution container, and administration set according to the therapy required. Then obtain an infusion pump.
- Label the container correctly and attach the administration set as appropriate.

Performing a venipuncture

- Dilate the vein, apply a tourniquet as appropriate, and prepare the access site.
- Stabilize the vein, and then position the venous access device with the bevel side up.
- Insert the device using a smooth, steady motion.
- Collect blood samples using appropriate equipment, and secure the venous access device.
- Document the procedure in the appropriate areas (such as the progress notes, intake and output flowsheets, or the patient's chart or medication sheet) according to your facility's policy.

Maintaining peripheral I.V. therapy

- Focus on preventing complications.
- Discontinue the infusion when therapy is completed.
- Change a gauze dressing every 48 hours.
- Change the I.V. solution container when due or every 24 hours.
- Change administration sets according to facility policy or every 72 hours.
- Change the I.V. site every 72 hours according to facility policy.
- Document dressing, tubing, and solution changes, and the condition of the venipuncture site.

Patients with special needs

- Infant I.V. sites include the hands, feet, antecubital fossa, dorsum of hand, and scalp. Scalp veins are used for infants ages 6 months and younger.
- Intraosseous access is used for fluid resuscitation, medication administration, and blood transfusions until a vein can be accessed.
- Veins in elderly patients are more fragile and less elastic. Remove the tourniquet promptly to prevent increased vascular pressure.

Peripheral I.V. therapy review *(continued)*

Complications of therapy

- Local complications include infiltration, phlebitis, cellulitis, catheter dislodgment, occlusion, vein irritation or pain at the I.V. site, severed or fractured catheter, hematoma, venous spasm, vasovagal reaction, thrombosis, thrombophlebitis, and damage to the nerves, tendons, or ligaments.
- Systemic complications include air embolism, allergic reactions, and septicemia.

- Document the time of removal, the catheter length and integrity, and the condition of the site. Also, record how the patient tolerated the procedure and any nursing interventions.

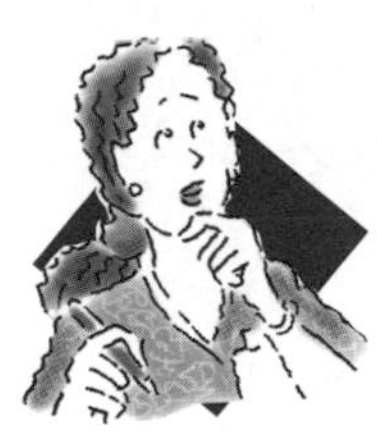

Quick quiz

1. The first step in performing a routine venipuncture is to:

A. prepare the venipuncture site.
B. dilate the vein.
C. use a local anesthetic.
D. attach the tubing to the device.

Answer: B. The sequence in performing the venipuncture is to dilate the vein and then prepare the site. An anesthetic may or may not be used.

2. When applying a transparent dressing, it's important to:

A. stretch the dressing as much as possible.
B. cover the site and the tubing.
C. tuck the dressing around and under the hub.
D. always use a gauze dressing with the transparent dressing.

Answer: C. Tucking the dressing in this manner will make the site occlusive to microorganisms. Stretching the dressing will cause itching, and the tubing should never be covered.

3. Which of the following is the preferred and most accessible site for a venous access device in the infant under age 6 months?

A. Foot
B. Hand
C. Antecubital fossa
D. Scalp

Answer: D. Although all of these sites are favorable, the scalp veins are the most accessible.

4. Your patient has swelling at the I.V. site, discomfort, burning, decreased skin temperature, and blanching around the site. These are signs of which of the following I.V. complications?

A. Phlebitis
B. Infiltration
C. Occlusion
D. Air embolism

Answer: B. Swelling at the I.V. site, discomfort, burning, decreased skin temperature, and blanching around the site may indicate infiltration.

5. Which peripheral venipuncture site should be used as a last resort when no other veins are available?

A. Cephalic vein
B. Median antebrachial vein
C. Metacarpal vein
D. Basilic vein

Answer: B. The median antebrachial vein should only be used as a last resort, when no other means are available. It rises from the palm and runs along the ulnar side of the forearm. All of the other veins listed are suitable for venipuncture.

6. An in-line filter may be used for which patient?

A. A patient receiving antibiotics I.V. every 6 hours
B. A patient with a history of phlebitis
C. A patient receiving normal saline solution
D. A patient scheduled for surgery

Answer: B. In-line filters aren't normally used because of the increased costs. However, you can expect to use an in-line filter for an immunosuppressed patient, when administering total parenteral nutrition, when using additives composed of many separate particles, and when the risk of phlebitis is high.

Scoring

☆☆☆ If you answered all six questions correctly, take a bow! At this juncture, fear no venipuncture.

☆☆ If you answered four to five questions correctly, congratulations! For the most part, you delivered the correct solutions.

☆ If you answered fewer than four questions correctly, don't get discouraged! Your quiz score is a peripheral matter. Review the chapter and try again.

3

Central venous therapy

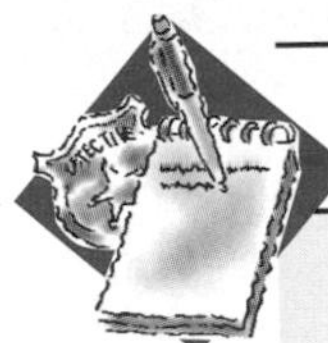

Just the facts

In this chapter, you'll learn:

- ♦ the purpose of central venous (CV) therapy
- ♦ CV therapy equipment
- ♦ patient preparation for CV access device insertion
- ♦ the nurse's role in access device insertion
- ♦ maintenance and discontinuation of CV therapy
- ♦ the proper care of a patient with an implanted port.

Understanding central venous therapy

In central venous (CV) therapy, drugs or fluids are infused directly into a major vein. CV therapy is used in various situations, including emergencies or when a patient's peripheral veins are inaccessible. It may be ordered when a patient:

- needs infusion of a large volume of fluid
- requires multiple infusions
- requires long-term infusion therapy
- needs infusion of irritating medications such as potassium
- needs infusion of fluids with high osmolarity such as total parenteral nutrition (TPN).

Bringing it on home

At one time, only patients in intensive care and specialty units received CV therapy. Today, patients in any unit or patients in home care and long-term care may receive CV therapy.

Benefits of central venous therapy

CV therapy offers many benefits, such as:

- access to the central veins
- rapid infusion of medications or large amounts of fluids
- a way to draw blood samples and measure CV pressure, an important indicator of circulatory function
- reduced need for repeated venipunctures, which decreases the patient's anxiety and preserves the peripheral veins
- reduced risk of vein irritation from infusing irritating or caustic substances.

By reducing the need for repeated venipunctures, CV therapy preserves peripheral veins.

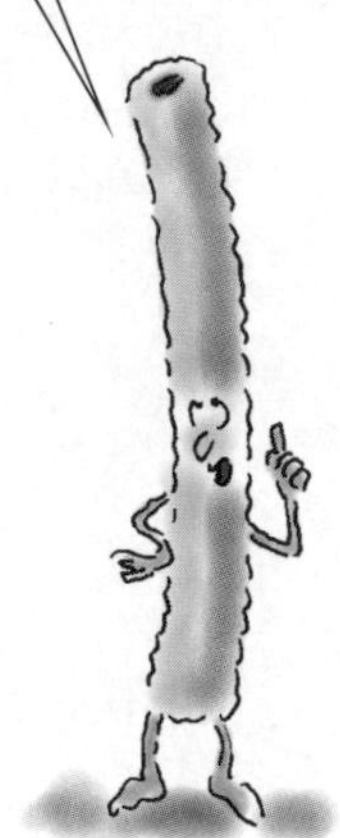

Risks of central venous therapy

Like any other invasive procedure, CV therapy has its drawbacks. It increases the risk of life-threatening complications, such as:

- pneumothorax
- sepsis
- thrombus formation
- perforation of the vessel and adjacent organs.

Using a CV access device also has disadvantages:

- It requires more time and skill to insert than a peripheral I.V. catheter.
- It costs more to maintain than a peripheral I.V. catheter.
- It carries a risk of air embolism.
- It carries a greater risk of infection than a peripheral I.V. catheter.

Venous circulation

The 5 L of blood in an average adult body really gets around. After delivering oxygen and nutrients throughout the body, depleted blood flows from the capillaries to ever-widening veins, finally returning to the right side of the heart before collecting a fresh supply of oxygen from the lungs.

CV circulation enters the right atrium through two major veins: the superior vena cava and the inferior vena cava.

Venous blood enters my right atrium through the superior and inferior venae cavae.

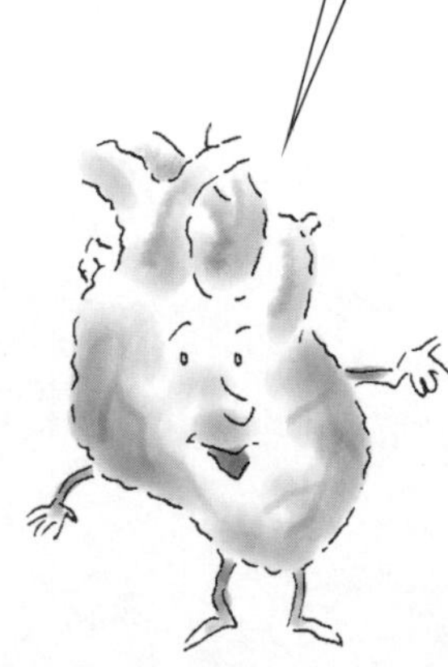

Going down...

Before flowing into the right atrium, venous return from the head, neck, and arms enters the superior vena cava through three main routes:

- internal and external jugular veins
- subclavian vein
- right and left brachiocephalic veins.

...and coming up

Venous return from the legs enters the inferior vena cava and returns blood to the right atrium through several routes, including the femoral venous system along with multiple accessory venous pathways throughout the abdomen.

Getting to the point

In CV therapy, a catheter is inserted with its tip in one of two places (depending on venous accessibility and the prescribed infusion therapy):

- superior vena cava
- inferior vena cava.

Blood flows unimpeded around the tip at about 2,000 ml/minute, allowing the rapid infusion of large amounts of fluid directly into the circulation. Because fluids are rapidly diluted by the venous circulation, highly concentrated or caustic fluids can be infused. (See *CV access device pathways*, page 84.)

Because blood flows very quickly and unimpeded around the CV access device's tip, fluids are rapidly diluted by the venous circulation, allowing for the infusion of highly concentrated or caustic solutions.

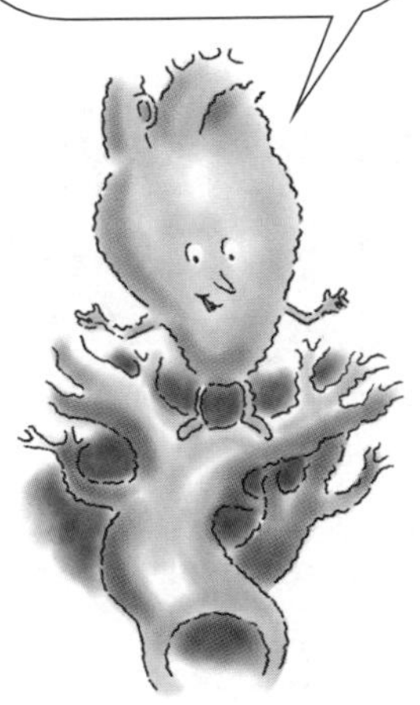

Taking a different route

In a variation of CV therapy, a catheter is inserted through a peripheral vein, and the catheter tip is passed all the way to the superior vena cava. For instance, a catheter inserted in the arm (at the antecubital fossa) enters the basilic vein and is threaded through the subclavian vein and the brachiocephalic vein to the superior vena cava. Catheters come with a variety of introducer and lumen sizes and variable lengths to help tailor the insertion to individual patients.

CV access devices

Selecting the appropriate CV access device for a patient depends on the type of therapy needed. Types of CV access devices include:

- nontunneled catheters
- tunneled catheters
- peripherally inserted central catheters (PICCs)
- implanted ports.

Nontunneled CV catheters

Nontunneled catheters are radiopaque, so placement can be checked by X-ray. They directly access the subclavian vein, and the catheter is advanced into the superior vena cava. They're usually designed for short-term use, such as brief continuation of I.V. therapy following a patient's hospitalization. They aren't appropriate for a patient starting long-term I.V. therapy.

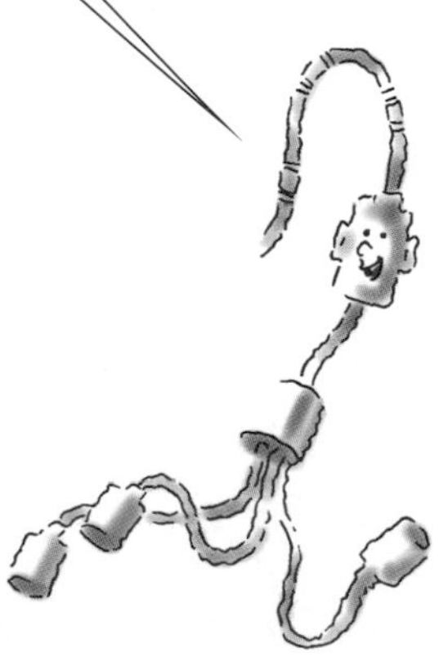

CV access device pathways

Usually, a central venous (CV) access device is inserted into the subclavian vein or the internal jugular vein. The access device should terminate in the superior vena cava. The illustrations below show several common pathways of the CV access device.

Inserted into the subclavian vein, this CV access device terminates in the superior vena cava.

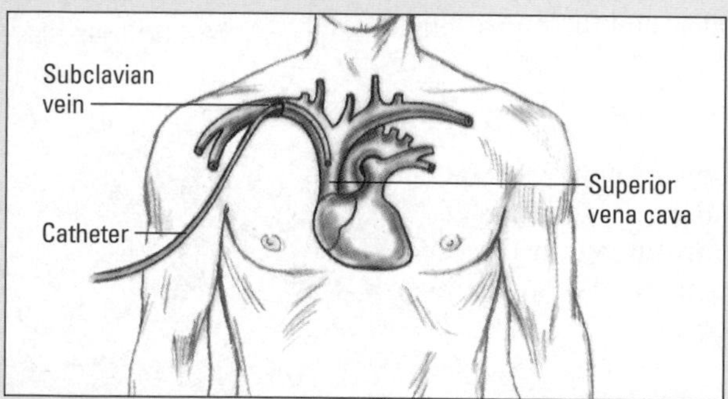

This CV access device enters the internal jugular vein and terminates in the superior vena cava.

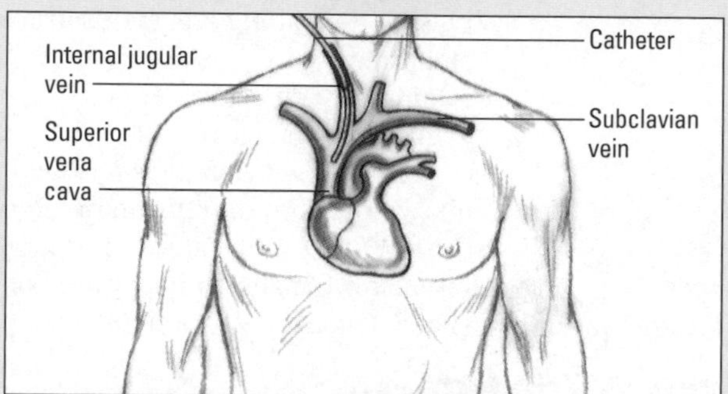

This catheter, peripherally inserted into the basilic vein, terminates in the superior vena cava.

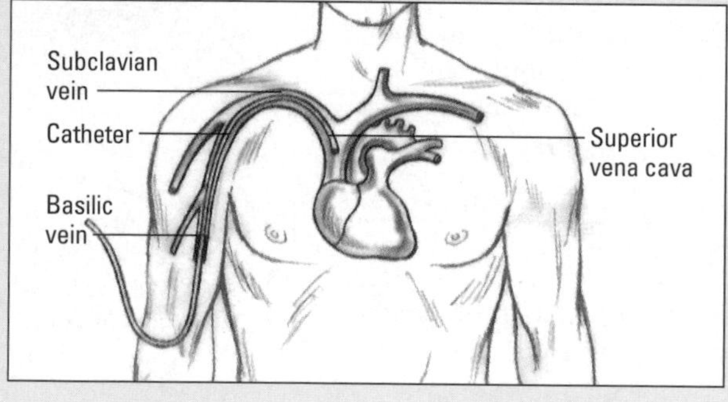

This CV access device enters the subclavian vein and terminates in the superior vena cava. Note that the catheter tunnels (shown by broken line) from the insertion site, through the subcutaneous tissue, to an exit site on the skin (usually located by the nipple). Also note how the position of the Dacron cuff helps hold the catheter in place.

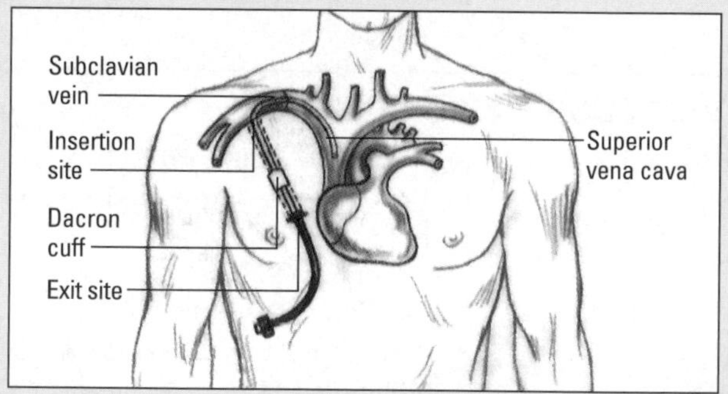

Need a change?

To avoid infection, nontunneled catheters are changed according to facility policy. The optimal time interval for removing the catheter is unknown; current standards recommend only changing the catheter when there is evidence of local or systemic complications caused by the catheter. Ongoing and frequent monitoring of the insertion site should be performed. If the insertion site appears red or if infection is suspected, stop using the access site as soon as possible and use an alternate site. Discuss culturing the site and catheter with the practitioner.

Tunneled CV catheters

Tunneled CV catheters are designed for long-term use. They're also radiopaque and usually made of silicone. Silicone is much less likely to cause thrombosis than polyurethane or polyvinyl chloride because it's more physiologically compatible. This compatibility minimizes irritation or damage to the vein lining.

Cuff link

A tunneled CV catheter has a cuff that encourages tissue growth within the tunnel. In about 7 to 10 days, the tissue anchors the catheter in place and keeps bacteria out of venous circulation. In most cases, the cuff is made of Dacron. An alternate type of cuff contains silver ions that provide antibacterial protection for about 3 months.

Tissue growth within a tunneled catheter keeps bacteria like me out of venous circulation.

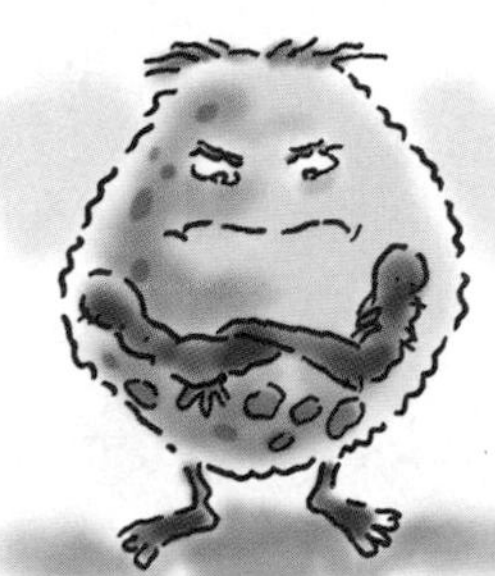

Tunnel tidbits

Tunneled catheters are better suited to home care patients than nontunneled catheters because they're designed for long-term use. They're used in patients who have poor peripheral venous access or who need long-term daily infusions, such as those with:

- cancer
- acquired immunodeficiency syndrome (AIDS)
- intestinal malabsorption
- anemia
- transplants
- bone or organ infections
- other chronic diseases.

Medications that are given by tunneled CV catheter include:

- antibiotics
- chemotherapy
- TPN
- blood products.

Tunnel types

Common tunneled catheters for long-term use include the Broviac, Hickman, and Groshong catheters. Tunneled catheters can be single-lumen, double-lumen, triple-lumen, or multilumen and can vary in size. The Broviac tunneled CV catheter has a small lumen. It's a good choice for a patient with small central veins, such as a child. (See *Guide to CV access devices*, pages 86 to 88.)

Peripherally inserted central catheters

One of the most commonly used catheters for peripheral CV therapy is the PICC. A PICC, also known as a long-arm or long-line catheter, is inserted through a peripheral vein, with the tip ending in the superior vena cava. If the catheter tip is located outside the vena cava, it's no longer considered a central catheter and should be removed.

Generally, PICCs are used when patients need infusions of caustic drugs (such as long-term antibiotic therapy) or solutions. They're also used in patients who need transfusions. PICCs are especially useful if the patient doesn't have reliable routes for short-term I.V. therapy.

Generally, PICCs are used when patients need infusions of caustic drugs or solutions.

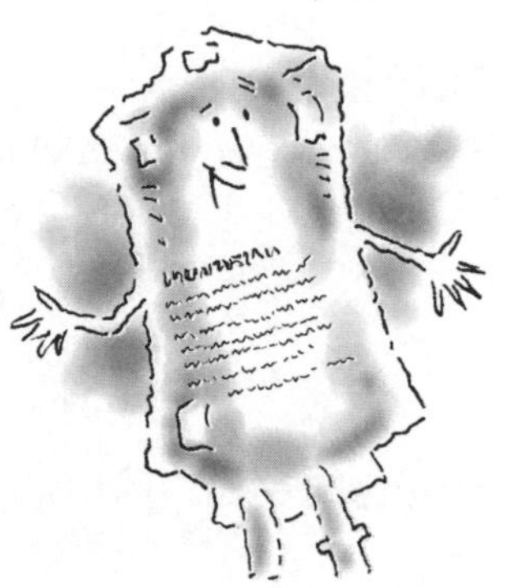

Why pick a PICC?

When a patient needs CV therapy for 5 days to several months or requires repeated venous access, a PICC may be the best choice. A PICC may also be ordered when a patient has a chest injury due to trauma or burns or respiratory problems due to chronic obstructive pulmonary disease (COPD) or other conditions.

Using a peripheral insertion site for a PICC helps prevent complications such as pneumothorax that may occur with a CV line that's inserted into the chest.

Guide to CV access devices

Types of central venous (CV) access devices differ in their design, composition, and indications for use. This chart outlines the advantages, disadvantages, and nursing considerations for several commonly used catheters.

Catheter description and indications	Advantages and disadvantages	Nursing considerations
Short-term, single-lumen catheter *Description* • Polyurethane or Silastic rubber • Approximately 8″ (20 cm) long • Variety of lumen gauges *Indications* • Short-term CV access • Emergency access • Patient who requires only a single lumen	*Advantages* • It can be inserted at bedside. • It's easily removed. • Stiffness aids central venous pressure (CVP) monitoring. *Disadvantages* • Catheter has limited functions. • Use limited to no more than 2 weeks.	• Assess frequently for signs of infection and clot formation.

Guide to CV access devices *(continued)*

Catheter description and indications	Advantages and disadvantages	Nursing considerations
Short-term, multilumen catheter *Description* • Polyurethane or Silastic rubber • Double, triple, or quadruple lumen at ¾″ (1.9-cm) intervals • Variety of lumen gauges *Indications* • Short-term CV access • Patient with limited insertion sites who requires multiple infusions	*Advantages* • It can be inserted at bedside. • It's easily removed. • Stiffness aids CVP monitoring. • It allows infusion of multiple solutions through the same catheter (for example, incompatible solutions). *Disadvantages* • Catheter has limited functions. • Use limited to no more than 2 weeks.	• Know the gauge and purpose of each lumen. • Use the same lumen for the same task (for example, to administer total parenteral nutrition or to collect a blood sample). 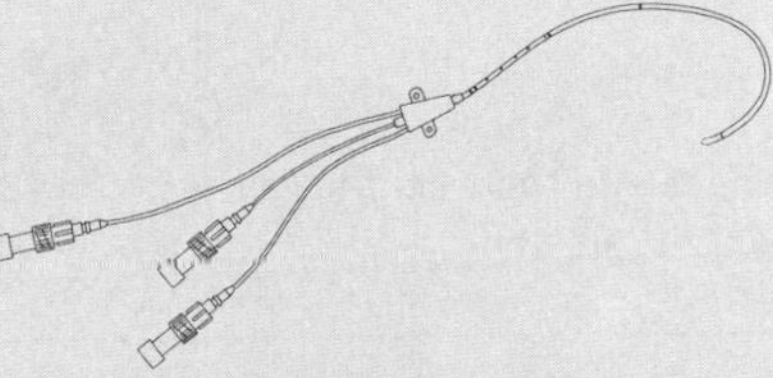
Groshong catheter *Description* • Silicone rubber • Approximately 35″ (88.9 cm) long • Closed end with pressure-sensitive three-way valve • Dacron cuff • Available with single or double lumen • Tunneled *Indications* • Long-term CV access • Patient with heparin allergy or risk of heparin-induced thrombocytopenia	*Advantages* • It's less thrombogenic than catheters made with polyvinylchloride. • Pressure-sensitive three-way valve eliminates heparin flushes. • Dacron cuff anchors catheter and prevents bacterial migration. *Disadvantages* • It requires surgical insertion. • It tears and kinks easily. • Blunt end makes it difficult to clear substances from its tip. • It must be removed by practitioner.	• Two surgical sites require dressing after insertion. • Handle the catheter gently. • Check the external portion frequently for kinks or leaks. (Repair kit is available.) • Observe frequently for kinks or tears. • Remember to flush the lumen with enough saline solution to clear the catheter, especially after drawing or administering blood. • Change the end caps weekly.
Hickman catheter *Description* • Silicone rubber • Approximately 35″ long • Open end with clamp • Dacron cuff 11¾″ (29.9 cm) from hub • Tunneled *Indications* • Long-term CV access • Home therapy 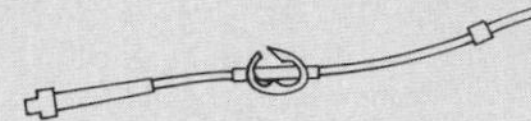	*Advantages* • Dacron cuff prevents excess motion and organism migration. • Clamps eliminate need for Valsalva's maneuver. *Disadvantages* • It requires surgical insertion. • Catheter has an open end. • It requires a practitioner for removal. • It tears and kinks easily.	• Two surgical sites require dressing after insertion. • Handle the catheter gently. • Observe frequently for kinks or tears. (Repair kit is available.) • Clamp the catheter whenever it becomes disconnected or open, using a clamp on the catheter. • Flush the catheter daily when not in use with 3 to 5 ml of heparin (10 units/ml) and before and after each use using the SASH (S=saline; A=additive; S=saline; H=heparin) protocol.

(continued)

Guide to CV access devices *(continued)*

Catheter description and indications	Advantages and disadvantages	Nursing considerations
Broviac catheter *Description* • Silicone rubber • Approximately 35″ long • Open end with clamp • Dacron cuff 11¾″ from hub • Tunneled *Indications* • Long-term CV access • Patient with small central vessels (pediatric, elderly)	*Advantages* • Small lumen ensures better comfort. *Disadvantages* • Small lumen may limit its uses. • It has a single lumen, which limits its functions (can't infuse multiple solutions at once). • In children, growth may cause the catheter tip to move its position outside the superior vena cava. • It must be removed by practitioner.	• Check facility policy before drawing or administering blood products. • Flush the catheter daily when not in use with 3 to 5 ml of heparin (10 units/ml) and before and after each use using the SASH protocol. 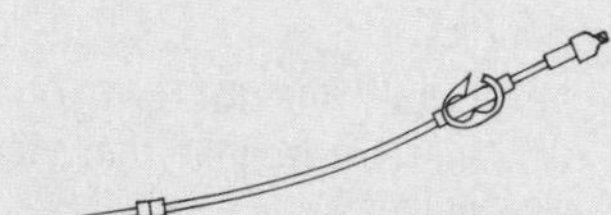
Hickman-Broviac catheter *Description* • Hickman and Broviac catheters combined in one catheter *Indications* • Long-term CV access • Patient who needs multiple infusions	*Advantages* • Double-lumen Hickman catheter allows sampling and administration of blood. • Broviac lumen delivers I.V. fluids, including TPN fluids. *Disadvantages* • It requires surgical insertion. • Catheter has an open end. • It requires a practitioner for removal. • It tears and kinks easily.	• Know the purpose and function of each lumen. • Label lumens to prevent confusion. • Flush the catheter when not in use with 3 to 5 ml of heparin (10 units/ml), and before and after each use using the SASH protocol. 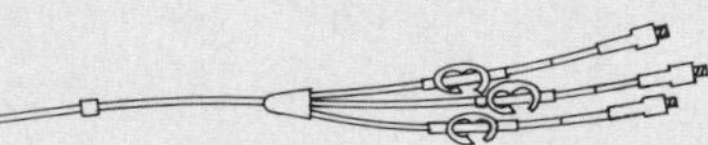
Long-line catheter *Description* • Peripherally inserted central catheter • Silicone rubber • 20″ to 24″ (51 cm to 61 cm) long; available in 14G, 16G, 18G, 20G, 22G, and 24G *Indications* • Long-term CV access • Patient with poor central access • Patient at high risk for complications from insertion at central access sites • Patient who needs CV access but faces or has had head and neck surgery	*Advantages* • It's peripherally inserted. • It can be inserted at bedside with minimal complications. • It may be inserted by a trained, skilled, competent registered nurse in most states. • Single, double, or triple lumen is available. *Disadvantages* • Catheter may occlude smaller peripheral vessels. • It may be difficult to keep immobile.	• Check frequently for signs of phlebitis and thrombus formation. • Insert the catheter above the antecubital fossa. • The catheter may alter CVP measurements. 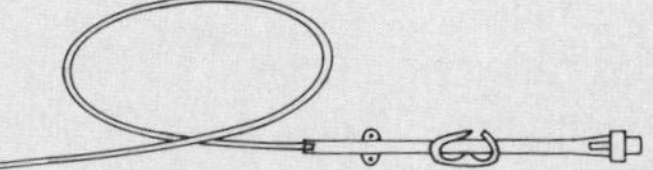

PICCs are commonly used in patients with such conditions as:

- AIDS
- cancer
- recurrent infections (such as osteomyelitis and endocarditis)
- sickle cell anemia
- women who require I.V. therapy because of severe morning sickness.

Infusions commonly given by a PICC include:

- analgesics
- antibiotics
- blood products
- chemotherapy
- immunoglobulins
- opioids
- TPN.

PICC specifics

PICCs are available in single-, double-, or triple-lumen configurations and with or without guide wires. A guide wire stiffens the catheter to ease its advancement through the vein, but it can damage the vein if used incorrectly.

The patient receiving PICC therapy must have a peripheral vein large enough to accept an introducer needle.

Catheter gauge depends on the size of the patient's vein and the type of fluid or medication to be infused. PICCs range from 14G to 24G in diameter and from 7¾″ to 23½″ (20 to 60 cm) in length. Other PICCs are configured for use in a neonate. If the patient is to receive blood or blood products through the PICC, you should use at least an 18G catheter. (See *Guide to PICCs*, pages 90 and 91.)

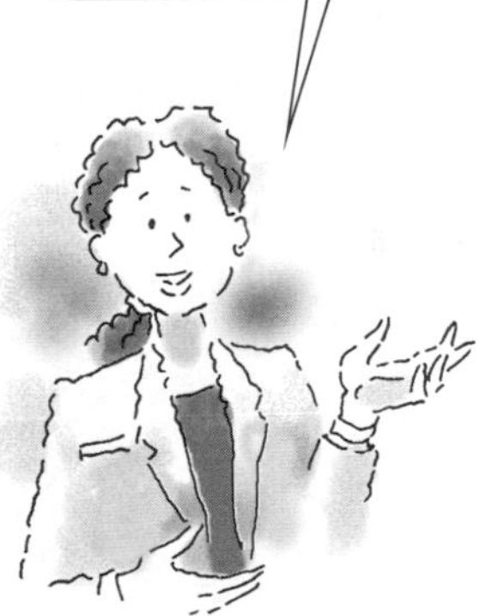

Don't pressure a PICC

Don't use a tuberculin syringe or a 3-ml syringe with a PICC to administer a medication or flush the catheter. These syringes create too much pressure (measured in pounds per square inch) in the line. Such excessive pressure can cause the device to burst. The appropriate syringe size is 10 ml.

PICCs permitted by practice acts

In many states, nurse practice acts allow registered nurses who are trained and skilled in the proper technique to insert PICCs. PICCs are widely used for home infusion therapy because they may be inserted at the bedside without a practitioner in attendance.

(Text continues on page 92.)

Guide to PICCs

Here are some of the peripherally inserted central catheters (PICCs) that are currently available.

Per-Q-Cath

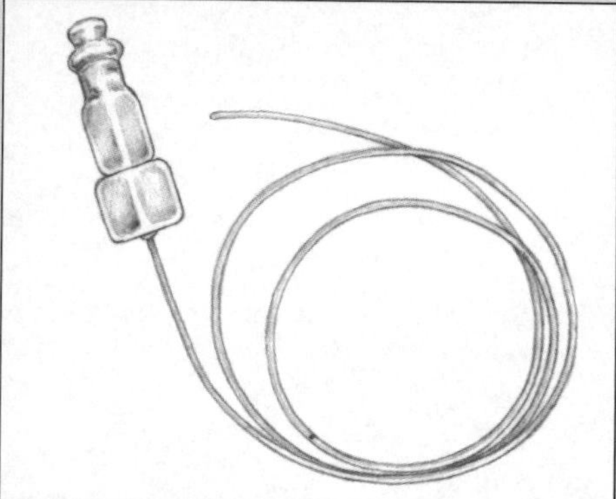

Dual-Lumen Per-Q-Cath

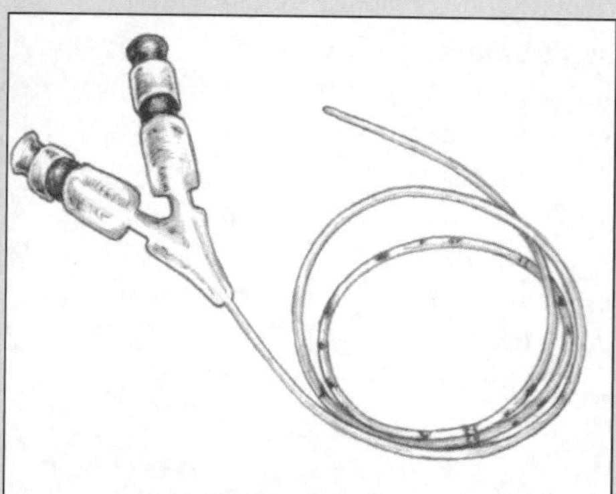

Per-Q-Cath and Dual-Lumen Per-Q-Cath are manufactured by Bard Access Systems. Features include:

- single lumen or double lumen
- gauges from 16G to 23G
- catheter length of 23″ (58 cm)
- insertion tray available
- repair kit available.

Groshong

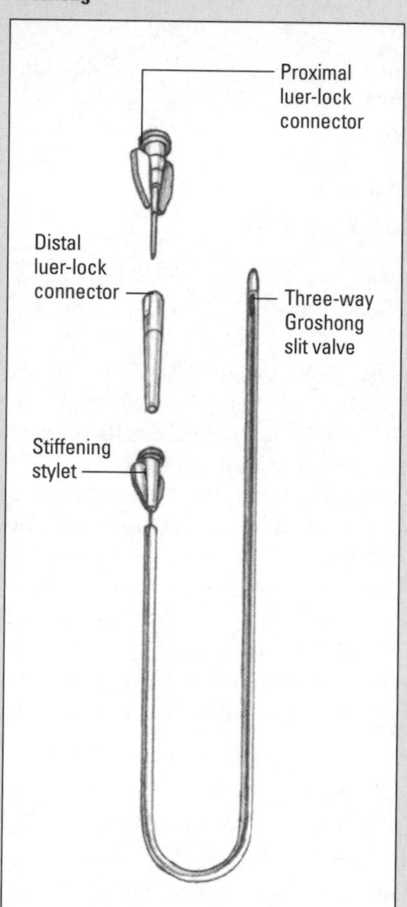

Groshong is manufactured by Bard Access Systems. Features include:

- single lumen or double lumen
- gauges from 18G to 20G
- catheter lengths from 22½″ to 23″ (57 to 58 cm).

Guide to PICCs *(continued)*

Arrow

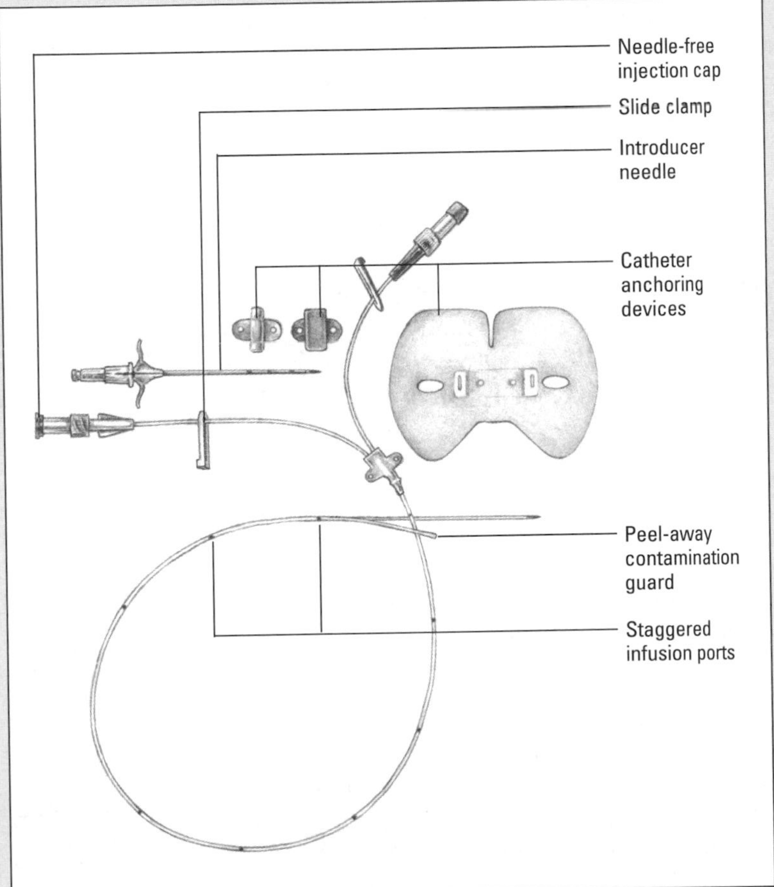

Arrow is manufactured by Arrow International. Features include:

- single, double, or triple lumen
- gauges from 18G to 20G
- polyurethane or silicone rubber (Silastic) catheter
- stylet-free insertion
- peel-away guard to maintain catheter sterility during insertion
- tip that deflects on contact with vessel walls to reduce intimal irritation during insertion
- anchoring device available on some.

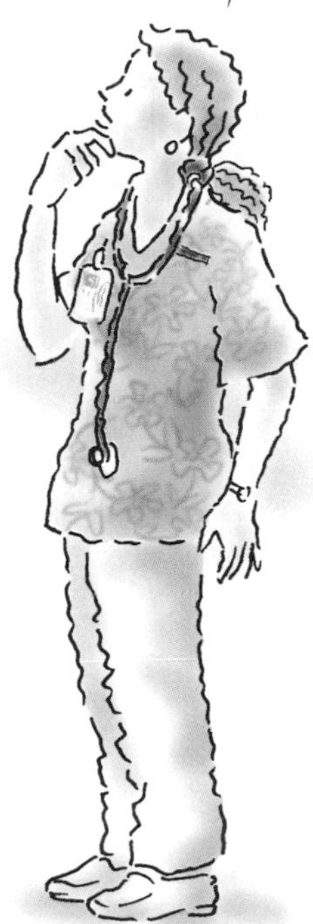

PICC imposter

The term PICC may be incorrectly used to describe an extended peripheral catheter. This catheter is more correctly known as a midline device. Technically, the midline device isn't a CV access device because its tip doesn't rest in the CV circulation but in the basilic, cephalic, or brachial vein.

A true PICC tip terminates in the superior or inferior vena cava. When caring for a patient with a PICC, make sure that you know where the catheter terminates and the entire length of the catheter, both indwelling and external.

PICC ups

PICCs have a definite upside:

- PICCs provide long-term access to central veins. A PICC can be left in place for long periods (unless complications develop) because the catheter is made of soft, physiologically compatible silicone or polyurethane. A single catheter may be used for an entire course of therapy.
- PICCs provide a safe, reliable route for infusion therapy and blood sampling.
- Some PICCs have antithrombogenic properties that minimize the risk of blood clots and phlebitis associated with other types of CV access devices.
- PICCs are extremely cost-effective compared with other long-term and short-term CV access devices.

PICC problems

A PICC may be unsuitable for a patient with bruises, scarring, or sclerosis from earlier multiple venipunctures at the intended PICC site. Bedside ultrasound should be used to assess whether a vein is suitable for a PICC. Also keep in mind that PICC therapy works best when it's introduced early in treatment; it shouldn't be considered a last resort.

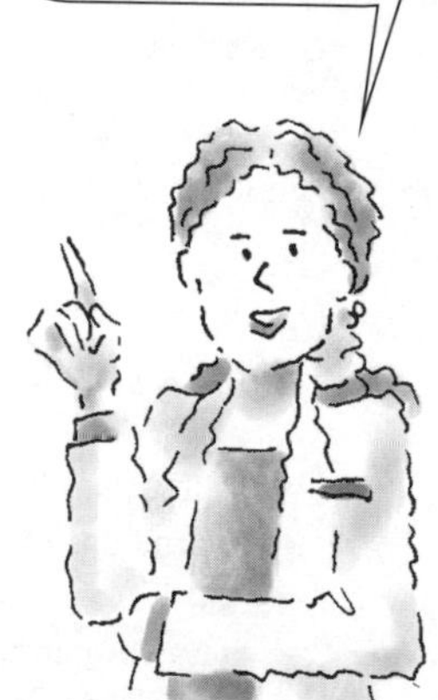

Implanted ports

As the number of chronically ill patients increases, so does the need for long-term I.V. therapy. When an external catheter isn't suitable, an implanted device may be used.

An implanted port functions like a long-term CV access device except that it has no external parts; it's implanted in a pocket under the skin. (See *Comparing implanted ports and long-term CV access devices.*)

The indwelling catheter that's attached to an implanted port is surgically tunneled under the skin until the catheter tip lies in the superior vena cava. The catheter may be threaded through the subclavian vein at the shoulder or through the jugular vein at the

Comparing implanted ports and long-term CV access devices

An implanted port offers the patient many of the advantages of a long-term central venous (CV) access device, along with an unobtrusive design that many patients find easier to accept. Both devices are indicated when poor venous access prohibits peripheral I.V. therapy. Deciding which device to use depends on the type and duration of treatment, the frequency of access, and the patient's condition. This chart shows how the two devices compare.

Type of treatment	Implanted port	Long-term CV access device
Continuous infusion of drugs or fluids	Yes, but maintaining continuous needle access eliminates the benefits of implantation	Yes
Self-administration of drugs or fluids	Yes, but it may be more difficult for the patient or family member to manage	Yes
Bolus injections of vesicant or irritant drugs by health care professionals	Yes	Yes
Duration of treatment		
Less than 3 months	No, because the high cost of implanting and removing the device precludes it	Yes
More than 3 months	Yes, but the cost of implantation and removal may exceed the cost benefit if treatment lasts less than 6 months	Yes
Frequency of access		
Three or more times per week	Yes, but it may minimize the advantage of having an implanted device	Yes
Less than once per week	Yes	No, because the high cost of maintaining the catheter precludes it
Patient concerns		
Negative effect on body image	No	Possibly
Negative reaction to needle punctures	Possibly	No
Ability to care for external catheter	Not needed	Needed
Cost of dressing changes and heparinization	Minimal	Considerable

base of the neck, for example. An implanted port is also suitable for epidural, intra-arterial, or intraperitoneal placement.

Implanted port: A safe harbor

Implanted devices are easier to maintain than external devices. They require heparinization only once per month to maintain patency. Implanted ports also pose less risk of infection because they have no exit site through which microorganisms can invade. Implanted ports offer several other advantages for patients, including:

- minimal activity restrictions
- few self-care measures to learn and perform
- few dressing changes (except when accessed and used to maintain continuous infusions or intermittent infusion devices).

Finally, because implanted ports create only a slight protrusion under the skin, many patients find them easier to accept than external venous access devices. A patient with an implanted port may shower, swim, and exercise without worrying about the device, as long as the device isn't accessed. The practitioner decides how soon after insertion the patient may undertake these activities.

For more information about implanted port insertion and infusions, turn to page 124.

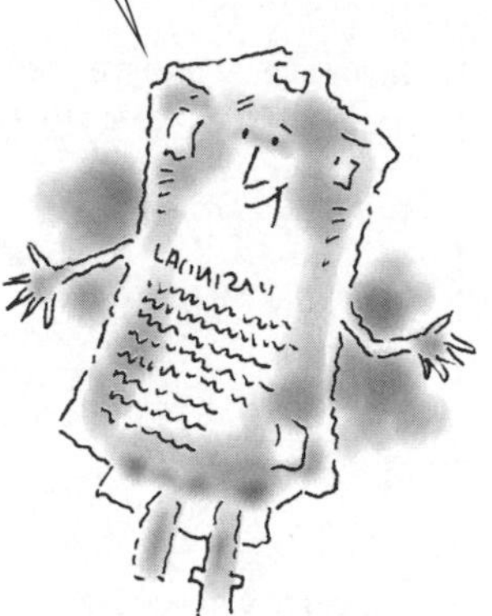

Out of sight, and out of reach

Because it's positioned under the skin, an implanted port may be more difficult for the patient to manage, especially for daily or frequent infusions. Accessing the device requires insertion of a specialized needle through subcutaneous tissue, which may be uncomfortable for patients who fear or dislike needle punctures.

Also, implanting and removing the port requires surgery and possible hospitalization, which can be costly. The comparatively high cost of an implanted port makes it worthwhile only for patients who require infusion therapy for at least 6 months. Another device, an implantable pump, may be used for patients who require continuous low-volume infusions. (See *Understanding implantable pumps.*)

Preparing for central venous therapy

The first step in preparing for CV therapy is selecting an insertion site for the catheter. You also need to prepare the patient physically and mentally. Depending on which procedure is to be used, you may then gather and prepare the appropriate equipment.

Selecting the insertion site

With the exception of PICC insertions, CV devices are usually inserted by a practitioner. If inserting a central line is an elective rather than an emergency procedure, you may collaborate with the patient and practitioner in selecting a site.

Understanding implantable pumps

An implantable pump is usually placed in a subcutaneous pocket made in the abdomen below the umbilicus. An implantable pump has two chambers separated by a filter. One chamber contains the I.V. solution, and the other contains a charging fluid. The charging fluid chamber exerts continuous pressure on the spring, forcing the infusion solution through the silicone outlet catheter into a central vein. The pump also has a domed septum that can be used to deliver bolus injections of medication. Generally, the pump is indicated for patients who require continuous low-volume infusions.

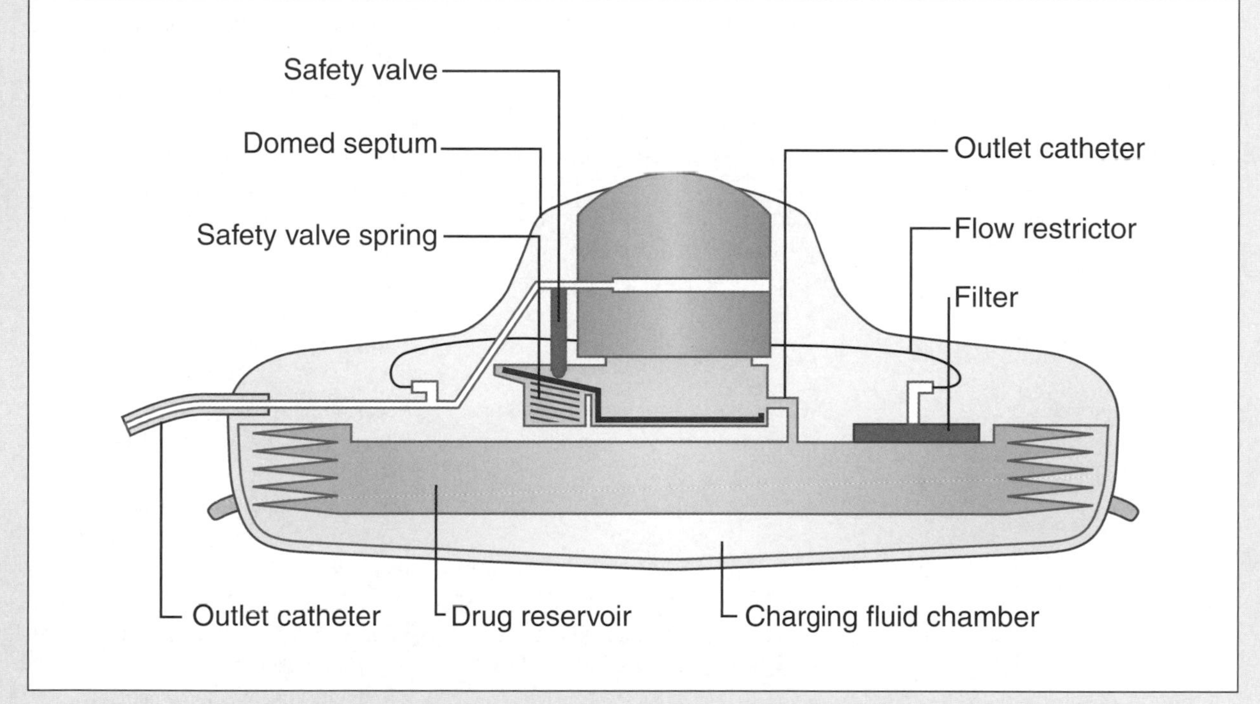

In CV therapy, the insertion site varies, depending on:

- type of catheter
- patient's anatomy and age
- duration of therapy
- vessel integrity and accessibility
- history of previous neck or chest surgery such as mastectomy
- presence of chest trauma
- possible complications.

Commonly used insertion sites include the subclavian, internal and external jugular, and brachiocephalic veins. Rarely, the femoral and brachial veins may be used. (See *Comparing CV insertion sites*, page 96.)

Comparing CV insertion sites

The chart below lists the most common insertion sites for a central venous (CV) access device and the advantages and disadvantages of each.

Site	Advantages	Disadvantages
Subclavian vein	• Easy and fast access • Easier to keep dressing in place • High flow rate, which reduces the risk of thrombus	• Proximity to subclavian artery (If artery is punctured during catheter insertion, hemorrhage can occur.) • Difficulty controlling bleeding • Increased risk of pneumothorax
Internal jugular vein	• Short, direct route to superior vena cava • Catheter stability, resulting in less movement with respiration • Decreased risk of pneumothorax	• Proximity to the common carotid artery (If artery is punctured during catheter insertion, uncontrolled hemorrhage, emboli, or impedance to flow can result.) • Difficulty keeping the dressing in place • Proximity to the trachea
External jugular vein	• Easy access, especially in children • Decreased risk of pneumothorax or arterial puncture	• Less direct route • Lower flow rate, which increases the risk of thrombus • Difficulty keeping the dressing in place • Tortuous vein, especially in elderly patients
Cephalic, basilic veins	• Least risk of major complications • Easy to keep the dressing in place	• Possible difficulty locating antecubital fossa in obese patients • Difficulty keeping elbow immobile, especially in children

Subclavian vein

The subclavian vein is one of the most common insertion sites for CV therapy. It affords easy access and a short, direct route to the superior vena cava and CV circulation.

The subclavian vein is a large vein with high-volume blood flow, making clot formation and vessel irritation less likely. The subclavian site also allows the greatest patient mobility after insertion.

Meet me in the angle of Louis

When using the subclavian site, the practitioner inserts the catheter into the vein percutaneously (through the skin and into the vessel with one puncture), threading it into the superior vena cava. This technique requires a venipuncture close to the apex of the lung and major vessels of the thorax.

As the catheter enters the skin between the clavicle and first rib, the practitioner directs the needle toward the angle of Louis, under the clavicle. The procedure may be difficult if the patient moves during insertion, has a chest deformity, or has poor posture.

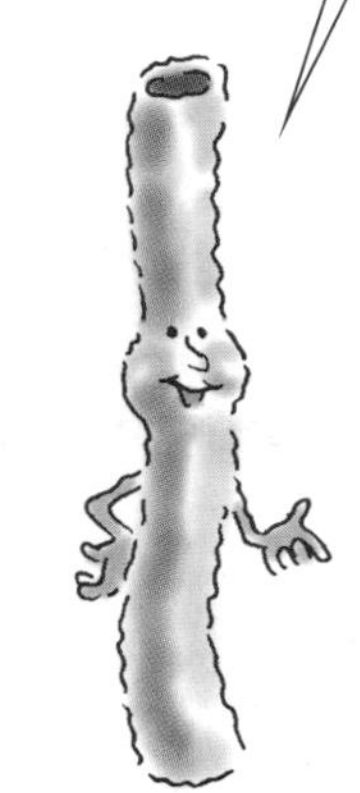

Internal jugular vein

The internal jugular vein provides easy access. In many cases, it's the preferred site. This insertion site is commonly used in children, but not infants.

Careful! It's close to the common carotid

The right internal jugular vein provides a more direct route to the superior vena cava than the left internal jugular vein. This site is also used for implanted port insertion. However, its proximity to the common carotid artery can lead to serious complications, such as uncontrolled hemorrhage, emboli, or impeded flow, especially if the carotid artery is punctured during catheter insertion (which can cause irreversible brain damage).

Using the internal jugular vein has other drawbacks. For example, it limits the patient's movement and may be a poor choice for home therapy because it's difficult to immobilize the catheter. Because of the location of the internal jugular vein, it's also difficult to keep a dressing in place.

Femoral veins

Femoral veins may be used if other sites aren't suitable. Although the femoral veins are large vessels, using them for catheter insertion entails some complications. Insertion may be difficult, especially in larger individuals, and carries the risk of puncturing the local lymph nodes.

Dress code

Dressing adherence is a big concern when selecting an insertion site. The femoral site inherently carries a greater risk of local infection because of the difficulty of keeping a dressing clean and intact in the groin area.

Straighten it out

When a femoral vein is used in CV therapy, the patient's leg needs to be kept straight and movement limited. Doing so prevents bleeding and keeps the catheter from becoming kinked internally or dislodged. Infection can also occur at the insertion site from catheter movement into and out of the incision.

Inserting a CV access device into a peripheral vein usually causes fewer traumatic complications, but it can lead to phlebitis or thrombus formation.

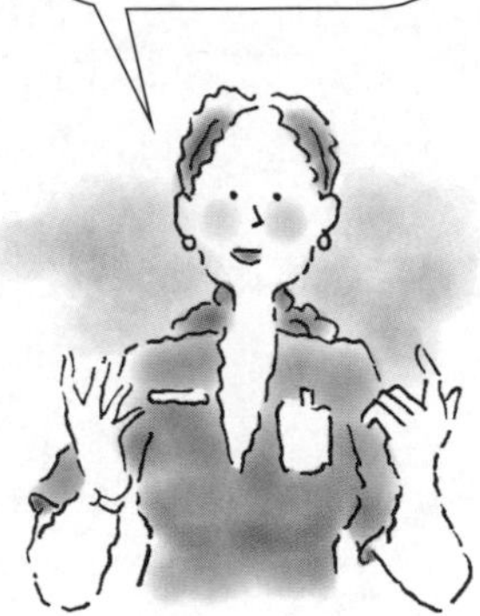

Peripheral veins

The peripheral veins most commonly used as insertion sites include:

- basilic
- cephalic
- external jugular
- median cubital of the antecubital fossa.

Far from internal organs

Because they're located far from major internal organs and vessels, peripheral veins cause fewer traumatic complications on insertion. However, accessing peripheral veins may cause phlebitis. The tight fit of the catheter in the smaller vessel allows only minimal blood flow around the catheter. Catheter movement may irritate the inner lumen or block it, causing blood pooling (stasis) and thrombus formation.

Vein pursuits

Although the cephalic vein is more accessible than the basilic vein, its sharp angle and location below the shoulder make it more difficult to thread a catheter through it. The larger, straighter basilic vein is usually the preferred insertion site. Bedside ultrasound may be used to locate the basilic vein and determine if the vein's condition is appropriate for catheter insertion.

The external jugular vein may provide a CV insertion site. Using the external jugular vein this way presents few complications. However, threading a catheter into the superior vena cava may be difficult because of the sharp angle encountered on entering the subclavian vein from the external jugular vein. For this reason, the catheter tip may remain in the external jugular vein. This position allows high-volume infusions but makes CV pressure measurements less accurate.

Accessing peripheral sites in the antecubital space may limit the patient's mobility because the device exits the skin at the bend of the elbow. Inserting the catheter above the antecubital space increases patient mobility and prevents kinking but makes it difficult to palpate the veins.

Dilution dilemma

External jugular veins shouldn't be used to administer highly caustic medications because blood flow around the tip of the catheter may not be strong enough to sufficiently dilute the solutions as they enter the vein.

Insertion site concerns

There are notable concerns in choosing an insertion site for a CV access device. Examples of these include:

- presence of scar tissue
- interference with the surgical site or other therapy
- configuration of the lung apices
- patient's lifestyle or daily activities.

Scar wars

In some patients, scar tissue from previous surgery or trauma may prohibit access to major blood vessels or make catheter insertion difficult. Alternatively, if the patient is facing surgery in the area of a central vein, another site may need to be chosen. A peripheral site, such as the basilic vein, or a central site on the side of the body unaffected by surgery are likely alternatives.

Tracheostomy treachery

An alternative site may be necessary if the patient is receiving other therapy that interferes with the insertion site. For example, if the patient has a tracheostomy, the internal or external jugular site should be avoided because the tracheostomy tapes come too close to these insertion sites. This proximity predisposes the patient to infection and may cause the catheter to dislodge.

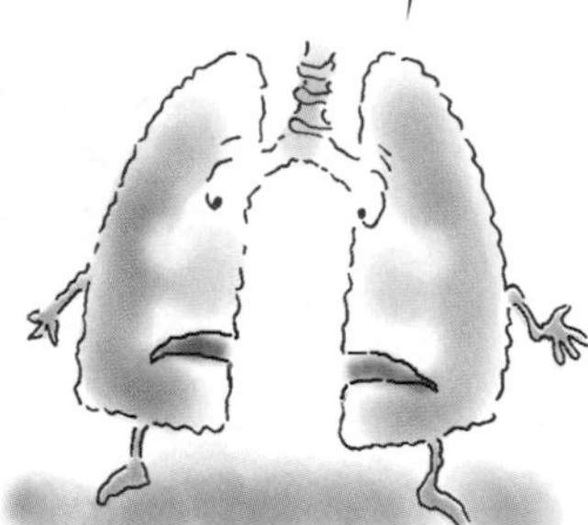

Look out for the lungs

Another site consideration is the location of the lung apices. In patients on mechanical ventilation — especially those receiving positive end-expiratory pressure therapy — intrathoracic pressures increase, which may elevate the lung apices and increase the chance of lung puncture and pneumothorax. Patients with COPD also have displaced lung apices, so consideration should be given to venous access sites outside the thorax in these patients.

Be practical and alert

Practical considerations play a role in site selection. For example, a home therapy patient with a PICC may have only one hand with which to work. A woman with a long-term tunneled catheter that exits near her bra straps would have a limited choice of clothing.

Be aware of the catheter's insertion site and the location of the catheter tip. That way, you can be alert for potential problems, such as thrombosis, catheter displacement, and infection.

Be aware of the insertion site and where my tip is located.

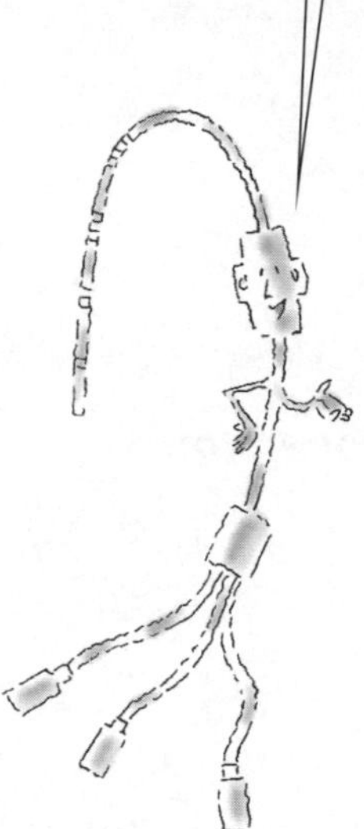

Preparing the patient

Accurate and thorough patient teaching increases the success of CV therapy. Before therapy begins, make sure that the patient understands the procedure and its benefits. Be sure to let him know what to expect during and after catheter insertion. Also, cover all self-care measures.

The primary responsibility for explaining the procedure and its goals rests with the practitioner. Your role may include allaying the patient's fears and answering questions about:

- movement restrictions
- cosmetic concerns
- management regimens.

Explaining the procedure

Ask the patient if he has ever received I.V. therapy before, particularly CV therapy. Evaluate the patient's learning capabilities and adjust your teaching technique accordingly. For example, use appropriate language when describing the procedure to a child. Also, ask the parents to help you phrase the procedure in terms their child understands. If time and resources permit, use pictures and physical models to enhance your teaching.

Getting all dressed up

If catheter insertion is to take place at the bedside, explain that sterile procedures require the staff to wear gowns, masks, and gloves. Tell your patient that he may need to wear a mask as well. If time allows, let your patient, especially a child, try on the mask.

The use of pictures and physical models can enhance your patient teaching. Remember to tailor your teaching to the patient's age and learning capabilities.

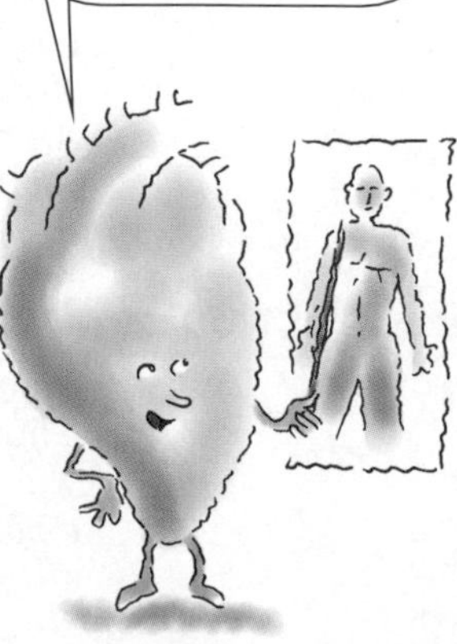

An important position

To minimize the patient's anxiety, explain how he'll be positioned during the procedure. If the subclavian or jugular vein will be used, he'll be in Trendelenburg's position for at least a short period, and a towel may be placed under his back between the scapulae. (In Trendelenburg's position, the head is low and the body and legs are on an inclined plane.)

Reassure the patient that he won't be in this position longer than necessary. Stress the position's importance for dilating the veins, which aids insertion and helps prevent insertion-related complications.

This may sting

Warn the patient to expect a stinging sensation from the local anesthetic and a feeling of pressure during catheter insertion.

Testing, testing

Explain any other tests that may be done. For example, the practitioner may obtain a venogram before the catheter insertion to check the status of the vessels, especially if the catheter is intended for long-term use. After catheter insertion, blood samples are commonly drawn to establish baseline coagulation profiles, and a chest X-ray is always done to confirm catheter placement.

Make sure the patient thoroughly understands self-care measures, and coordinate your teaching with the home-therapy coordinator or discharge planner.

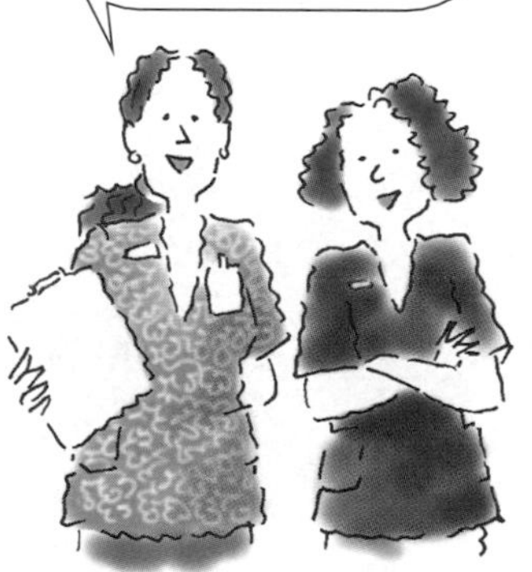

Explaining self-care measures

In explaining self-care measures to your patient, make sure that you cover the following topics:

- Teach the patient Valsalva's maneuver, and have him demonstrate it to you at least twice. This maneuver helps prevent air embolism. The patient may need to perform it in the future whenever the catheter is open to the air. This training is especially important when the patient is taking care of his catheter at home.
- If the catheter is to be in place long-term or will be managed at home, thoroughly explain all care procedures, such as how to change the dressing and how to flush the device. Ask the patient to demonstrate the various techniques and procedures, and include other family members, as appropriate. A home-therapy coordinator or discharge planner should coordinate teaching and follow-up assessments before and after catheter insertion.

Preparing the equipment

Besides the I.V. solution, infusion equipment typically includes an administration set with tubing containing an air-eliminating in-line filter if TPN is being infused. An infusion pump should also be used when solutions are administered through a CV access device.

Getting equipped

When you're assisting with an insertion at the patient's bedside, first collect the necessary equipment. Most facilities use pre-assembled disposable trays that include the CV access device.

Although most trays include the necessary equipment, be sure to check. If you don't have a preassembled tray, gather the following items:

- linen-saver pad
- clippers
- sterile gauze pads
- chlorhexidine
- local anesthetic
- 3-ml syringe with 25G needle for introduction of anesthetic
- sterile syringe for blood samples
- sterile towels or drapes
- suture material
- sterile dressing
- CV access device.

You also need to obtain extra syringes and blood sample containers if the practitioner wants venous blood samples to be drawn during the procedure.

Gowns, masks, caps, and gloves are standard issue for a bedside CV access device insertion.

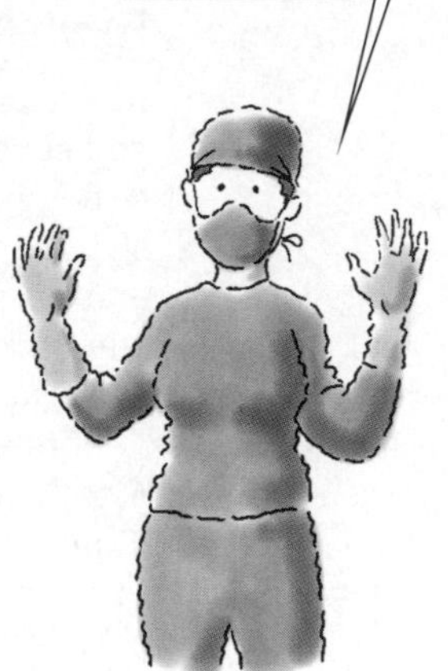

Mask, gown, and gloves required

Make sure that everyone participating in the insertion has a cap, mask, gown, and gloves. You may also need such protection for the patient, especially if there's a risk of site contamination from oral secretions or if the patient is unable to cooperate.

Some assembly required

To set up the equipment, follow these steps:

- Attach the tubing to the solution container.
- Prime the tubing with the solution.
- Prime and calibrate any pressure monitoring setups.

Aseptic, air-free, secure, and sealed

In addition, take the following precautions:

- All priming must be done using strict aseptic technique.
- All tubing must be free from air.
- After you have primed the tubing, recheck all the connections to make sure that they're secure.
- Make sure that all open ends are covered with sealed caps.

Performing central venous therapy

Although specific steps may vary, the same basic procedure is used whether catheter insertion is done at the bedside or in the operating room. Before the practitioner inserts the catheter, you need to:

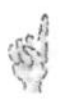

 position the patient

 prepare the insertion site.

Gonna be sedated?

Some patients may require sedation for the catheter to be placed. Such patients must be carefully monitored by staff trained in this procedure.

A rolled towel or blanket may be helpful when positioning the patient, to promote visibility of anatomic landmarks and prevent puncture of the lung apex and adjacent vessels.

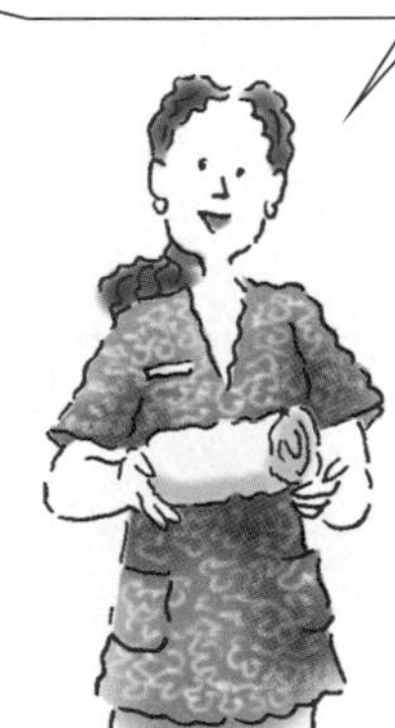

Positioning the patient

After you have assembled the equipment, position the patient to make him as comfortable as possible.

Visible and accessible

Position the patient in Trendelenburg's position (for insertion in the subclavian or internal jugular veins). This position distends neck and thoracic veins, making them more visible and accessible. Filling the veins also lessens the chance of air emboli because the venous pressure is higher than atmospheric pressure.

On a roll

If the subclavian vein is to be used, you may need to place a rolled towel or blanket between the patient's scapulae. Doing so allows for more direct access and may prevent puncture of the lung apex or adjacent vessels.

If a jugular vein is to be used, place a rolled blanket under the opposite shoulder to extend the neck and make anatomic landmarks more visible.

Preparing the insertion site

Prepare the insertion site by taking these steps:

Place a linen-saver pad under the site to prevent soiling the bed.

Make sure that the skin is free from hair because the follicles can harbor microorganisms. (See *Removing hair from a CV insertion site.*)

Prepare the intended venipuncture site with chlorhexidine. Use a back-and-forth motion to prepare the skin. Don't wipe the same area twice, and be sure to discard each sponge after each complete cycle. Be sure to let the solution dry completely before proceeding with vascular access device insertion.

Sterile drape style

After the site is prepared, the practitioner places sterile drapes around it and, possibly, around the patient's face as well. (This makes the patient's mask unnecessary.) If the patient's face is draped, you can help ease anxiety by uncovering his eyes. The drapes should provide a work area at least as large as the length of the catheter or guide wire.

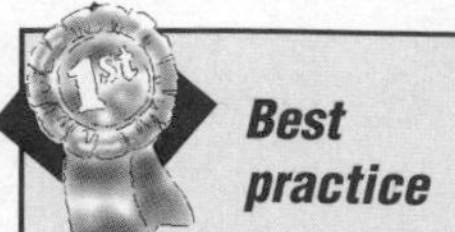

Best practice

Removing hair from a CV insertion site

Infection-control practitioners and the Infusion Nurses Society recommend clipping the hair close to the skin rather than shaving.

Irritation, open wounds, infection
Shaving may cause skin irritation and create multiple, small, open wounds, increasing the risk of infection. To avoid irritation, clip the patient's hair with single-patient-use clipper blades.

Rinse, wash, and remove
After you remove the hair, rinse the skin with saline solution to remove hair clippings. You may also need to wash the skin with soap and water before the actual skin prep to remove surface dirt and body oils.

Inserting the catheter

During catheter insertion, you may be responsible for monitoring the patient's tolerance of the procedure and providing emotional support. The practitioner usually prepares the equipment, which comes with a CV access kit and requires aseptic technique. In some cases, radiologic techniques, such as fluoroscopy or injectable dyes, may be used to assist with catheter placement.

Blood samples

You may obtain venous blood samples after the catheter is inserted. You'll need a sterile syringe that's large enough to hold all of the needed blood such as a 10-ml syringe. Place the blood in the proper sample container or, using a needleless system, access a saline lock at the end of the port with a Vacutainer. This device draws blood directly into the appropriate tube.

Patient participation

Each time the catheter hub is open to air—such as when the syringe is changed—tell the patient to perform Valsalva's maneuver or clamp the port to decrease the risk of air embolism.

Catheter inserted. Now what?

After the catheter is inserted, your primary responsibilities are monitoring the patient and administering therapy. You'll also need to apply a dressing to the insertion site and document your interventions and all information related to the catheter insertion.

Monitoring the patient

After the catheter has been inserted, monitor the patient for complications. Make sure that you tailor your assessment and interventions to the particular catheter insertion site. For example, if the site is close to major thoracic organs, as with a subclavian or internal jugular vein site, you should closely monitor the patient's respiratory status, watching for dyspnea, shortness of breath, and sudden chest pain.

Be aware that catheter insertion can cause arrhythmias if the device inadvertently enters my right atrium or right ventricle.

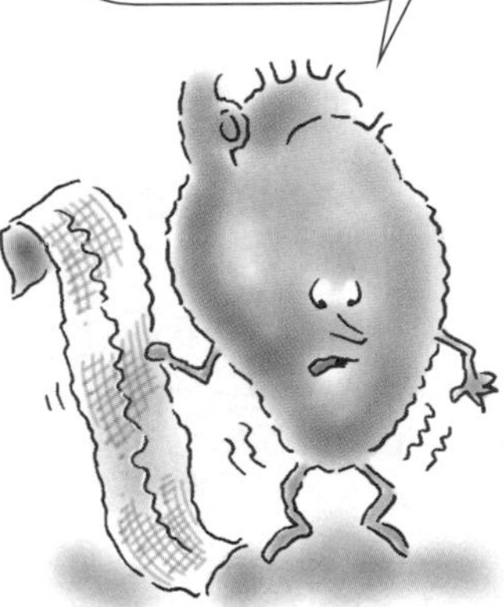

Arrhythmia alert

Inserting the catheter can cause arrhythmias if the catheter enters the right atrium (irritating the node) or right ventricle (irritating the cardiac muscle). For this reason, make sure that you monitor the patient's cardiac status. (Arrhythmias usually abate as the catheter is withdrawn.) If the patient isn't attached to a cardiac monitor, palpate the radial pulse to detect rhythm irregularities.

Suture in his future

When the proximal end of the catheter rests on the sterile drape, the practitioner will use one or two sutures to secure the catheter to the skin. Most short-term catheters have preset tabs to hold the sutures.

X-ray vision

Finally, a chest X-ray is ordered to confirm the location of the catheter tip before starting infusions. The line should be capped and flushed with normal saline solution until an X-ray confirms placement. After confirmation, begin the infusion by connecting the I.V. tubing or intermittent cap to the catheter hub. Adjust the flow rate as prescribed.

Poor positioning poses problems

A catheter may be positioned poorly, especially if it's inserted into the internal or external jugular veins. This may cause several problems. It can:

- make dressing changes difficult
- make maintaining an occlusive dressing impossible
- cause the catheter to kink.

Applying a dressing

Maintain sterile technique and place a sterile dressing over the insertion site of a short-term catheter or exit site of the PICC or tunneled catheter. To apply the dressing, follow these steps:

1. Clean the site with chlorhexidine using the same method as the initial skin preparation.

2. Cover the site with a transparent semipermeable dressing.

3. Seal the dressing with nonporous tape, checking that all edges are well secured. Label the dressing with the date and time, your initials, and the length of the catheter outside the body.

A successful application

After you apply the dressing, place the patient in a comfortable position and reassess his status. Elevate the head of the bed 45 degrees to help the patient breathe more easily. Remember to keep the site clean and dry to prevent infection. Also remember to keep the dressing occlusive to prevent contamination.

Prevent infection: Keep the insertion site clean and dry and the dressing occlusive.

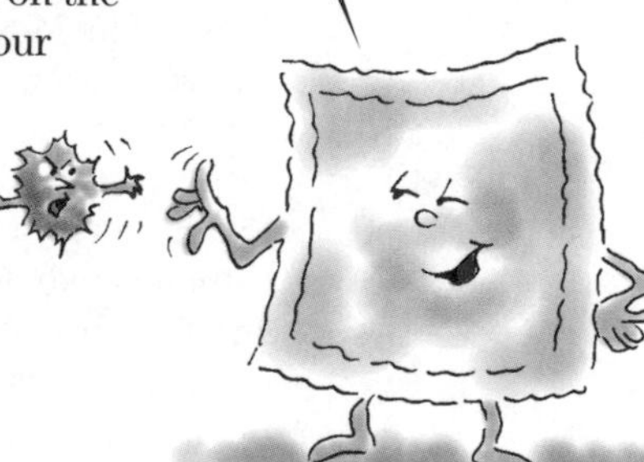

Documenting access device insertion

Record all pertinent information in the nurses' notes and on the I.V. flow sheet, if your facility uses one. Make sure that your documentation includes:

- type of access device used
- location of insertion
- catheter tip position as confirmed by X-ray
- patient's tolerance of the procedure
- blood samples taken.

A measure of migration

Some facilities recommend documenting the length of catheter remaining outside the body so other nurses can compare the measurements, checking for catheter migration.

Maintaining central venous infusions

One of your primary responsibilities is maintaining CV infusions. Doing so includes meticulous care of the CV access device insertion site as well as the catheter and tubing.

Routine care

Expect to perform the following care measures:

- Change the transparent semipermeable dressing weekly or whenever it becomes moist, loose, or soiled.
- Change the I.V. tubing and solution.
- Flush the catheter.
- Change the infusion cap.
- Administer a secondary infusion or obtain blood samples, if needed.
- Record your assessment findings and interventions according to your facility's policy.

Changing dressings

To reduce the risk of infection, always wear gloves and a mask when changing the dressing. The patient should also wear a mask. If the patient can't tolerate a facial mask, have him turn his head away from the catheter during the dressing change.

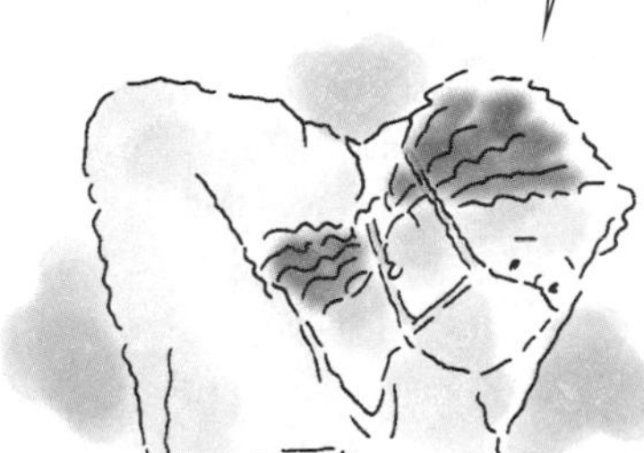

Getting equipped

Many facilities use a preassembled dressing-change tray that contains all the necessary equipment. If your facility doesn't use this type of tray, gather the necessary equipment, including:

- chlorhexidine swabs
- transparent semipermeable dressing
- sterile drape
- sterile gloves and masks
- clean gloves
- bag to dispose of old dressing.

A different brand of dressing

Expect to change your patient's central venous access device dressing every 48 hours if it's a gauze dressing and at least every 7 days if it's transparent. Dressings should be changed immediately if they become soiled, moist, or loose, or if the integrity of the dressing is compromised. (See *Changing a CV dressing*, page 108.)

Changing solutions and tubing

Change the I.V. solution every 24 hours and tubing every 72 hours or as directed by your facility's policy, maintaining strict aseptic technique. You don't need to wear a mask unless there's a contamination risk, for example, if you have an upper respiratory tract infection.

Changing a CV dressing

After you assemble all needed equipment, follow the step-by-step technique below to safely change a central venous (CV) dressing.

Getting ready

- Wash your hands. Then place the patient in a comfortable position.
- Prepare a sterile field. Open the bag, placing it away from the sterile field but still within reach.

Out with the old

- Put on clean gloves and remove the old dressing.
- Inspect the old dressing for signs of infection. You may want to culture discharge at the site or on the old dressing. If not, discard the dressing and gloves in the bag. Be sure to report an infection to the practitioner immediately and to document it in the nurses' notes.
- Check the position of the catheter and the insertion site for signs of infiltration or infection, such as redness, swelling, tenderness, or drainage.

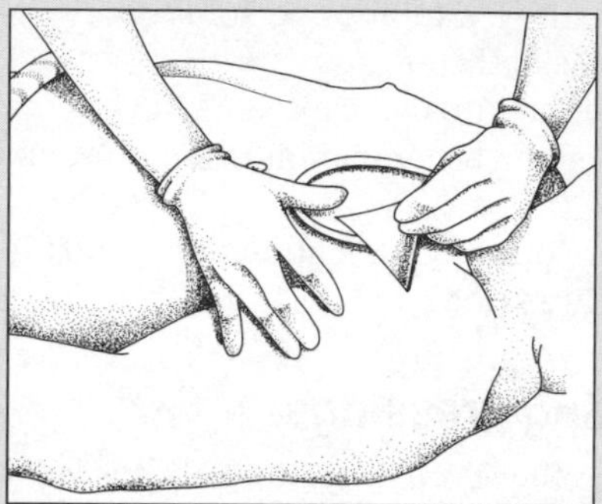

Remove the old dressing.

In with the new

- Put on sterile gloves and clean the skin around the catheter with chlorhexidine using a back-and-forth or side-to-side motion.
- Re-dress the site with a transparent semipermeable dressing.
- If the access device isn't sutured to the skin, use a catheter securement device or sterile tape or sterile surgical strips to help secure it. If you're using sterile tape or sterile surgical strips, avoid placing them directly on the catheter insertion site. A catheter securement device is the preferred method for securing an access device, other than sutures; it should be changed whenever you change the dressing.

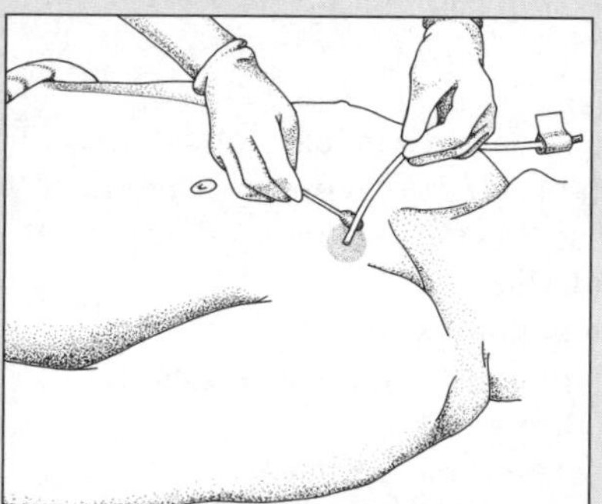

Clean the insertion site.

Write it down

- Label the dressing with the date, time, and your initials.
- Discard all used items properly; reposition the patient comfortably.

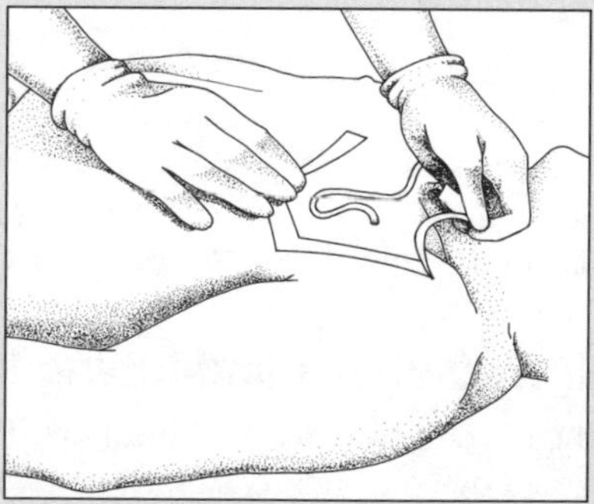

Re-dress the site.

If possible, change the solution and tubing at the same time. You may not be able to do this if, for example, the tubing is damaged or the solution runs out before it's time to change the tubing.

Open air prevention

To prevent air embolism, have the patient perform Valsalva's maneuver and clamp the port each time the catheter hub is open to air.

Switching solutions

To change the solution, follow these steps:

1. Gather a solution container and an alcohol swab.
2. Wash your hands.
3. Put on gloves.
4. Stop or pause the electronic infusion device.
5. Remove the cap and seal from the solution container.
6. Clamp the CV line.
7. Remove the spike quickly from the solution container, and reinsert it into the new container.
8. Hang the new container and restart the electronic infusion device.

Turning over the tubing

To change the tubing, gather an I.V. administration set, an extension set, an alcohol wipe, and gloves. (For instructions on what to do next, see *Changing CV tubing*, page 110.)

Flushing the access device

Flush the CV access device with saline solution routinely, according to your facility's policy, to maintain patency. When the system is maintained as an intermittent infusion device, the flushing procedure varies, depending on:

- facility policy
- type of catheter used
- medication administration schedule.

Changing CV tubing

After assembling the needed equipment, follow these guidelines to safely and quickly change the central venous (CV) tubing:

- Wash your hands.
- Stop the I.V. infusion device and clamp the access device.
- Remove the old spike from the container and hang it on the I.V. pole. Place the cover of the new spike loosely over the old one.
- Keeping the old spike in an upright position above the patient's heart level, insert the new spike into the I.V. container.
- Prime the system. Hang the new I.V. container and primed set on the pole, and grasp the new adapter in one hand. Then stop the flow rate in the old tubing.
- Put on gloves.
- Place a sterile gauze pad under the cannula hub.
- Gently disconnect the old tubing. (If you have trouble disconnecting the old tubing, use a hemostat to hold the hub securely while twisting the tubing to remove it. Or use one hemostat on the access device and another on the hard plastic end of the tubing. Then pull the hemostats in opposite directions. Don't clamp the hemostats shut because this could crack the tubing adapter or the venipuncture device.)
- Remove the protective cap from the new tubing, and connect the new adapter to the hub.
- Unclamp the access device and restart the I.V. infusion device.

How often? How much?

All lumens of an access device must be flushed regularly. Most facilities use a heparin flush solution available in premixed 10-ml multidose vials. Recommended concentrations vary from 10 to 100 units of heparin per milliliter. The Infusion Nurses Society recommends flushing with heparin at established intervals to help maintain patency of intermittently used central venous access devices. Normal saline solution should be used instead of heparin to maintain patency in two-way valved devices, such as the Groshong type, because research suggests that heparin isn't always needed to keep the line open.

The recommended frequency for flushing central venous access devices varies from once every 8 hours to once weekly. The recommended amount of flushing solution also varies as different catheters require different amounts of solution. Most facilities recommend using 3 to 5 ml of solution to flush the catheter, although some facility policies call for as much as 10 ml of solution. The size of syringe used for flushing also varies according to the catheter's manufacturer instructions.

Mismatched medications

A heparin or normal saline solution flush should also be performed before and after the administration of incompatible medications.

Flushing made simple

To flush the catheter, follow these steps:

1. Put on gloves.
2. Clean the cap with an alcohol swab (using a 70% alcohol solution).
3. Allow the cap to dry.
4. Inject the recommended or prescribed type and amount of flush solution.

To prevent blood backflow and possible clotting in the line, continue with these steps:

5. Maintain positive pressure by keeping your thumb on the plunger of the syringe.
6. Engage the clamping mechanism on the access device.
7. Withdraw the syringe.

Changing caps

CV access devices used for infrequent infusions have intermittent injection caps similar to saline lock adapters used for peripheral I.V. infusion therapy. These caps must be a luer-lock type to prevent inadvertent disconnection and an air embolism. They contain a small amount of empty space, so there's no need to preflush the cap before connecting it.

The frequency of cap changes varies according to facility policy and how often the cap is used. However, it's recommended that caps be changed at least every 7 days.

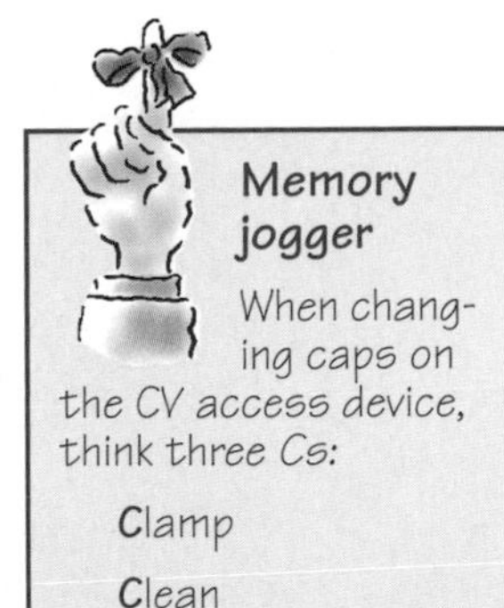

Memory jogger

When changing caps on the CV access device, think three Cs:

Clamp

Clean

Connect.

Integrity check

The integrity of an injection cap should be checked before and after each use. If at any time the integrity is compromised, or blood appears in the cap, the cap should be changed. Remember, always use strict sterile technique when changing the cap.

Clamp, clean, and connect

To change the cap, follow these steps:

1. Close the clamping mechanism on the catheter.

2. Clean the connection site with an alcohol swab.

3. Instruct the patient to perform Valsalva's maneuver while you quickly disconnect the old cap and connect the new cap, using aseptic technique. If the patient can't perform Valsalva's maneuver, time the disconnect maneuver with the patient's respiratory cycle and remove the cap during the expiratory phase.

Infusing secondary fluids and drawing blood

To add other fluids to the patient's CV infusion, make sure that solutions running in the same line are compatible and connections are luer-locked. Secondary I.V. lines may be piggybacked into a side port or Y-port of a primary infusion line instead of being connected directly to the catheter lumen. However, if there's no primary infusion prescribed, the medication may be infused through the CV access device.

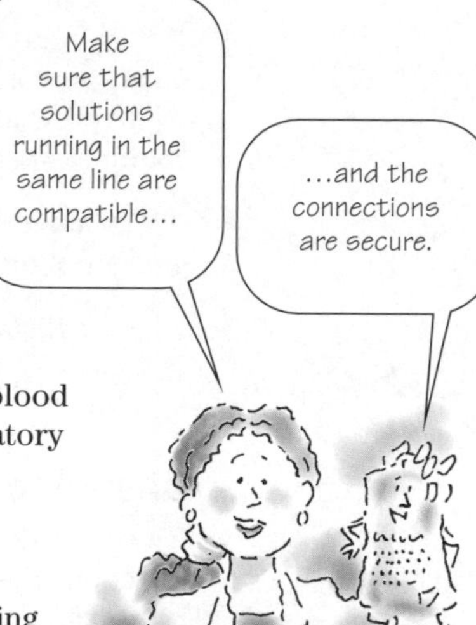

You may use the CV access device to obtain ordered blood samples, especially if the patient requires frequent laboratory work. (See *Drawing blood from a CV access device.*)

Documentation

Record your assessment findings and interventions according to your facility's policy. Include such information as:

- the type, amount, and rate of infusion
- dressing changes, including the type, appearance, and location of the catheter and site
- how the patient tolerated the procedure
- tubing and solution changes
- cap changes
- flushing procedures, including any problems encountered, and the amount and type of solution used
- the blood samples collected, including the type and amount.

Drawing blood from a CV access device

After assembling your equipment, use these step-by-step instructions to safely draw blood from a central venous (CV) access device. Keep in mind that a CV access device should only be used to draw blood when no other venipuncture options are available.

- Wash your hands and put on gloves.
- Clamp the catheter lumen, and clean the injection surface with an alcohol pad.
- Attach an empty 10-ml syringe to the hub. Release the clamp, and aspirate the discard volume to clear the catheter of dead space and blood diluted by the flush solution.
- Clamp the catheter and remove the syringe for discard.
- Wipe the injection surface with alcohol, and connect the empty syringe or blood collection tube to the catheter. Release the clamp, and withdraw the blood sample. If using a blood collection tube with a rubber diaphragm, swab the area with alcohol before use.
- Clamp the catheter and remove the syringe or blood collection tube.
- Wipe the injection surface with alcohol, and connect the syringe with normal saline solution.
- Open the clamp and flush with solution. Close the clamp.
- Repeat the flushing procedure with a heparin flush solution according to facility policy if the patient doesn't have a continuous infusion prescribed.
- If you've used a syringe instead of a blood collection tube, attach a needle to the syringe with the blood sample and inject the blood into the appropriate blood collection tube after wiping it with an alcohol swab.
- Label the specimens with the patient's name, his room number, and the date and time of collection.

Special care

Besides performing routine care measures during CV infusions, be prepared to:

- prevent or handle common problems that may arise during infusion, such as a damaged or kinked catheter, fluid leaks, and clot formation at the catheter's tip
- tailor your interventions to meet the special infusion requirements of pediatric, elderly, and home therapy patients
- manage potential traumatic complications, such as pneumothorax, and systemic complications such as sepsis. (See *Managing common problems in CV therapy*, page 115.)

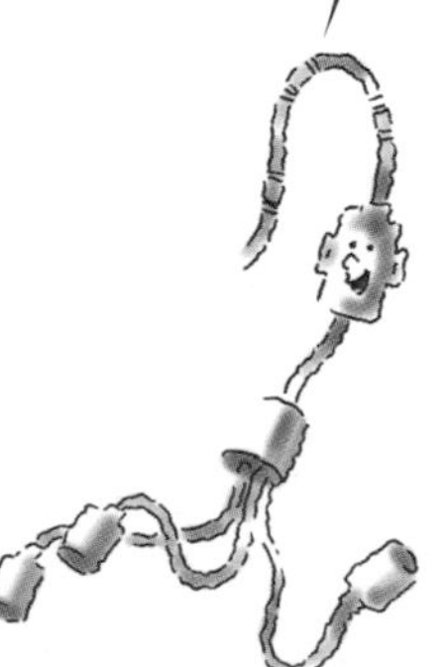

Common infusion problems

During CV infusions, problems arising from the catheter may call for special care measures.

Catheter breakdown

A serrated hemostat will eventually break down silicone rubber and tear the catheter, causing blood to back up and fluid to leak from the device. If air enters the catheter through the tear, an air embolism could result. Prevent catheter tears by using nonserrated clamps. If the catheter or part of the catheter breaks, cracks, or becomes nonfunctional, the practitioner may replace the entire catheter with a new one or use a repair kit if available.

Working out the kinks

The catheter can become kinked or pinched either above or beneath the skin. Kinks beneath the skin are detected by X-ray and are usually located between the clavicle and the first rib. The catheter may need to be unsutured and repositioned or replaced.

Never attempt to straighten kinks in stiff catheters, such as those made from polyvinyl chloride. These catheters fracture easily. Fractured particles may enter the circulation and act as an embolus. The practitioner may try to unkink a long-term catheter, which is made of pliable silicone rubber. The unkinking is done under guided fluoroscopy using aseptic technique.

You may be able to prevent external catheter kinks by taping and positioning the catheter properly. For example, looping the extension tubing once and securing it with tape adjacent to the dressing prevents the catheter from being pulled if the tubing gets entangled. Doing so also helps prevent the catheter from moving or telescoping at the insertion site, a major cause of catheter-related infections and site irritations.

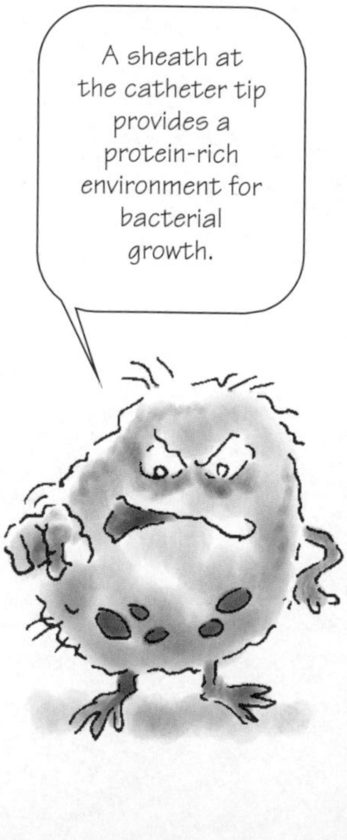

Meet the sheath

If you have difficulty withdrawing blood or infusing fluid, there may be a fibrin sheath at the tip of the catheter. This type of sheath impedes the flow of blood and provides a protein-rich environment for bacterial growth.

Occasionally, this sheath forms so that fluids infuse easily while blood aspiration is difficult or impossible. The fibrin sheath may be removed surgically or dissolved by instilling a thrombolytic agent. The agent may be instilled by a practitioner trained in the procedure.

This procedure is usually recommended for long-term CV catheters because they're difficult and costly to replace. However, attempting to salvage a device isn't always appropriate or possible.

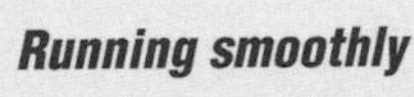

Running smoothly

Managing common problems in CV therapy

Maintaining central venous (CV) therapy requires being prepared to handle potential problems. This chart tells you how to recognize and manage some common problems.

Problem	Possible causes	Nursing interventions
Fluid won't infuse	• Closed clamp • Displaced or kinked catheter • Thrombus	• Check the infusion system and clamps. • Change the patient's position. • Have the patient cough, breathe deeply, or perform Valsalva's maneuver. • Remove the dressing and examine the external portion of the catheter. • If a kink isn't apparent, obtain an X-ray order. • Try to withdraw blood. • Try a gentle flush with saline solution. (The practitioner may order a thrombolytic flush.)
Unable to draw blood	• Closed clamp • Displaced or kinked catheter • Thrombus or fibrin sheath • Catheter movement against vessel wall with negative pressure	• Check the infusion system and clamps. • Change the patient's position. • Have the patient cough, breathe deeply, or perform Valsalva's maneuver. • Remove the dressing and examine the external portion of the catheter. • Obtain an X-ray order to check catheter tip placement.
Fluid leaking at the site	• Displaced or malpositioned catheter • Tear in catheter • Fibrin sheath	• Check the patient for signs of distress. • Change the dressing and observe the site for redness. • Notify the practitioner. • Obtain an X-ray order to check catheter tip placement. • Prepare for a catheter change, if necessary. • If the tear occurred in a Hickman, Groshong, or Broviac catheter, obtain a repair kit.
Disconnected catheter	• Patient moved • Not securely connected to tubing	• Apply a catheter clamp, if available. • Place a sterile syringe in the catheter hub. • Change the I.V. extension set. Don't reconnect the contaminated tubing. • Clean the catheter hub with chlorhexidine if the patient has an iodine allergy. Don't soak the hub. • Connect clean I.V. tubing or a heparin lock plug to the site. • Restart the infusion.

Patients with special needs

There are a few additional considerations involved in caring for pediatric, elderly, and home therapy patients.

Across the generation gap

Essentially the same access devices are used in both pediatric and elderly patients. However, four possible differences include:

- catheter length
- lumen size
- insertion sites
- amount of fluid infused.

In infants, for example, the jugular vein is the preferred insertion site, even though it's much more difficult to maintain than other sites. Usually, the practitioner and the patient's family select a mutually acceptable site if the catheter will be used for long-term therapy.

Because pediatric patients are smaller, they require shorter catheters with a smaller lumen than that needed for adults. As pediatric patients grow, a larger catheter is required.

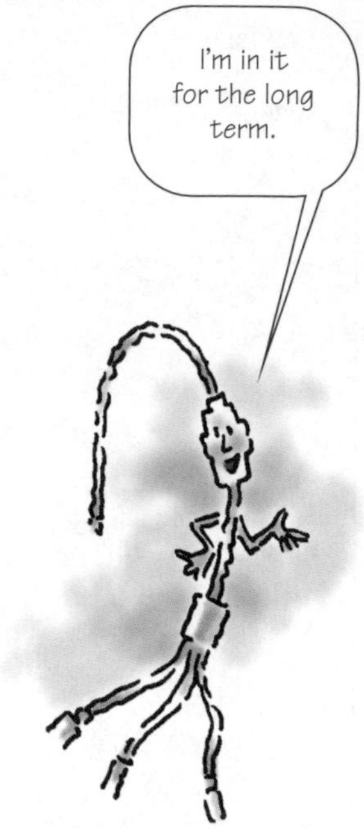

I'm in it for the long term.

Homework

Long-term CV access devices allow patients to receive fluids, medications, and blood infusions at home. These catheters have a much longer life because they're less thrombogenic and less prone to infection than short-term devices.

The care procedures used in the home are the same as those used in the hospital, including aseptic technique. A candidate for home CV therapy must have:

- a family member or friend who can assist in safe and competent administration of I.V. fluids
- a suitable home environment
- a telephone
- transportation
- the ability to prepare, handle, store, and dispose of the equipment.

To ensure your patient's safety, patient teaching begins well before he's discharged. After discharge, a home-therapy coordinator provides follow-up care. This care helps ensure compliance until the patient or caregiver can independently provide catheter care and infusion therapy at home. The home therapy patient can learn to care for the catheter himself and to infuse his own medications and solutions.

Traumatic and systemic complications

Complications can occur at any time during CV therapy. Traumatic complications, such as pneumothorax, typically occur on insertion but may not be noticed until after the procedure is completed. Systemic complications such as sepsis typically occur later in therapy. (See *Risks of CV therapy*, pages 118 to 120.)

Yikes! Insertion of a catheter into subclavian or internal jugular veins may cause pneumothorax.

Traumatic topic: Pneumothorax

Pneumothorax, the most common traumatic complication of catheter insertion, is associated with the insertion of a CV access device into the subclavian or internal jugular vein. It's usually discovered on the chest X-ray that confirms catheter placement if the patient doesn't have symptoms immediately.

Pneumothorax may be minimal and may not require intervention (unless the patient is on positive-pressure ventilation). A thoracotomy is performed and a chest tube inserted if pneumothorax is severe enough to cause signs and symptoms, such as:

- chest pain
- dyspnea
- cyanosis
- decreased or absent breath sounds on the affected side.

Sneaky signs and symptoms

Initially, the patient may be asymptomatic; signs of distress gradually show up as pneumothorax gets larger. For this reason, you need to monitor the patient closely and auscultate for breath sounds for at least 8 hours after catheter insertion.

If unchecked, pneumothorax may progress to tension pneumothorax, a medical emergency. The patient exhibits such signs as:

- acute respiratory distress
- asymmetrical chest wall movement
- possibly, a tracheal shift away from the affected side.

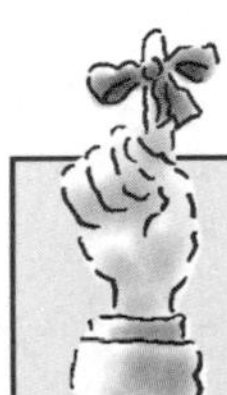

Memory jogger

Use the mnemonic **ACT** to remember the signs and symptoms of tension pneumothorax so that you can "act" fast to protect your patient:

Acute respiratory distress

Chest wall motion that's asymmetrical

Tracheal shifting.

(Text continues on page 120.)

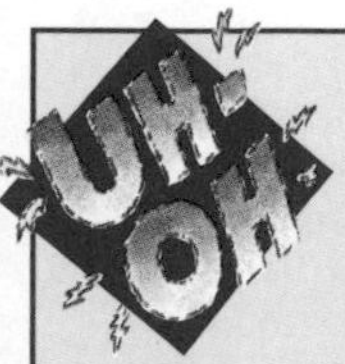

Warning!

Risks of CV therapy

As with any invasive procedure, central venous (CV) therapy poses risks, including pneumothorax, air embolism, thrombosis, and infection. This chart outlines how to recognize, manage, and prevent these complications.

Signs and symptoms	Possible causes	Nursing interventions	Prevention
Pneumothorax, hemothorax, chylothorax, or hydrothorax			
• Chest pain • Dyspnea • Cyanosis • Decreased breath sounds on affected side • Decreased hemoglobin because of blood pooling (occurs with hemothorax) • Abnormal chest X-ray	• Lung puncture by catheter during insertion or exchange over a guide wire • Large blood vessel puncture with bleeding inside or outside lung • Lymph node puncture with lymph fluid leakage • Infusion of solution into chest area through perforated catheter	• Stop the infusion and notify the practitioner. • Remove the catheter or assist with its removal. • Administer oxygen as ordered. • Set up and assist with chest tube insertion. • Document interventions.	• Position the patient's head down with a towel roll between scapulae to dilate and expose the internal jugular or subclavian vein as much as possible during catheter insertion. • Assess for early signs of fluid infiltration, such as swelling in the shoulder, neck, chest, and arm area. • Ensure immobilization with adequate patient preparation and restraint during the procedure; active patients may need to be sedated or taken to the operating room for catheter insertion. • Confirm CV access device position by X-ray.
Air embolism			
• Respiratory distress • Unequal breath sounds • Weak pulse • Increased central venous pressure (CVP) • Decreased blood pressure • Churning murmur over precordium • Change in or loss of consciousness	• Intake of air into CV system during catheter insertion or tubing changes; inadvertent opening, removal, cutting, or breaking of catheter	• Clamp the catheter immediately. • Cover the catheter exit site. • Turn the patient on his left side, head down, so that air can enter the right atrium, preventing it from entering the pulmonary artery. • Don't have the patient perform Valsalva's maneuver. (Large intake of air worsens the situation.) • Administer oxygen. • Notify the practitioner. • Document interventions.	• Purge all air from tubing before hookup. • Teach the patient to perform Valsalva's maneuver during catheter insertion and tubing changes (bear down or strain and hold breath to increase CVP). • Use air-eliminating filters proximal to the patient. • Use an infusion-control device with air detection capability. • Use luer-lock tubing for all connections.

Risks of CV therapy *(continued)*

Signs and symptoms	Possible causes	Nursing interventions	Prevention
Thrombosis			
• Edema at puncture site • Ipsilateral swelling of arm, neck, and face • Pain along vein • Fever, malaise • Tachycardia • Erythema	• Sluggish flow rate • Hematopoietic status of patient • Preexisting limb edema • Infusion of irritating solutions • Irritation of tunica intima • Repeated use of same vein or long-term use • Vein irritation during insertion	• Notify the practitioner. (Catheter may need to be removed.) • Possibly, infuse a thrombolytic to dissolve the clot. • Verify thrombosis with diagnostic studies. • Apply warm, wet compresses locally. • Don't use the limb on the affected side for subsequent venipuncture. • Document interventions.	• Maintain flow through the catheter at a steady rate with an infusion pump, or flush at regular intervals. • Verify that the catheter tip is in superior vena cava before using the catheter. • Dilute irritating solutions. • Use a 0.22-micron filter for infusions.
Local infection			
• Redness, warmth, tenderness, and swelling at insertion or exit site • Possible exudate of purulent material • Local rash or pustules • Fever, chills, malaise	• Failure to maintain aseptic technique during catheter insertion or care • Failure to comply with dressing change protocol • Wet or soiled dressing remaining on site • Immunosuppression • Irritated suture line	• Monitor temperature frequently. • Culture the site. • Re-dress aseptically. • Treat systemically with antibiotics or antifungals, depending on the culture results and the practitioner's orders. • Anticipate and assist with catheter removal, if necessary. • Document interventions.	• Maintain strict aseptic technique. Use gloves, masks, and gowns when appropriate. • Adhere to dressing change protocols. • Teach the patient about restrictions (bathing, swimming), if applicable. (Patients with adequate white blood cell counts can do these activities if the practitioner allows.) • Change a wet or soiled dressing immediately. • Change the dressing more frequently if the catheter is located in the femoral area or near a tracheostomy. • Complete tracheostomy care after catheter care.

(continued)

Risks of CV therapy *(continued)*

Signs and symptoms	Possible causes	Nursing interventions	Prevention
Systemic infection			
• Fever, chills without other apparent reason • Leukocytosis • Nausea, vomiting • Malaise • Elevated urine glucose level	• Contaminated catheter or infusate • Failure to maintain aseptic technique during solution hookup • Frequent opening of catheter or long-term use of single I.V. access • Immunosuppression	• Draw central and peripheral blood cultures; if cultures match, the catheter is primary source of sepsis and should be removed. • If cultures don't match but are positive, the catheter may be removed or the infection may be treated through the catheter. • Treat the patient with antibiotic regimen, as ordered. • Culture the tip of the catheter if removed. • Assess for other sources of infection. • Monitor vital signs closely. • Document interventions.	• Examine infusate for cloudiness and turbidity before infusing. • Check the fluid container for leaks. • Monitor urine glucose level in a patient receiving total parenteral nutrition; if greater than 2+, suspect early sepsis. • Use strict sterile technique for hookup and disconnection of fluids. • Use a 0.22-micron filter (or a 1.2-micron filter for 3-in-1 TPN solutions). • Keep the system closed as much as possible. • Teach the patient aseptic technique.

A chest tube must be inserted immediately before respiratory and cardiac decompensation occur.

Let's talk puncture at this juncture

The second most common life-threatening complication is arterial puncture. Arterial puncture may lead to hemothorax and internal bleeding, which may not be detected immediately. A hemothorax is treated like pneumothorax, except that the chest tube is inserted lower in the chest to help evacuate the blood.

Left untreated, internal bleeding caused by arterial puncture leads to hypovolemic shock. Signs and symptoms include:

- increased heart rate
- decreased blood pressure
- cool, clammy skin
- obvious swelling in the neck or chest
- mental confusion (especially if the common carotid arteries are involved)
- formation of a hematoma (a large, blood-filled sac), which causes pressure on the trachea and adjacent vessels.

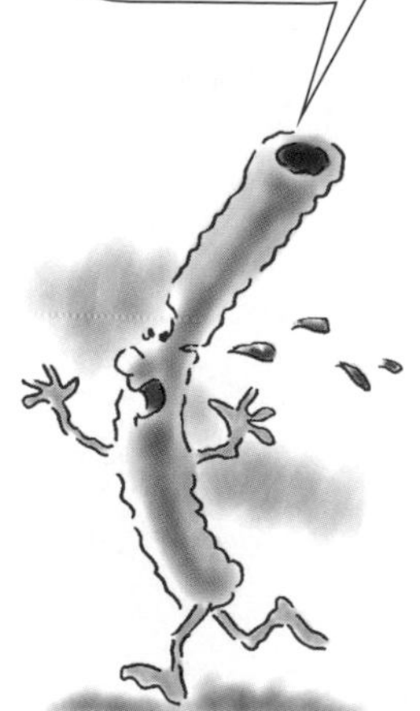

Rare but risky

There are a few additional, but rare, complications of CV therapy:

- Tracheal puncture is associated with insertion of a catheter into the subclavian vein.
- Development of a fistula between the brachiocephalic vein and the subclavian artery may result from perforation by the guide wire on insertion into the vessel.
- Chylothorax results when a lymph node is punctured and lymph fluid leaks into the pleural cavity.
- Hydrothorax (or infusion of solution into the chest), thrombosis, and local infection are also potential complications of CV therapy.

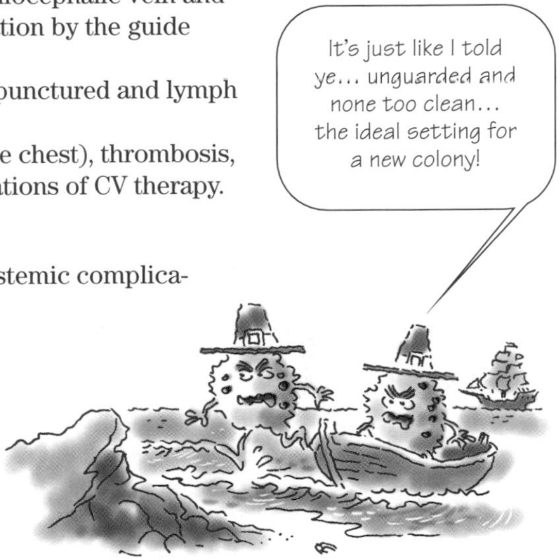

Sepsis is systemic and serious

Catheter-related sepsis is the most serious systemic complication. It may lead to:

- septic shock
- multisystem organ failure
- death.

Most sepsis attributed to CV access devices is caused by skin surface organisms, such as *Staphylococcus epidermidis*, *S. aureus*, and *Candida albicans*.

Strict aseptic technique and close observation are the best defense against sepsis. Regularly check the catheter insertion site for signs of localized infection, such as redness, drainage, and tenderness along the catheter path. If the patient shows signs of generalized infection, such as unexplained fever, draw blood cultures from a peripheral site as well as from the device itself according to facility protocol.

Out with the old, in with the new

If catheter-related sepsis is suspected, the catheter may be removed and a new one inserted in a different site. Culture the catheter tip after removal. Administer antibiotics, as ordered, and draw blood for repeat cultures after the antibiotic course is complete.

PICC-specific complications

PICC therapy causes fewer and less severe complications than other CV lines. Pneumothorax is extremely rare because the insertion site is peripheral. Catheter-related sepsis is usually related to site contamination.

Phlebitis — mechanical or bacterial

Mechanical phlebitis — painful inflammation of a vein — may be the most common PICC complication. It may occur during the first 72 hours after PICC insertion and is more common when a large-gauge catheter is used.

If the patient develops mechanical phlebitis, apply warm, moist compresses to his upper arm; elevate the extremity; and restrict activity to mild exercise. If the phlebitis continues or worsens, remove the catheter, as ordered.

Bacterial phlebitis can occur with PICCs; however, this usually occurs later in the infusion therapy. If drainage occurs at the insertion site and the patient's temperature increases, notify the practitioner. The catheter may need to be removed.

Deeds for those who bleed

Expect minimal bleeding from the PICC insertion site for the first 24 hours. Bleeding that persists needs additional evaluation. A pressure dressing should be left in place over the insertion site for at least 24 hours. After that, if there's no bleeding, the dressing can be changed and a new transparent dressing applied without a gauze pressure dressing.

One way to treat pain at the PICC insertion site is to apply a warm compress.

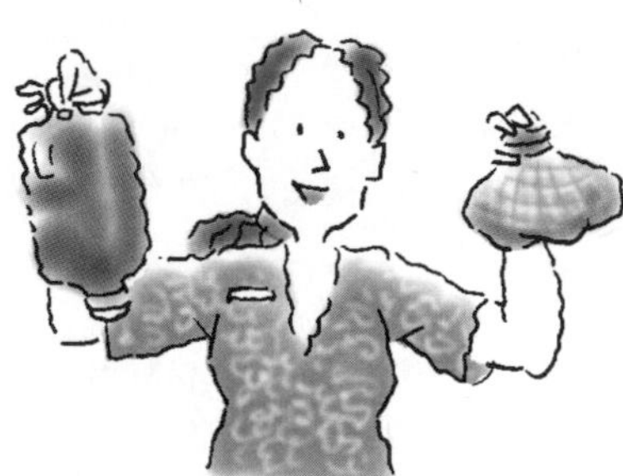

Tame the pain

Some patients complain of pain at the PICC insertion site, usually because the device is located in an area of frequent flexion. Pain may be treated by:

- applying warm compresses
- restricting activities until the patient becomes adjusted to the presence of the PICC.

Spared of air (embolisms)?

Air embolism in PICC therapy is less common than in traditional CV access devices because the line is inserted below the level of the heart.

Discontinuing central venous therapy

You or the practitioner may remove the catheter, depending on your state's nurse practice act, your facility's policy, and the type of catheter. Long-term catheters and implanted devices are always removed by the practitioner. However, PICC lines may be removed by a qualified nurse.

Discontinue continuous, implement intermittent

You may receive an order to discontinue continuous infusion therapy and begin intermittent infusion therapy. If so, follow the same procedure used for peripheral I.V. therapy. (See Chapter 2, *Peripheral I.V. therapy*.)

Removing the catheter

Begin catheter removal with a couple of precautions:

First, check the patient's record or other documentation (such as the nurses' notes, practitioner's notes, or the written X-ray report) as directed by facility policy for the most recent placement confirmed by an X-ray to trace the catheter's path as it exits the body.

Then make sure that backup assistance is available if a complication, such as uncontrolled bleeding, occurs during catheter removal. This complication is common in patients with coagulopathies.

Remember... bearing down or straining while holding your breath? It's done to increase central venous pressure during catheter changes and withdrawal, whenever the catheter is open to air, to prevent air emboli.
Valsalva's maneuver?

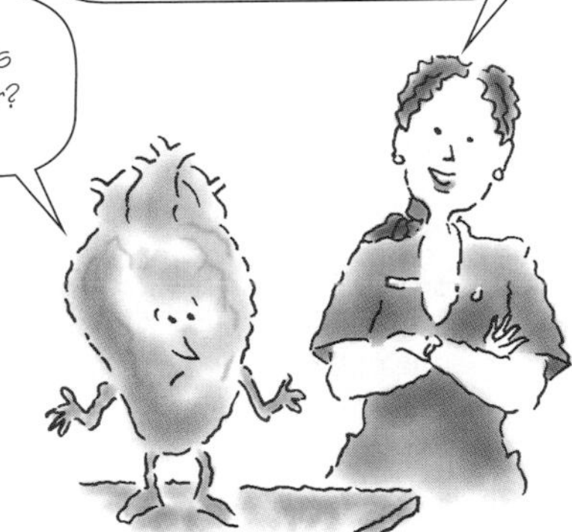

Patient preparation

Before you remove the catheter, explain the procedure to the patient. Tell him that he'll need to turn his face away from the site and perform Valsalva's maneuver when the catheter is withdrawn. If necessary, review the maneuver with him.

Getting equipped

Before removing the catheter, gather the necessary equipment, including:

- sterile gauze
- clean gloves
- sterile gloves
- forceps
- sterile scissors
- antimicrobial swab
- antibiotic ointment
- alcohol swabs
- sterile transparent semipermeable dressing
- tape.

If you're sending the catheter tip for culture, you also need a sterile specimen container. (See *Removing a CV catheter*, page 124.)

Note this

After removing the catheter, be sure to document:

- patient tolerance
- condition of the catheter, including the length
- time of discontinuation of therapy
- cultures ordered and sent
- dressings applied
- other pertinent information.

Removing a CV catheter

After assembling your equipment, follow the step-by-step guidelines listed below to safely remove a central venous (CV) catheter.

Getting ready

- Place the patient in a supine position to prevent emboli.
- Wash your hands and put on clean gloves.
- Turn off all infusions.
- Remove the old dressing.
- Inspect the site for signs of drainage or inflammation. Clean the site with an antimicrobial swab.
- Remove your gloves and put on sterile gloves.

Removing the catheter

- Clip the sutures and, using forceps, remove the catheter in a slow, even motion. Have the patient perform Valsalva's maneuver as the catheter is withdrawn to prevent air emboli.
- Apply pressure with a sterile gauze pad immediately after removing the catheter.
- Apply antibiotic ointment to the insertion site to seal it.
- Place a transparent semipermeable dressing over the site. Label the dressing with the date and time of the removal and your initials.
- Inspect the catheter and measure the length to see if any pieces broke off during the removal. If so, notify the practitioner immediately and monitor the patient closely for signs of distress. If a culture is to be obtained, use sterile scissors to clip approximately 1″ (2.5 cm) off the distal end of the catheter, letting it drop into the sterile specimen container.
- Properly dispose of the I.V. tubing and equipment you used.

Monitoring the patient

Insidious bleeding may develop after removing the catheter. Remember that some vessels, such as the subclavian vein, aren't easily compressed. By 72 hours, the site should be sealed and the risk of air emboli should be past; however, you may still need to apply a dry dressing to the site.

Make a notation on the nursing care plan to recheck the patient and insertion site frequently for the next few hours. Check for signs of respiratory decompensation, possibly indicating air emboli, and for signs of bleeding, such as blood on the dressing, decreased blood pressure, increased heart rate, paleness, or diaphoresis.

Noteworthy

Document the time and date of the catheter removal and any complications that occurred, such as catheter shearing, bleeding, or respiratory distress. Also record the length of the catheter and signs of blood, drainage, redness, or swelling at the site.

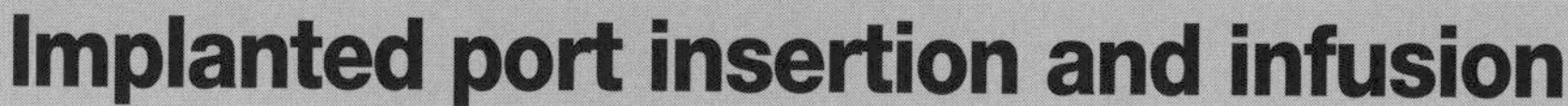

Implanted port insertion and infusion

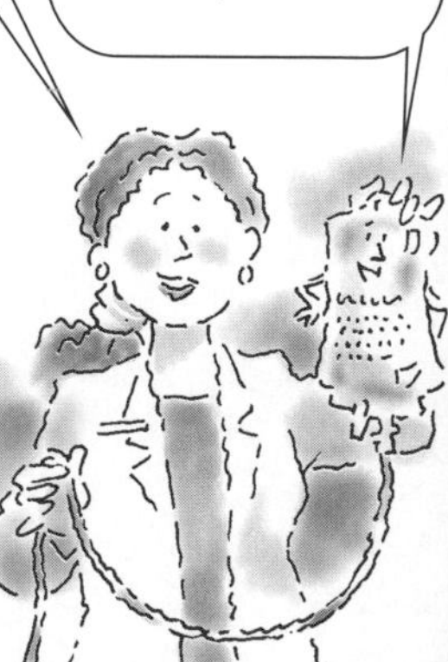

Positioned securely under the skin, an implanted port consists of a silicone catheter attached to a titanium or plastic reservoir covered by a self-sealing silicone rubber septum. Inserting an implanted port requires surgery. The device may be placed in the arm, chest, abdomen, flank of the chest, or thigh.

When to tap a port

Usually, you'll use an implanted port to deliver intermittent infusions. For example, you may use one to deliver:

- chemotherapy
- I.V. fluids
- pain control
- medications
- blood products.

Implanted ports may also be used to deliver TPN. When administering TPN, you'll need to closely monitor the access site to assess skin integrity. Implanted ports may also be used for long-term antibiotic therapy or to obtain blood samples.

On punctures and patients

To reduce the number of punctures to an implanted port, an intermittent infusion device or lock may be used.

Implanted ports should be used cautiously in patients with a high risk of developing an allergic reaction or infection.

Selecting the equipment

The implanted port selected for a patient depends on:

- the type of therapy needed
- how often the port must be accessed. (Typically, implanted ports are used for intermittent infusions and only require access during the prescribed therapy.)

The selection of infusion equipment will depend partly on the type of implanted port selected and the insertion site. Generally, you'll use the same infusion equipment as in peripheral I.V. and CV therapy, including an infusion solution and an administration set with tubing.

Depending on the patient's size and the type of therapy, an implanted port catheter with one or two lumens may be chosen.

Port variations

Implanted ports come in two basic types:

- top entry
- side entry.

In a top-entry implanted port, the needle is inserted perpendicular to the reservoir. In a side-entry implanted port, the needle is inserted almost parallel to the reservoir. Top-entry implanted ports are more commonly used. (See *A close look at a top-entry implanted port*, page 126.)

Material matters

The implanted port reservoir may be made of:

- titanium
- stainless steel
- molded plastic.

The type of reservoir used depends on the patient's therapeutic needs. For example, a patient undergoing magnetic resonance imaging should have a device made of titanium or plastic, instead of stainless steel, to avoid distorting test results.

A close look at a top-entry implanted port

An implanted port is typically used to deliver intermittent infusions of medication, chemotherapy, and blood products. It offers several advantages over external central venous (CV) therapy. Because the device is completely covered by the patient's skin, the risk of extrinsic contamination is reduced. In addition, patients may prefer this type of CV access device because it doesn't alter the body image and requires less routine catheter care.

The implanted port consists of a catheter connected to a small reservoir. A septum designed to withstand multiple punctures seals the reservoir. To access the port, a special noncoring needle is inserted perpendicular to the reservoir.

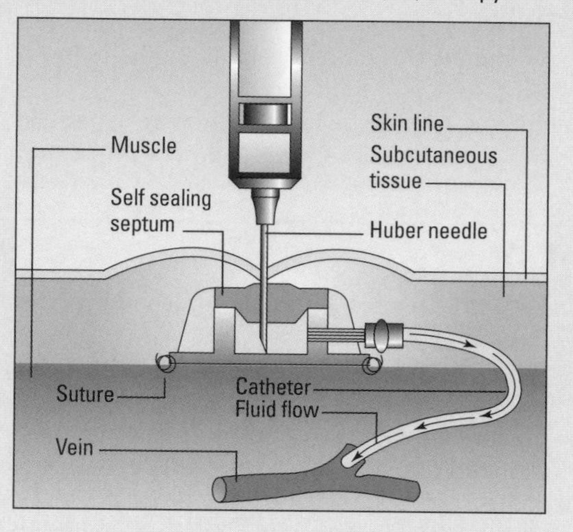

Noncoring needles needed

To avoid damaging the port's silicone rubber septum, use only noncoring needles. A noncoring needle has an angled or deflected point that slices the septum on entry, rather than coring it as a conventional needle does. When the noncoring needle is removed, the septum reseals itself. (See *A close look at noncoring needles.*)

Noncoring needles come with metal or plastic hubs in straight or right-angle configurations, with or without an extension set. Each configuration comes in various lengths (depending on the depth of septum implantation) and gauges (depending on the rate of infusion). (See *Choosing the right implanted port needle.*)

Implanted ports require special needles to access the device. Also, different gauges are needed for infusion of solutions, blood infusion or withdrawal, and flushing.

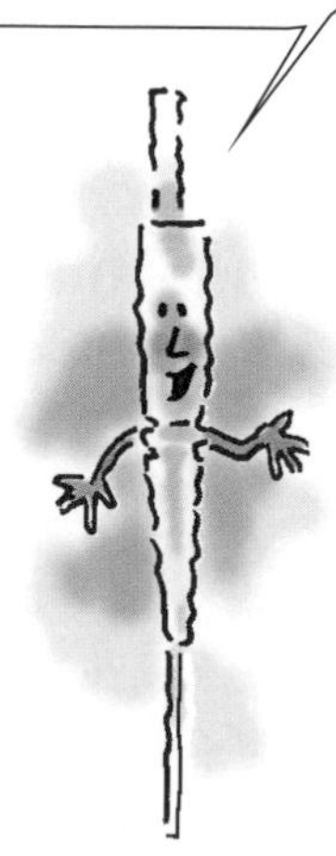

Continuous port access

An over-the-needle catheter allows continuous access to the port. This style of catheter is more comfortable for the patient and there's less risk of the device migrating out of the septum.

In an over-the-needle catheter, a solid-spike introducer and flexible catheter are passed through the silicone septum. Then the introducer is removed and the flexible Teflon catheter is positioned along the contour of the patient's chest wall.

A close look at noncoring needles

Unlike a conventional hypodermic needle, a noncoring needle has a deflected point, which slices the port's septum instead of coring it. Noncoring needles come in two types: straight and right angle.

Generally, expect to use a right-angle needle with a top-entry port and a straight needle with a side-entry port. When administering a bolus injection or continuous infusion, you'll also use an extension set.

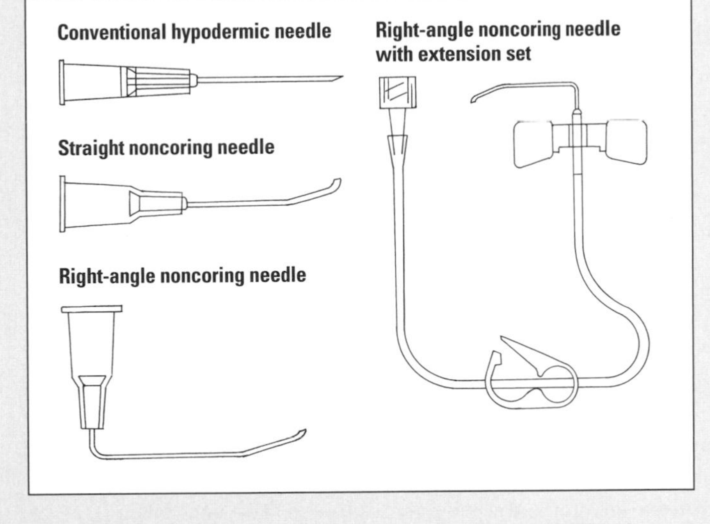

Choosing the right implanted port needle

When choosing an implanted port needle, the size of the needle will be determined by the therapy being delivered:

- 19G needles for blood infusion or withdrawal
- 20G needles for most infusions (other than blood infusion or withdrawal), including total parenteral nutrition
- 22G needles for flushing.

Remember that you should use only noncoring needles with a VAP.

Right angle vs. straight

A right-angle noncoring needle is most commonly used; rarely, a longer needle, such as a straight 2″ noncoring needle, is used to access a deeply implanted port.

You can use either a straight needle or a right-angle needle to inject a bolus into a top-entry port. For continuous infusions, however, experts recommend using a right-angle needle because it's easily secured to the patient. Side-entry ports are designed for use with straight noncoring needles only.

Implanted port insertion

A doctor inserts the implanted port, usually using local anesthesia with conscious sedation. Occasionally, general anesthesia may be used.

It begins with an incision

Inserting the implanted port involves the following steps:

1. The doctor makes a small incision and introduces the catheter into the superior vena cava through the subclavian, jugular, or cephalic vein. Fluoroscopy is used to verify placement of the catheter tip.

2. The doctor then creates a subcutaneous pocket over a bony prominence on the chest wall and tunnels the catheter to the pocket.

Next, the doctor connects the catheter to the reservoir, places the reservoir in the pocket, and flushes it with heparinized saline solution.

Finally, the doctor sutures the reservoir to the underlying fascia and closes the incision.

You may then apply a dressing to the wound site, according to your facility's policy and procedures. When the insertion site is healed, use routine dressing practices when the implanted port is in use.

Preparing the patient

Because implanted port insertion is a surgical procedure, teaching should cover preoperative and postoperative considerations.

Pre-op pointers

Use these pointers to guide your teaching before implanted port insertion:

- Make sure that the patient understands the procedure, its benefits, and what's expected of him after the insertion. Be prepared to supplement information provided by the doctor. You'll also need to allay the patient's fears and answer questions about movement restrictions, cosmetic concerns, and maintenance regimens. Clear explanations help ensure the patient's cooperation.
- Explain to the patient the purpose of a venogram, which may be ordered to determine the best vessel to use. The venogram is performed while the patient is under anesthesia.
- Describe how the patient will be positioned during the procedure.

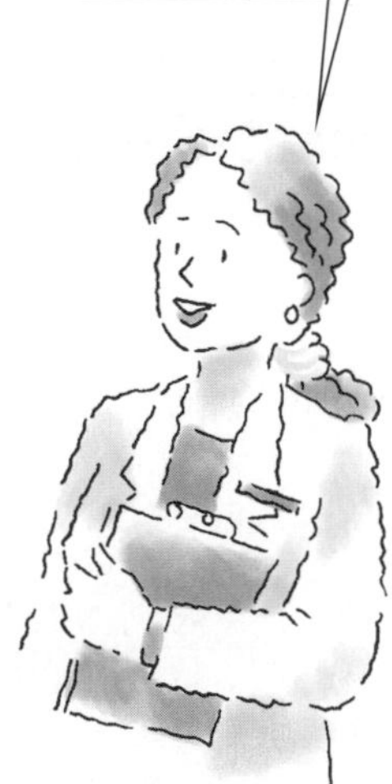

Obtaining consent

Most facilities require a signed informed consent form before an invasive procedure. Tell the patient he'll be asked to sign a consent form and explain what it means.

The doctor obtains consent; occasionally, you may witness the patient's signature. Before the patient signs, make sure that he understands the procedure. If not, delay signing until you or the doctor clarifies the procedure and the patient demonstrates understanding.

Post-op pointers

Discuss the following postoperative care topics:

- Remind the patient that, after the device is in place, he'll have to keep scheduled appointments to have the port heparinized. Another option is to teach him or a family member how to heparinize the port.
- Tell the patient to report signs and symptoms of systemic infection (fever, malaise, and flulike symptoms) and local infection (redness, tenderness, and drainage at the port or tunnel track site).
- The patient may need to receive prophylactic antibiotics before undergoing dental or surgical procedures to prevent contamination and colonization of the implanted port. Tell him to inform his dentist or practitioner that he has an implanted device. Tell the patient to carry identification material pertaining to specific care protocols, serial number, and model of the implanted port.
- Teach the patient to recognize and report signs and symptoms of infiltration, such as pain or swelling at the site, especially if he'll be receiving continuous infusions. Stress the need for immediate intervention to avoid damaging the tissue surrounding the port, especially if the patient is receiving vesicant medications.

Monitoring the patient

After the implanted port is inserted, observe the patient for several hours. The device can be used immediately after placement. However, swelling and tenderness may persist for about 72 hours, making the device initially difficult to palpate and uncomfortable for the patient.

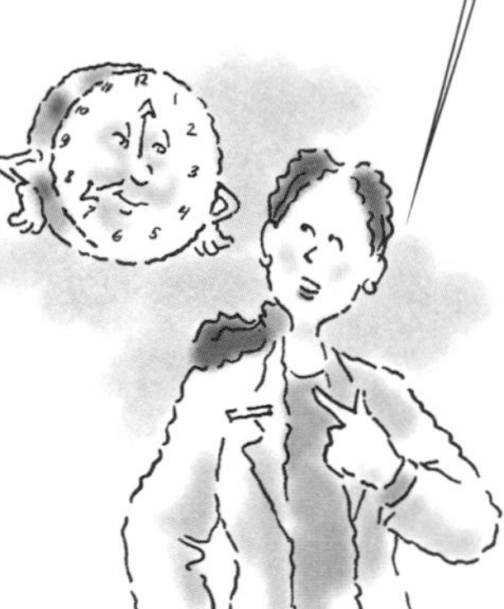

Site lines

The incision requires routine postoperative care for 7 to 10 days. Assess the insertion site for signs of:

- infection
- clotting
- redness
- device rotation or port housing movement
- skin irritation.

Implanted port infusion

To administer an infusion using an implanted port, the doctor may first access the port with the appropriate needle in the operating room. When you're ready to initiate infusion therapy, you'll need to set up the equipment and prepare the site.

Preparing the equipment

To set up infusion equipment, follow these steps:

 Attach the tubing to the solution container.

 Prime the tubing with fluid.

If setting up an intermittent system, obtain two syringes—one with 10 ml of normal saline solution and the other with 5 ml of heparin solution (100 units/ml).

Prime the noncoring needle and extension set with the saline solution from the syringe. (Prime the tubing and purge it of air using strict aseptic technique.)

After priming the tubing, recheck all the connections for tightness. Make sure that all open ends are covered with sealed caps.

If your facility doesn't have an implantable port access kit, you'll need to gather the necessary equipment.

Preparing the site

To prepare the needle insertion site, obtain an implantable port access kit, if your facility uses them. If a kit isn't available, gather the necessary equipment, including:

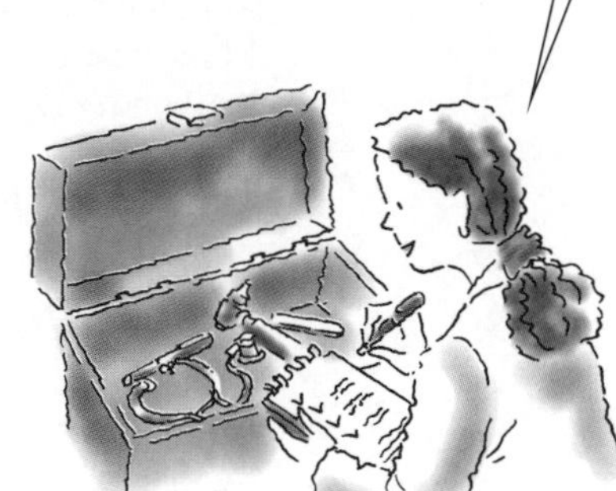

- sterile gloves
- three alcohol swabs
- three chlorhexidine swabs
- sterile 3″ × 3″ gauze pad
- sterile 1″ × 1″ gauze pad
- transparent dressing
- tape
- mask
- sterile drape.

Clear the field

When you're ready to prepare the access site, take the following precautions:

- Establish a sterile field for the sterile supplies, and inspect the area around the port for signs of infection or skin breakdown.
- An ice pack may be placed over the area for several minutes to numb the site. You may also apply a local anesthetic cream over the injection port, and cover it with a transparent dressing for about 1 hour. Be sure to remove this cream completely before putting on sterile gloves and preparing the access site.

Wash up and get started

To prepare the access site, follow these steps:

1. Wash your hands thoroughly and put on sterile gloves.

2. Clean the area with an alcohol swab, starting at the center of the port and working outward with a firm back-and-forth, or swiping, motion. Repeat this procedure twice more, allowing the alcohol to dry thoroughly.

3. Clean the area with a chlorhexidine swab using a back-and-forth scrubbing motion. Repeat this procedure twice. Most importantly, allow the chlorhexidine to dry completely.

4. If facility policy calls for a local anesthetic, check the patient's record for possible allergies. As indicated, anesthetize the insertion site by injecting 0.1 ml of lidocaine (Xylocaine), without epinephrine, intradermally.

If using transdermal analgesia, remember to apply it about 1 hour before the access procedure.

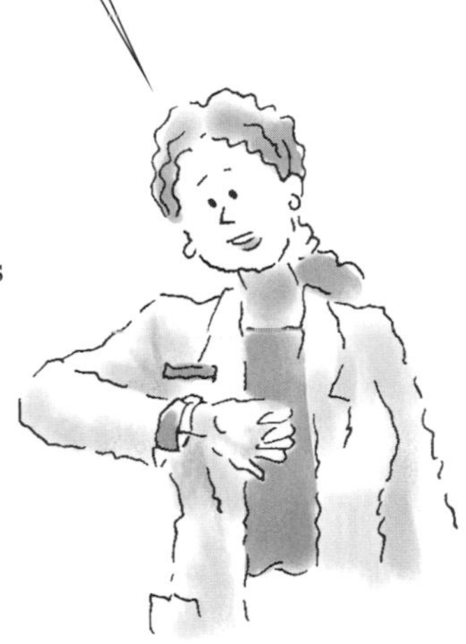

Accessing the site

When accessing a top-entry implanted port, you'll usually use a right-angle noncoring needle and a 10-ml syringe filled with saline solution. Follow the instructions in *How to access a top-entry implanted port*, page 132.

Side entrance

To gain access to a side-entry port, follow the same procedure used to access a top-entry port. However, insert the needle parallel to the reservoir instead of perpendicular to it.

Save time, decrease discomfort, prolong port life

While the patient is hospitalized, an intermittent infusion cap may be attached to the end of the extension set. This provides ready access for administering intermittent infusions.

Besides saving valuable nursing time, an accessed implanted port reduces the discomfort of reaccessing the port. It also prolongs the life of the port septum by decreasing the number of needle punctures.

Giving a bolus injection

To give a bolus injection, you need:

- 10-ml syringe filled with saline solution
- syringe containing the prescribed medication

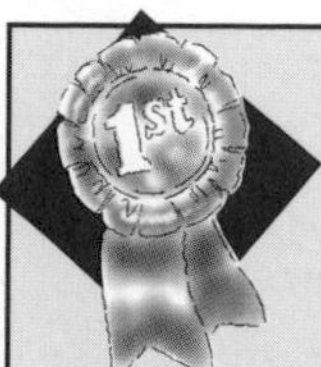

Best practice

How to access a top-entry implanted port

After assembling your equipment, use the following step-by-step guidelines to safely and securely access a top-entry implanted port:

- Palpate the area over the port to locate the septum. Optimally, the patient should be sitting up with his back supported.
- Anchor the port between your thumb and the first two fingers of your non-dominant hand. Then, using your dominant hand, aim the needle at the center of the device in between your thumb and first finger.
- Insert the needle perpendicular to the port septum, as shown. Push the needle through the skin and septum until you reach the bottom of the reservoir.
- Check the needle placement by aspirating for a blood return.
- If you can't obtain blood, remove the needle and repeat the procedure. Inability to obtain blood might indicate that the catheter is malfunctioning. If you can't obtain a blood return, notify the practitioner: A fibrin sheath on the distal end of the catheter may be blocking the opening.
- Flush the device with normal saline solution. If you detect swelling or if the patient reports pain at the site, remove the needle and notify the practitioner.

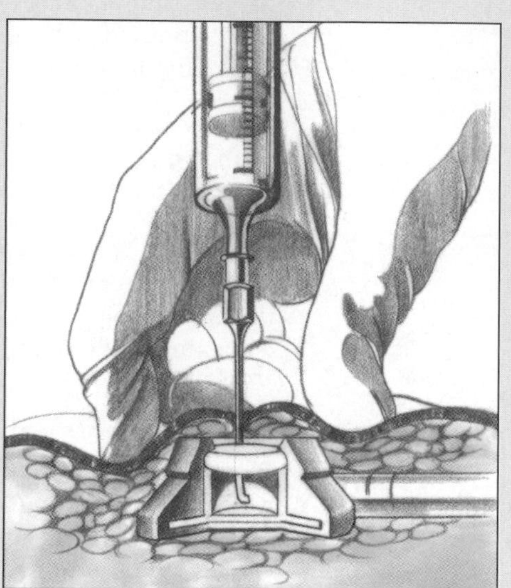

- syringe filled with the appropriate heparin flush solution (optional). (See *How to administer a bolus injection by implanted port.*)

Starting a continuous infusion

To prepare for a continuous infusion with an implanted port, gather the necessary equipment, including:

- prescribed I.V. solution or medication
- I.V. administration set with an air-eliminating filter, if ordered
- 10-ml syringe filled with saline solution
- adhesive tape
- sterile 2″ × 2″ gauze pad
- sterile tape or surgical strips
- transparent semipermeable dressing.

Make sure that the access needle is attached with an extension set that has a clamp, and you're ready to administer the infusion. (See *How to administer a continuous implanted port infusion,* page 134.)

How to administer a bolus injection by implanted port

Follow the step-by-step instructions below to safely and accurately give a bolus injection via an implanted port.

Attach, check, clamp, and connect

- Attach a 10-ml syringe filled with saline solution to the end of the extension set, and remove all the air. Then attach the extension set to a noncoring needle.
- Check for a blood return. Then flush the port with saline solution, according to your facility's policy. If no blood is obtained, notify the practitioner.
- Clamp the extension set and remove the saline solution syringe.
- Connect the medication syringe to the extension set. Open the clamp and inject the drug, as ordered.

Examine, clamp, and flush

- Examine the skin surrounding the needle for signs of infiltration, such as swelling or tenderness. If you note these signs, stop the injection and intervene appropriately.
- When the injection is complete, clamp the extension set and remove the medication syringe.
- Open the clamp and flush with 5 ml of saline solution after each drug injection to minimize drug incompatibility reactions.
- Flush with heparin solution, as your facility's policy directs.

Write it down

Document the injection according to your facility's policy. Include the following information: the type and amount of medication injected, the time of the injection, the appearance of the site, the patient's tolerance of the procedure, and any pertinent nursing interventions.

Maintaining implanted port infusions

To maintain infusion therapy with an implanted port, perform such care measures as:

- flushing the port with the appropriate heparin solution if the implanted port is used intermittently
- assessing the site at established intervals
- changing the dressing per the facility's protocol or whenever the dressing's integrity is compromised
- managing common equipment problems and patient complications
- discontinuing therapy when ordered, or converting the implanted port to an intermittent system to keep the device patent until it's needed again.

Flushing an implanted port

Follow these guidelines to determine when to flush an implanted port:

- If your patient is receiving a continuous or prolonged infusion, flush the port after each infusion and change the transparent dressing and needle every 7 days. However, any dressing should be changed immediately if its integrity is compromised. You'll also need to change the tubing and solution, as you would for a long-term CV infusion.

How to administer a continuous implanted port infusion

Follow the step-by-step instructions below to administer a continuous implanted port infusion safely and accurately.

Assemble, remove, flush, connect, and begin

- Assemble the equipment.
- Remove all the air from the extension set by priming it with an attached syringe of saline solution. Now attach the extension set to a noncoring needle.
- Flush the port system with saline solution. Clamp the extension set, and remove the syringe.
- Connect the administration set, and secure the connections, if necessary.
- Unclamp the extension set and begin the infusion.

Adjust and examine

- Place a gauze pad under the needle hub if it doesn't lie flush with the skin, as shown below left.
- To help prevent needle dislodgment, secure the needle to the skin with sterile tape or sterile surgical strips, as shown below right.
- Apply a transparent semipermeable dressing over the needle insertion site.
- Examine the site carefully for infiltration. If the patient complains of burning, stinging, or pain at the site, discontinue the infusion and intervene appropriately.

Obtain, clamp, and attach

- When the solution container is empty, obtain a new I.V. solution container, as ordered, with primed I.V. tubing.
- Clamp the extension set, and remove the old I.V. tubing.
- Attach the new I.V. tubing with the solution container to the extension set. Open the clamps, and adjust the infusion rate.

Write it down

Document the infusion according to your facility's policy, including the following information: the type, amount, rate, and time of infusion; the patient's tolerance of the procedure; the appearance of the site; and any pertinent nursing interventions.

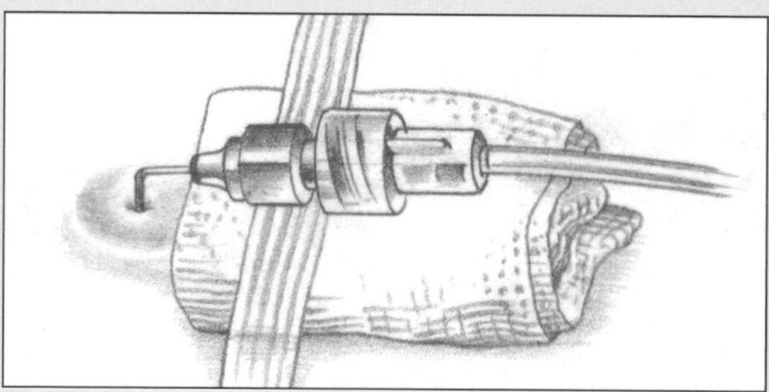

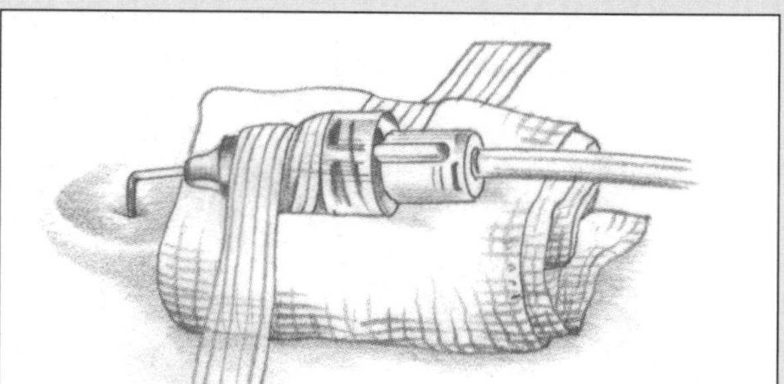

- If your patient is receiving an intermittent infusion, flush the port after each infusion and periodically with saline and heparin solutions.
- To help prevent clot formation in the device, flush the implanted port with heparin solution after each saline solution flush. When the port isn't accessed, flush it once every 4 weeks.

Getting equipped

To flush the implanted port, first gather the necessary equipment, including:

- 22G noncoring needle with an extension set
- 10-ml syringe filled with sterile normal saline solution
- 10-ml syringe filled with 5 ml of heparin flush solution (100 units/ml). Label each syringe carefully so you don't confuse them.

Ready, set, flush

Prepare the injection site, as described in the previous section. Then follow these steps:

1. Attach the 10-ml syringe of normal saline solution to the extension set and noncoring needle, applying gentle pressure to the plunger to expel all air from the set.
2. Palpate the area over the port to locate it, and then access the port.
3. Aspirate a blood return, and flush the port with normal saline solution to confirm patency. Then flush with the heparin solution.
4. While stabilizing the port with two fingers, withdraw the noncoring needle.

Obtaining blood samples

You can obtain blood samples from an implanted port with:

- a syringe
- an evacuated tube. (See *How to obtain a blood sample from an implanted port*, page 136.)

Clearing the implanted port

If clotting threatens to occlude the implanted port, making flushing and infusions sluggish, the practitioner may order a thrombolytic agent to clear the port and catheter.

To clear the implanted port, gather the necessary equipment, including:

- 20G or 22G noncoring needle with an extension set
- syringe filled with a thrombolytic
- empty 10-ml syringe
- two 10-ml syringes filled with saline solution
- syringe filled with heparin flush solution.

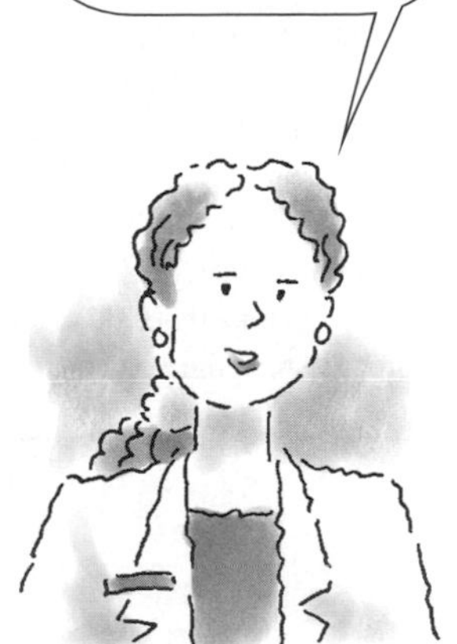

Clear the way

Follow these steps to clear the port and catheter:

1. Palpate the area over the port, and access the implanted port as described.
2. Check for blood return.
3. Flush the port with 5 ml of saline solution, and clamp the extension tubing.
4. Attach the syringe containing the thrombolytic and unclamp the extension tubing.

How to obtain a blood sample from an implanted port

After assembling your equipment, follow the step-by-step guidelines below to safely obtain a blood sample from an implanted port.

Syringe technique

To obtain a blood sample with a syringe, first gather the following equipment: a 19G, 20G, or 22G noncoring needle with an extension set; two 10-ml syringes filled with saline solution; a 10-ml sterile syringe; blood sample tubes; and a sterile syringe filled with heparin flush solution.

Prepare the site, then follow these steps:

- Attach one of the 10-ml syringes with saline solution to the noncoring needle and extension set. Remove all air from the set.
- Palpate the area over the port to locate it. Then access the port.
- Flush the port with 5 ml of saline solution.
- Withdraw at least 5 ml of blood, and then clamp the extension set and discard the syringe.
- Connect a 10-ml sterile syringe to the extension set; unclamp the set.
- Aspirate the desired amount of blood into the 10-ml syringe.
- After obtaining the sample, clamp the extension set, remove the syringe, and attach the second 10-ml syringe filled with saline solution. Unclamp the extension set.
- Immediately flush the port with 10 ml of saline solution. (Solution concentrations and amounts may vary according to facility policy.)
- Clamp the extension set, remove the saline syringe, and attach a sterile heparin-filled syringe. Perform the heparin flush procedure.
- Transfer the blood into appropriate blood sample tubes.

Evacuated tube technique

To obtain a blood sample using an evacuated tube, first gather the following equipment: a 19G, 20G, or 22G noncoring needle with an extension set; a luer-lock injection cap; two 10-ml syringes with saline solution; alcohol swabs; an evacuated tube and holder (disposable tubes come with the needleless device already attached); blood sample tubes (label one "Discard"); and a sterile syringe filled with heparin flush solution.

Prepare the site; then follow these steps:

- Attach the luer-lock injection cap to the noncoring needle extension set, using sterile technique. Remove all air from the set with the saline-filled syringe.
- Palpate the area over the port to locate it. Then access the port.
- Flush the port with 5 ml of saline solution to ensure correct noncoring needle placement. Remove the saline solution syringe.
- Wipe the injection cap with an alcohol swab.
- Insert the evacuated tube needleless device into the injection cap.
- Insert the blood sample tube labeled "Discard" into the evacuated tube holder.
- Allow the tube to fill with blood; remove the tube and discard.
- Insert another tube and allow it to fill with blood. Repeat this procedure until you obtain the necessary amount of blood.
- Remove the evacuated tube needleless device from the injection cap.
- Insert the 10-ml saline-filled syringe, and immediately flush the port with 10 ml of saline solution; then remove the syringe.
- Next, attach the heparin-filled syringe and perform the heparin flush procedure.
- After you have flushed the port with saline solution and heparin, clamp the extension set.

Obtaining blood samples during therapy

You may be ordered to obtain blood samples either before administering a bolus injection or during a continuous infusion. If you'll be administering a bolus injection, use the syringe method to obtain the blood sample, but don't flush with heparin solution.

If the patient is already receiving a continuous infusion, shut off the infusion and clamp the extension set. Then disconnect the extension set, maintaining aseptic technique. Follow the procedure for obtaining a blood sample with a syringe, up to and including the saline solution flush procedure. After the catheter is flushed with saline solution, clamp the extension set and remove the syringe. Reconnect the I.V. extension set. Then unclamp it and adjust the flow rate.

Instill the thrombolytic solution using a gentle pull-push motion on the syringe plunger to mix the solution in the access equipment, port, and catheter.

Clamp the extension set, and leave the solution in place for 15 minutes (up to 30 minutes in some facilities).

Then attach an empty 10-ml syringe, unclamp the extension set, and aspirate the thrombolytic and clot with the 10-ml syringe. Discard this syringe. Doing so will prevent the accidental injection of the thrombolytic into the systemic circulation.

If the clot can't be aspirated, wait 15 minutes and try again. You can safely instill a thrombolytic solution as many as three times in a 4-hour period if the patient's platelet count is greater than 20,000/ml. Repeat the procedure only once in a 4-hour period if the patient's platelet count is less than 20,000/ml.

After the blockage is cleared, flush the catheter with at least 10 ml of saline solution, and then flush with heparin solution, as described above.

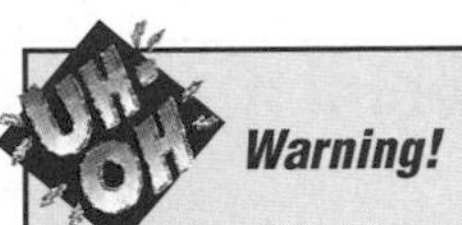

Thrombolytics may be forbidden

Because thrombolytic agents increase the risk of bleeding, they may be contraindicated in patients who have had surgery within the past 10 days; who have active internal bleeding, such as GI bleeding; or who have experienced central nervous system damage, such as infarction, hemorrhage, trauma, surgery, or primary or metastatic disease within the past 2 months.

Thrombolytics aren't for *everyone*

Treatment with a thrombolytic agent is contraindicated in patients with such conditions as:

- active bleeding
- intracranial neoplasms
- hypersensitivity to thrombolytic agents
- liver disease
- stroke in the past 2 months. subacute bacterial endocarditis, or visceral tumors (see *Thrombolytics may be forbidden*).

Documenting implanted port infusions

Record your assessment findings and interventions according to your facility's policy. Include such information as:

- type, amount, rate, and duration of the infusion
- appearance of the site
- development of problems, as well as the steps taken to resolve them
- needle gauge and length and dressing changes for continuous infusions
- blood samples obtained, including the type and amount
- patient-teaching topics covered and the patient's response to the procedure.

Special precautions

Routine care measures are subject to a few glitches. Be prepared to handle common problems that may arise during an infusion with an implanted port. Problems may include the inability to:

- flush the port
- withdraw blood from the port
- palpate and access the port. (See *Managing common implanted port problems.*)

A big exception for small patients

Generally, the procedures for implanting and maintaining an implanted port are the same for pediatric, elderly, and adult patients, with one big exception: For pediatric patients, general anesthesia may be used during insertion depending on the situation.

Usually, when a child undergoes implanted port insertion, general anesthesia is used.

Homework

A home care patient requires thorough teaching about procedures and follow-up visits from a home care nurse to ensure compliance, safety, and successful treatment.

If the patient is to access the port himself, explain that the most uncomfortable part of the procedure is inserting the needle into the skin. After the needle has penetrated the skin, the patient will feel some pressure but little pain. Eventually, the skin over the port may become less sensitive to frequent needle punctures. Until then, the patient may want to use a topical anesthetic.

All the way back

Stress the importance of pushing the needle into the port until the needle bevel touches the back of the port. Many patients tend to stop short of the back of the port, leaving the needle bevel in the rubber septum. This can cause blockage or slow the infusion rate.

Recognizing risks

A patient with an implanted port faces risks similar to those associated with a traditional CV access device, such as infection and infiltration. Teach the patient or caregiver how to recognize signs and symptoms of these complications. Make sure that they know how to intervene or how to reach the home health agency. (See *Complications of implanted port therapy,* page 140.)

Interrupting implanted port therapy

When interrupting implanted port therapy, remove the access needle from the port only after it has been flushed for maintenance.

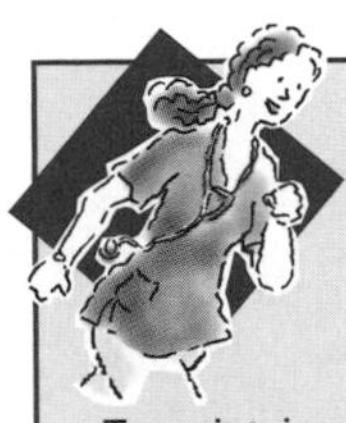

Running smoothly

Managing common implanted port problems

To maintain an implanted port, you must be able to handle common problems. This chart outlines problems you may encounter, their possible causes, and the appropriate nursing interventions needed.

Problem and possible causes	Nursing interventions
Inability to flush or withdraw blood	
Kinked tubing or closed clamp	• Check the tubing or clamp.
Incorrect needle placement or needle that won't advance through septum	• Regain access to the device. • Teach a home care patient to push down firmly on the noncoring needle device in the septum and to verify needle position by aspirating for blood return.
Clot formation	• Assess patency by trying to flush the port while the patient changes position. • Notify the practitioner; obtain an order for thrombolytic instillation. • Teach the patient to recognize clot formation, to notify the practitioner if it occurs, and to avoid forcibly flushing the port.
Kinked catheter, catheter migration, or port rotation	• Notify the practitioner immediately. • Tell the patient to notify the practitioner if he has difficulty using the port.
Catheter lodged against vessel wall	• Reposition the patient. • Teach the patient to change his position to free the catheter from the vessel wall. • Raise the arm that's on the same side as the catheter. • Roll the patient to his opposite side. • Have the patient cough, sit up or take a deep breath. • Infuse 10 ml of normal saline solution into the catheter. • Regain access to the implanted port using a new needle.
Inability to palpate the port	
Deeply implanted port	• Note portal chamber scar. • Use deep palpation technique. • Ask another nurse to try locating the implanted port. • Use a 1½" to 2" noncoring needle to gain access to the implanted port.

Although there's usually little or no bloody drainage when the access needle is removed, take these precautions:

- Wear gloves.
- Dispose of the needle properly.
- Place a small dressing temporarily over the implanted port site.

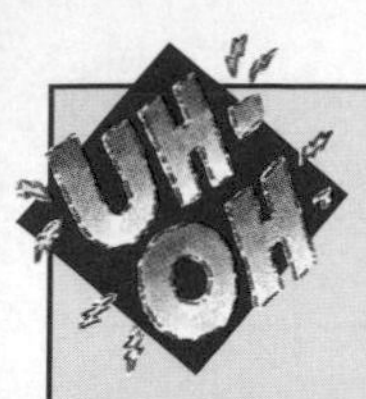

Warning!

Complications of implanted port therapy

This chart lists common complications of implanted port therapy as well as their signs and symptoms, causes, nursing interventions, and preventive measures.

Signs and symptoms	Possible causes	Nursing interventions	Prevention
Site infection or skin breakdown			
• Erythema, swelling, and warmth at the port site • Oozing or purulent drainage at port site or pocket • Fever	• Infected incision or pocket • Poor postoperative healing	• Assess the site daily for redness; note any drainage. • Notify the practitioner. • Administer antibiotics, as prescribed. • Apply warm soaks for 20 minutes four times per day, as ordered.	• Teach the patient to inspect for and report redness, swelling, drainage, or skin breakdown at the port site.
Extravasation			
• Burning sensation or swelling in subcutaneous tissue	• Needle dislodged into subcutaneous tissue • Needle incorrectly placed in port • Needle position not confirmed; needle pulled out of septum • Rupture of catheter along tunneled route • Use of vesicant drugs	• Don't remove the needle. • Stop the infusion. • Notify the practitioner; prepare to administer the antidote, if prescribed.	• Teach the patient how to gain access to the device, verify placement of the device, and secure the needle before initiating the infusion.
Thrombosis			
• Inability to flush port or administer infusion	• Frequent blood sampling • Infusion of packed red blood cells (RBCs)	• Notify the practitioner; obtain an order to administer a thrombolytic agent according to facility policy.	• Flush the port thoroughly right after obtaining a blood sample. • Administer packed RBCs as a piggyback with saline solution and use an infusion pump; flush with saline solution between units.
Fibrin sheath formation			
• Blocked port and catheter lumen • Inability to flush port or administer infusion • Possibly swelling, tenderness, and erythema in neck, chest, and shoulder	• Adherence of platelets to catheter	• Notify the practitioner; prepare to administer thrombolytic.	• Use the port only to infuse fluids and medications; don't use it to obtain blood samples. • Administer only compatible substances through the port.

Discontinuing implanted port therapy

To prepare to discontinue therapy, first gather the necessary equipment, including:

- 10-ml syringe filled with normal saline solution
- 10-ml syringe filled with 5 ml of sterile heparin flush solution (100 units/ml)
- sterile gloves
- sterile 2″ × 2″ gauze pad and tape.

Be sure to label the syringes so you don't mix up the heparin and saline solution flushes. Then, follow these steps:

- After shutting off the infusion, clamp the extension set and remove the I.V. tubing.
- Attach the syringe filled with saline solution using aseptic technique.
- Unclamp the extension set, flush the device with the saline solution, and remove the saline solution syringe.
- Attach the heparin syringe, flush the port with the heparin solution, and clamp the extension set.

Removing the noncoring needle

After flushing the port with heparin solution, remove the noncoring needle by following these steps:

1. First, put on gloves.
2. Place the gloved index and middle fingers from the nondominant hand on either side of the port septum.
3. Stabilize the port by pressing down with these two fingers, maintaining pressure until the needle is removed.
4. Using your gloved, dominant hand, grasp the noncoring needle and pull it straight out of the port.
5. Apply a dressing as indicated.
6. If no more infusions are scheduled, remind the patient that he'll need a heparin flush in 4 weeks.

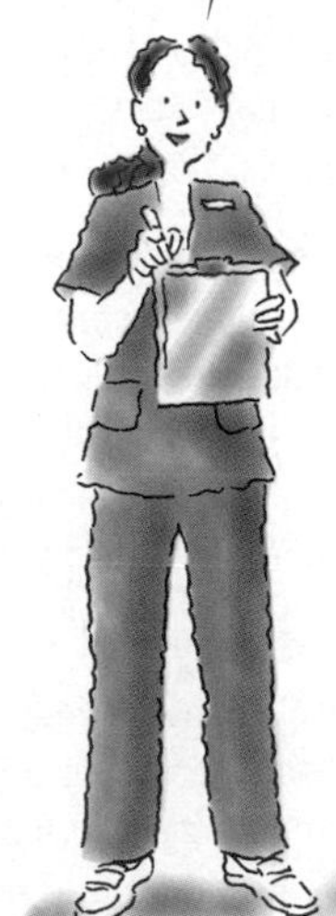

Document

After removing the noncoring needle, document the following:

- removal of the infusion needle
- status of the site
- use of the heparin flush
- patient's tolerance of the procedure
- your teaching efforts
- problems you encountered and resolved.

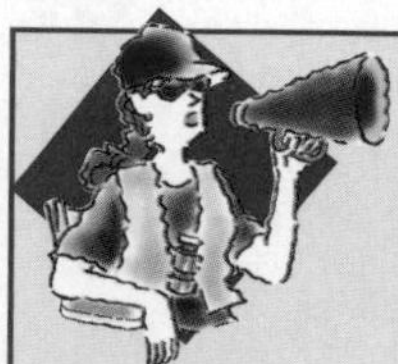

That's a wrap!

Central venous therapy review

Benefits
- Provides access to the central veins
- Permits rapid infusion of medications or large amounts of fluids
- Allows clinicians to draw blood samples and measure CV pressure
- Reduces the need for repeated venipunctures
- Reduces the risk of vein irritation

Drawbacks
- Increases the risk of life-threatening complications

Catheter types and uses
- Nontunneled: designed for short-term use
- Tunneled: designed for long-term use
- PICCs: used when the patient requires infusions of caustic drugs or solutions
- Implanted ports: inserted when an external catheter isn't suitable

Common CV insertion sites
- Subclavian vein
- Internal or external jugular vein
- Cephalic vein
- Basilic vein

Insertion site considerations
- Presence of scar tissue
- Possible interference with surgical site or other therapy
- Configuration of lung apices
- Patient's lifestyle and daily activities

Before insertion
- Explain the procedure to the patient.
- Place the patient in Trendelenburg's position.
- Prepare the insertion site: clip hair and clean the site with chlorhexidine.
- Assist with sterile drape application.
- Conscious sedation may be used; if so, the patient requires close observation.

During insertion
- Monitor patient tolerance.
- Assist as needed.
- Provide support to the patient.

After insertion
- Monitor for complications.
- Apply a transparent semipermeable dressing.
- Document the insertion.

Complications of CV therapy
- Pneumothorax, hemothorax, chylothorax, hydrothorax
- Air embolism
- Thrombus formation
- Perforation of vessel and adjacent organs
- Local infection
- Systemic infection

Complications of implanted port therapy
- Infection at injection site
- Skin breakdown
- Extravasation
- Thrombosis
- Fibrin sheath formation

Infusion maintenance
- Change the transparent semipermeable dressing whenever it becomes moist, loose, or soiled.
- Change the I.V. solution and tubing every 24 hours according to facility protocol.
- Flush the catheter with a 2- or 3-way valve daily to every 8 hours (if not in use) or according to facility protocol.

Central venous therapy review *(continued)*

- Change the gauze dressing at least every 48 hours.
- Change the intermittent injection caps at least every 7 days.

Implanted port insertion and maintenance

- Explain the procedure to the patient and make sure he's signed a consent form.
- Monitor the patient during and after implantation for complications (infection, clotting, skin irritation).
- Change the dressing whenever its integrity is compromised.
- Flush every 4 weeks if not accessed.

What to document

- Status of the site
- Type of needle used
- Type of device used
- Procedure performed
- Patient's tolerance of the procedure
- Problems encountered and nursing interventions performed
- Type of dressing used
- Patient teaching performed and patient's understanding of teaching

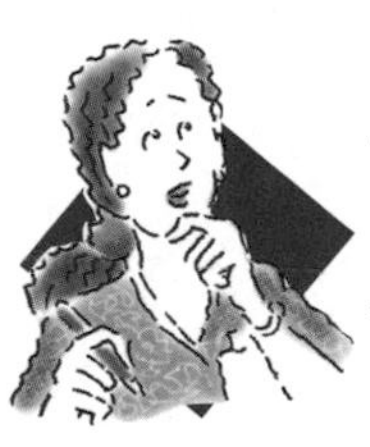

Quick quiz

1. In CV therapy, an access device is inserted with its tip in the:
 A. inferior vena cava or right atrium.
 B. superior or inferior vena cava.
 C. superior vena cava or right atrium.
 D. right atrium or right ventricle.

Answer: B. Depending on venous accessibility and the prescribed infusion therapy, a CV access device is inserted with its tip in the superior or inferior vena cava.

2. The advantages of CV therapy include:
 A. ability to rapidly infuse fluids, draw blood specimens, and measure CV pressure.
 B. minimal or no complications on insertion.
 C. increased patient mobility.
 D. decreased risk of infection.

Answer: A. CV therapy provides access to central veins as well as the ability to rapidly infuse medications or fluids, draw blood specimens, and measure CV pressure.

3. Which vein is the most commonly used CV insertion site?

A. Femoral
B. Brachial
C. Cephalic
D. Subclavian

Answer: D. The subclavian vein is the most common CV insertion site. It provides easy access and a direct route to the superior vena cava and CV circulation.

4. Nursing responsibilities when preparing a patient for CV therapy include:

A. explaining the procedure and care measures of the therapy.
B. selecting the site.
C. obtaining consent.
D. inserting the device.

Answer: A. When preparing a patient for CV therapy, the nurse should explain the procedure and its care measures and answer the patient's questions.

5. Which catheter would be most appropriate for pediatric patients?

A. Broviac tunneled catheter
B. Hickman-Broviac tunneled catheter
C. PICC
D. Groshong tunneled catheter

Answer: A. The Broviac tunneled catheter is more appropriate for use in individuals with small central veins, such as pediatric patients.

6. When drawing a specimen, what amount of blood is discarded from an implanted port?

A. 1 ml
B. 2 ml
C. 3 ml
D. 5 ml

Answer: D. You should discard 5 ml of blood before drawing the specimen.

Scoring

☆☆☆ If you answered six questions correctly, right on! You took a central route to understanding this chapter.

☆☆ If you answered four or five questions correctly, good job! You followed the text right to the heart of the matter.

☆ If you answered fewer than four questions correctly, don't fret! Instead, center yourself and reaccess the material.

I.V. medications

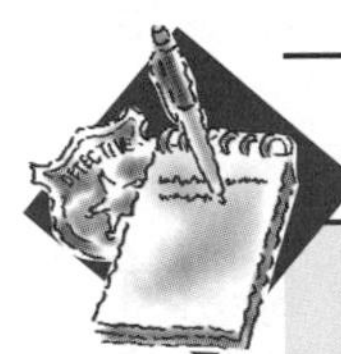

Just the facts

In this chapter, you'll learn:

- ♦ the purpose of I.V. medications
- ♦ advantages and disadvantages of I.V. medications
- ♦ dosage calculation for I.V. dosages and administration rates
- ♦ the preparation of I.V. medications
- ♦ administration of I.V. medications by direct injection and by intermittent or continuous infusion
- ♦ advantages and disadvantages of patient-controlled analgesia devices
- ♦ common complications of I.V. medication therapy
- ♦ proper care techniques for pediatric and elderly patients receiving I.V. medications.

Understanding I.V. medications

Hospitalized patients receive about 50% of their medications by the I.V. route. I.V. medications may be given by:

- direct injection
- intermittent infusion
- continuous infusion.

Did you know that about half of all medications administered to patients in the hospital are given by the I.V. route?

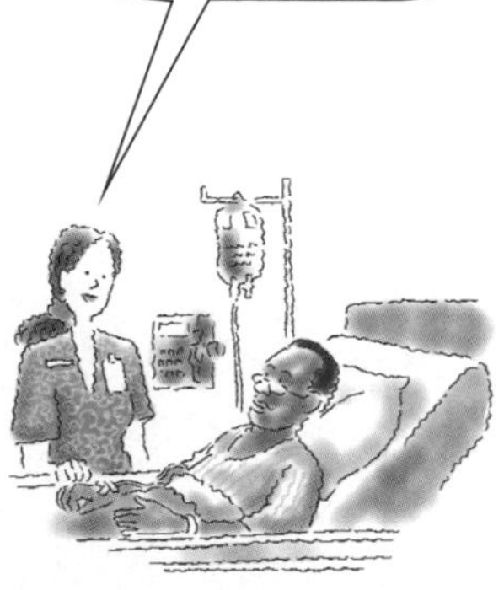

Entering the I.V. league

An I.V. medication may be ordered when:

- a patient needs a rapid therapeutic effect
- the medication can't be absorbed by the GI tract, either because it has a high molecular weight or is unstable in gastric juices

- the patient may receive nothing by mouth
- an irritating drug would cause pain or tissue damage if given intramuscularly (I.M.) or subcutaneously (subQ)
- a controlled administration rate is needed.

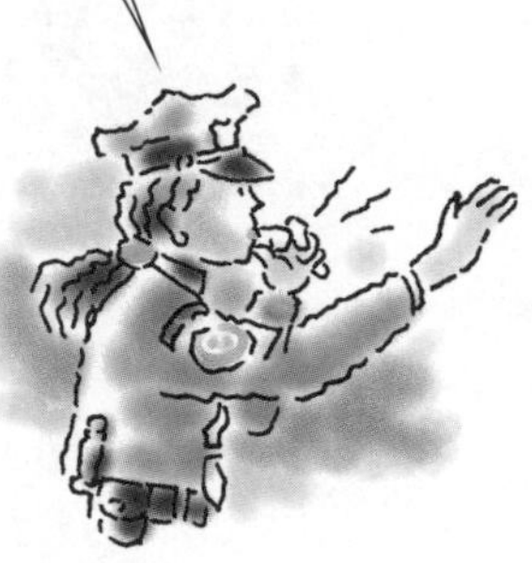

Benefits

Compared with the oral, subQ, and I.M. routes, the I.V. route has many advantages, including:

- rapid response
- effective absorption
- accurate titration
- less discomfort.

The I.V. route also provides an alternative when the oral route must be bypassed, such as when your patient is unconscious or uncooperative or can take nothing by mouth.

Stopping power

In addition, if an adverse reaction occurs, I.V. drug delivery can be stopped immediately. With other routes, absorption would continue until the drug was physically removed by vomiting, gastric suctioning, or dialysis.

Rapid response

I.V. medications go directly into the patient's circulation, rapidly achieving therapeutic blood levels. This difference in absorption explains why, for drugs such as propranolol, I.V. doses are much smaller than oral doses.

Effective absorption

Drug absorption covers the progress of a drug from the time it's administered through the time it passes through the tissues, until it becomes available for use by the body. Absorption of subQ, I.M., and orally administered drugs may be less effective.

The aim is to be effective, not erratic

Absorption may be erratic with subQ and I.M. drug administration because the complex systems of muscle and skin delay drug passage. Giving drugs I.V. avoids this problem because the active drug reaches systemic circulation immediately, causing the drug to achieve therapeutic levels quickly.

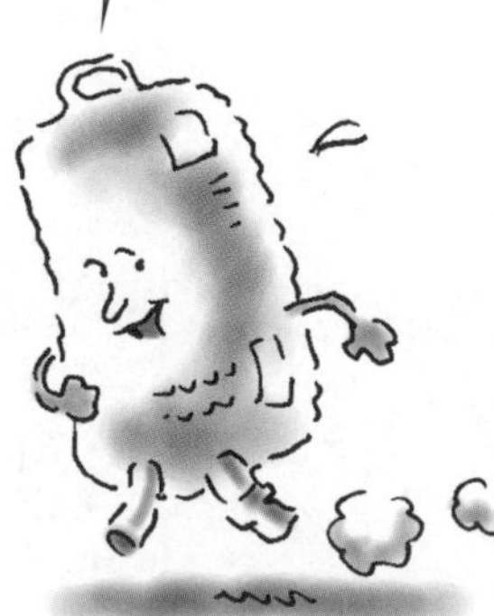

Bypassing the first-pass

Some oral medications are unstable in gastric juices and digestive enzymes, making absorption uncertain. Some oral medications may also interact with food or other medications which may alter absorption. Absorption problems also occur with oral medications that are metabolized by the liver.

In the liver, significant amounts of the drug are processed and eliminated before they reach the bloodstream. This process—known as *first-pass metabolism*—may be so rapid and extensive (in the case of lidocaine, for example) that it precludes oral administration.

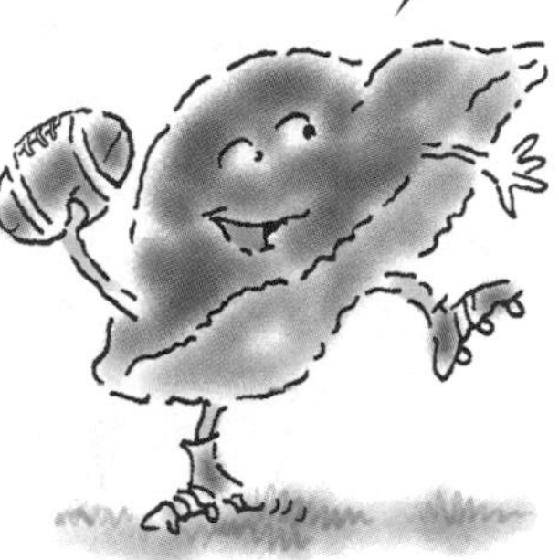

Accurate titration

Because gastric absorption isn't a factor with I.V. therapy, you can accurately titrate doses by adjusting the concentration of the infusate and the administration rate.

Less discomfort

I.V. administration prevents the pain and discomfort of I.M. and subQ injections. However, some I.V. medications can cause venous irritation.

Diluting discomfort

You may sometimes reduce venous irritation by further diluting an I.V. medication in a larger volume of solute.

Risks

Like all administration routes, the I.V. route has certain risks. These include:

- solution and drug incompatibilities
- poor vascular access in some patients
- immediate adverse reactions.

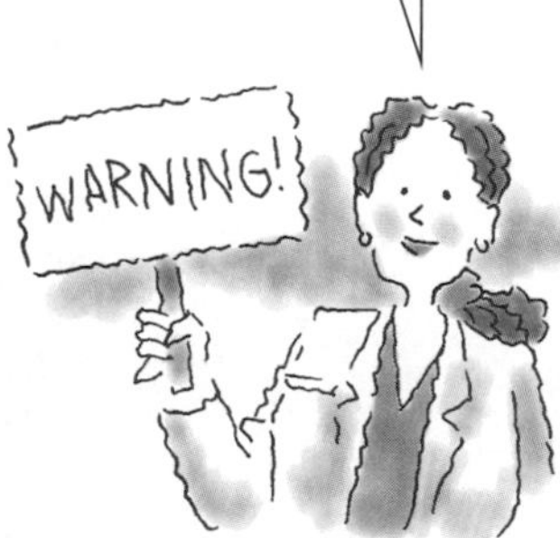

Incompatibility

To successfully mix medication in a solution for infusion, two things must be compatible: drug and diluent. If you aren't sure about the compatibility of a mixture, ask the pharmacist or check an up-to-date compatibility chart.

When drugs and solutions don't get along

Most I.V. drugs are compatible with commonly used I.V. solutions. The more complex the solution, however, the greater the risk of incompatibility. In addition, an I.V. solution that contains divalent cations (such as calcium) has a higher incidence of incompatibility.

Incompatibility problems are also common in mixtures containing:
- other electrolytes
- mannitol
- bicarbonate
- nutritional solutions.

Can you be more specific?

Specific incompatibilities fall into three categories:

 physical

 chemical

 therapeutic. (See *Factors affecting drug compatibility.*)

Physical incompatibility

A physical incompatibility (also called a *pharmaceutical incompatibility*) occurs more commonly with multiple additives.

Signs of physical incompatibility can be seen in the solution and include:
- precipitation
- haze
- gas bubbles
- cloudiness.

Study I.V. solutions for signs of physical incompatibility — precipitates, haze, bubbles, and cloudiness.

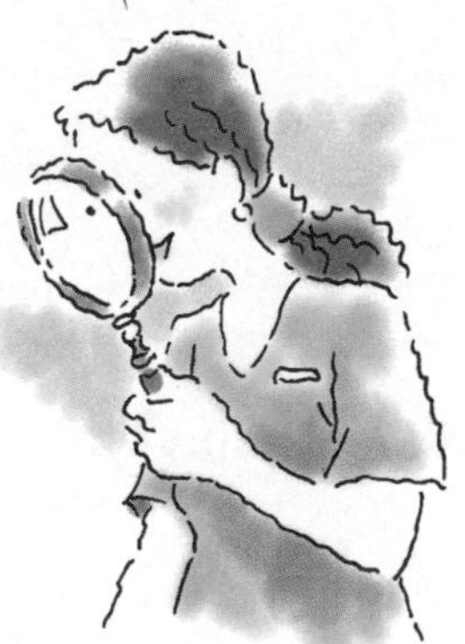

Expect some precipitation

The presence of calcium in a solution (such as lactated Ringer's solution) commonly increases the likelihood that a precipitate might form if the solution is mixed with another drug.

So degrading

Other physical incompatibilities occur as a result of drug degradation such as the degradation of norepinephrine when added to sodium bicarbonate.

Chemical incompatibility

With chemical incompatibility, mixing two drugs alters the integrity and potency of active ingredients. When a drug loses more than 10% of its potency, it's considered incompatible with whatever caused the loss of potency. Decomposition of a drug indicates a chemical incompatibility. Factors commonly associated with chemical incompatibility include:
- drug concentration
- pH of the solution
- volume of solution used to mix medications

Factors affecting drug compatibility

Incompatibility is an undesirable chemical or physical reaction between a drug and a solution or between two or more drugs. The following factors can affect the compatibility of an I.V. drug or solution.

Order of mixing

Mixing order is a concern when you're adding more than one drug to an I.V. solution. Chemical changes occur after each drug is added. A drug that's compatible with the I.V. solution alone may be incompatible with the mixture of the I.V. solution and another drug. Changing the order in which the drugs are mixed may prevent incompatibility.

Drug concentration

The higher the drug concentration, the more likely an incompatibility will develop. Gently invert the container after adding each drug to evenly disperse it throughout the solution, preventing a high-concentration buildup. Do this before starting an infusion and before adding another drug to the container.

Contact time

The longer two or more drugs are together, the more likely an incompatibility will occur. For example, amikacin and acyclovir become incompatible when combined for 4 or more hours. You should know if two drugs are incompatible before deciding how to give them. Suppose, for example, that your patient is receiving a continuous heparin infusion, and gentamicin sulfate is ordered. Because these two drugs have an immediate incompatibility, you shouldn't piggyback the gentamicin into the heparin solution. If you do, your patient won't receive a therapeutic dose of gentamicin.

Temperature

Higher temperatures promote chemical reactions. The higher the temperature of an admixture, the greater the risk of incompatibility. For this reason, prepare the admixture immediately before administering it, or refrigerate it until needed.

Light

Prolonged exposure to light can affect the stability of certain drugs. Nitroprusside sodium and amphotericin B, for example, must be protected from light during administration to maintain their stability.

pH

Generally, drugs and solutions that are to be mixed should have similar pH values to avoid incompatibility. The pH of each I.V. solution is listed on the manufacturer's label. You'll find the pH of each drug on the package insert.

- length of time that the medications are in contact with each other
- temperature
- light.

Acid and alkali actions

The most common chemical incompatibility involves the reaction between acidic and alkaline drugs and solutions. For example, mixing heparin solutions with intermittent aminoglycoside infusions commonly creates a chemical incompatibility, leading to such reactions as precipitate formation, color change, or gas bubbles.

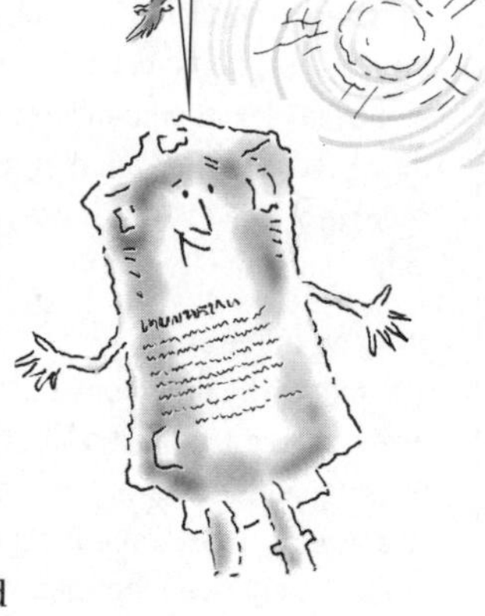

Light plight

Bright light, such as sunlight, may provide the energy needed for a chemical reaction. To avoid such a reaction, certain drugs must be protected from light. Examples of drugs that need protection from light when they're diluted are amphotericin B and nitroprusside sodium.

Therapeutic incompatibility

A therapeutic incompatibility may occur when two or more drugs are administered concurrently. Concurrent administration may happen when a patient is prescribed two antibiotics—for example, chloramphenicol and penicillin. Chloramphenicol reportedly antagonizes the antibacterial effects of penicillin. Therefore, penicillin should be infused at least 1 hour before chloramphenicol.

Poor vascular access

In an emergency, you may find that normally accessible veins have collapsed from vasoconstriction or hypovolemia. Venipuncture may also be difficult in patients who require frequent or prolonged I.V. therapy. You may find that these patients have developed small, scarred, inaccessible veins from repeated venipunctures or infusions of irritating drugs.

Alternate routes

If peripheral venous access isn't possible, the practitioner may use a central vein, commonly by the subclavian route. If venipuncture isn't possible, drugs may be given I.M. or subQ. However, these routes can be used only if the volume to be infused is small and the drugs cause little or no tissue irritation.

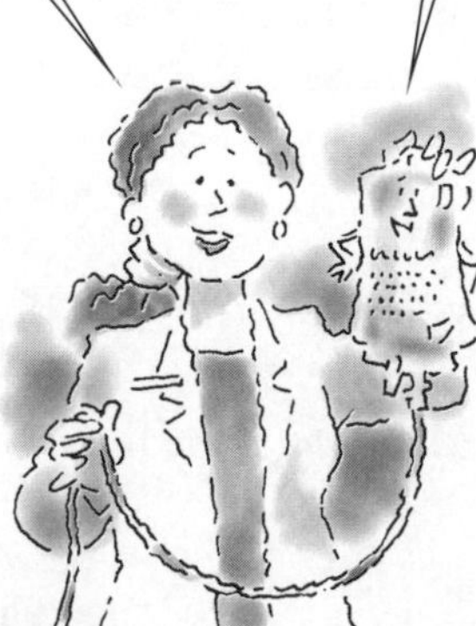

Adverse reactions

Because I.V. drugs quickly produce high blood levels, severe adverse reactions may occur immediately. The type of adverse reaction depends largely on the type of drug that's infused.

Don't get crossed-up

Hypersensitivity to I.V. drugs, although uncommon, can occur immediately or any time after administration. Keep cross-sensitivity in mind; if a patient is hypersensitive to a particular drug, he may be hypersensitive to chemically similar drugs. The most severe hypersensitivity reaction is anaphylaxis. Penicillin and its synthetic derivatives make up one of the drug families that's most likely to produce anaphylaxis.

Be on guard for adverse reactions any time you give a drug I.V.

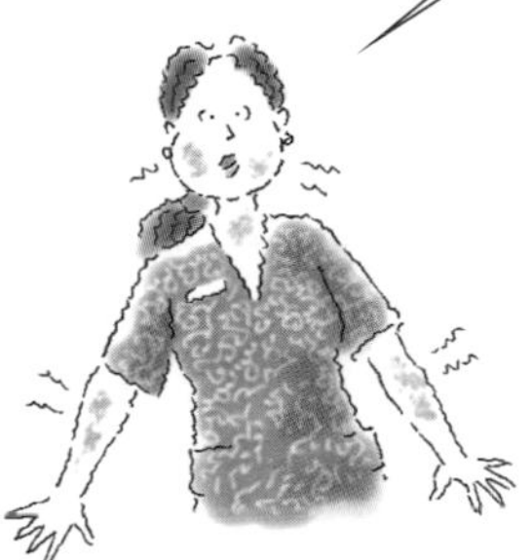

Perilous preservatives

Your patient may suffer from an adverse reaction to the preservative in a drug or I.V. solution. Sulfites, for example, can cause sensitivity reactions, particularly in patients with asthma. Large amounts of benzyl alcohol may cause seizures in neonates; therefore, all solutions administered to neonates must be preservative-free.

An intolerance that turns things topsy-turvy

You may encounter patients who have an inherent inability to tolerate certain chemicals. They can experience another kind of adverse reaction, called an *idiosyncratic reaction.* For example, a tranquilizer may cause excitation rather than sedation. Idiosyncratic reactions are more common in children and elderly patients.

Calculating I.V. drug dosages

In many cases, you must calculate an ordered dosage and verify that the dosage is within the recommended range.

Weighing in

With some drugs (I.V. immune globulin, for instance), dosage is based on the patient's weight in kilograms. To convert a patient's weight from pounds to kilograms, simply divide the number of pounds by 2.2. (Remember, 2.2 lb = 1 kg.)

Coming to the surface

With other drugs (such as chemotherapeutic agents), the dosage may be based on the patient's body surface area (BSA). One method for determining BSA is to use a nomogram. (See *Using a nomogram for children*, page 152, and *Using a nomogram for adults*, page 153.)

Calculating administration rates

Typically, an order for I.V. medication prescribes the number of milliliters to infuse over a specified period. For instance, an order may call for 1,000 ml of dextrose 5% in half-normal saline solution every 8 hours.

To find out how many milliliters to administer in 1 hour, divide the total volume by the number of hours required to deliver the infusion.

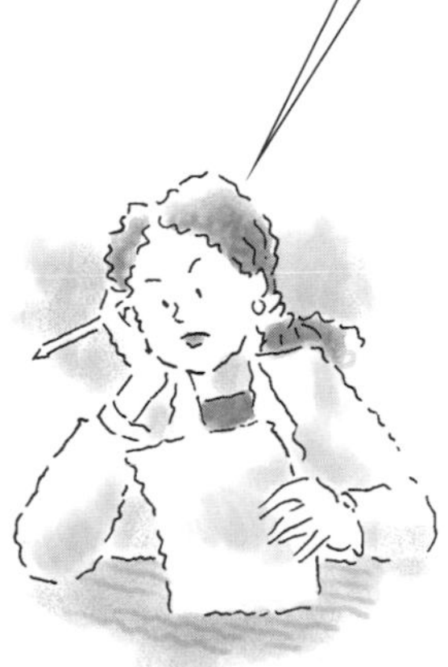

To make sure that you deliver the drug solution evenly, you must determine how many milliliters to give in 1 hour. To do so, just divide the total volume of the infusion by the number of hours

Using a nomogram for children

To estimate a child's body surface area (BSA) with a nomogram, find the child's weight in the right column and his height in the left column. Mark these two points, and then draw a line between them. The point where the line intersects the surface area column in the middle gives you the BSA in square meters (m²).

On this nomogram, the child's height is 36″ (91.4 cm) and his weight is 55 lb (24.9 kg). A straight line drawn between the two columns intersects the center column at 0.8. That tells you that this patient's BSA is 0.8 m².

If the child is of average size, you can determine BSA from weight alone by using the shaded area.

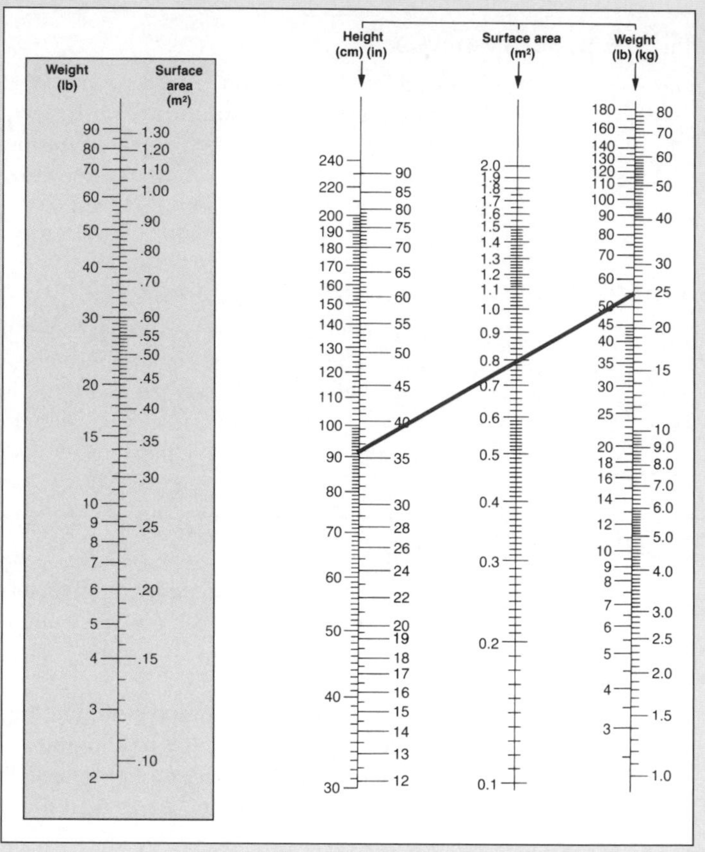

the infusion is to take. In this case, divide 1,000 ml by 8 hours to determine that you must give 125 ml/hour.

Additional orders

Additional I.V. orders affect your calculations. Suppose the patient who's receiving 1,000 ml of dextrose 5% in half-normal saline solution every 8 hours also needs to receive gentamicin 80 mg once every 8 hours by intermittent infusion. There are two possible ways to handle this:

- After determining that the patient can tolerate the extra volume, you may simply incorporate the antibiotic fluid into the total daily intake.

Using a nomogram for adults

To estimate an adult's body surface area (BSA) with a nomogram, find your patient's weight in the right column and his height in the left column. Mark these two points; then draw a line between them. The point where the line intersects the middle column gives you the BSA in square meters (m^2).

On this nomogram, the patient's height is 5′ 3″ (160 cm) and her weight is 110 lb (49.9 kg). A straight line drawn between the two columns intersects the center column at 1.50. That tells you this patient's BSA is 1.5 m^2.

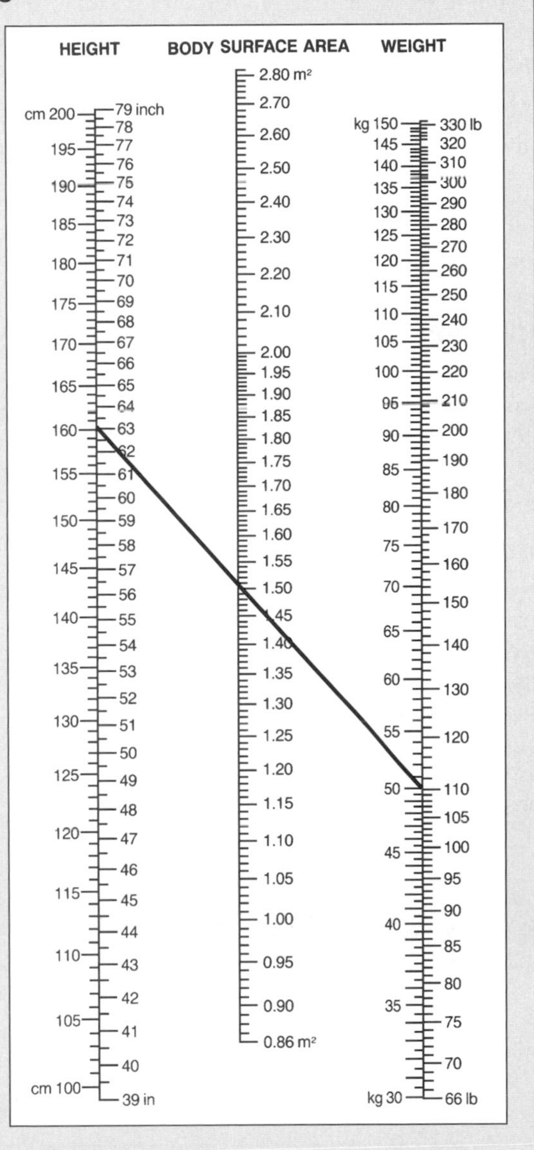

After determining that gentamicin and the primary infusate (dextrose 5% in half-normal saline solution) are compatible, you may recalculate the infusion rate for the primary infusion after the antibiotic has been administered.

Ready, set, recalculate

If you need to recalculate the infusion rate, some simple subtraction and division are needed. To recalculate the infusion rate for the previous example, use these two steps:

1. Subtract the time needed to give the gentamicin from the total time. For example, if you administer the gentamicin over 1 hour, there are 7 hours left to give the primary solution.

2. Divide 1,000 by 7 to find that you must deliver the primary solution at a rate of 143 ml/hour.

Remember, when using an administration set instead of an infusion pump, you must convert milliliters per hour to drops per minute.

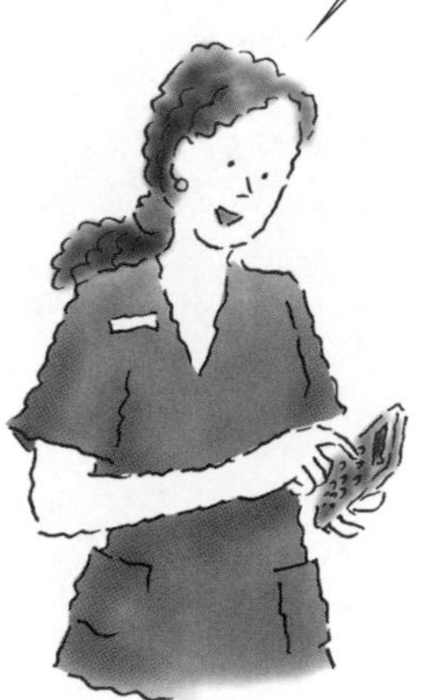

Equipment considerations

Your calculations may also depend on the delivery equipment. If you're using an infusion pump, simply set the rate for the desired milliliters per hour rate. However, if you're using an administration set, you have to convert milliliters per hour to drops per minute (gtt/minute).

Don't drop this formula

To convert milliliters per hour to drops per minute, you must know the number of drops per milliliter that the particular I.V. tubing delivers. Microdrip tubings deliver 60 gtt/ml, but macrodrip tubings vary. To find drops per milliliter information, check the product wrapper or box; then use this formula:

$$\text{Drip rate in drops/minute} = \frac{\text{Total milliliters}}{\text{Total minutes}} \times \text{Drop factor in drops/ml}$$

Administering I.V. medications

Before you give an I.V. medication to your patient, you need to prepare the medication for delivery and select the right equipment.

Preparing medications

Most I.V. drug solutions are prepared in the pharmacy by pharmacists or pharmacy technicians. Occasionally, however, you have to prepare I.V. drug solutions yourself.

Safety first

When you're preparing a medication for I.V. administration, be sure to take some basic safety measures:

- Maintain aseptic technique. Always wash your hands before mixing, and avoid contaminating any part of the vial, ampule, syringe, needle, needleless device, or container that must remain sterile. When you're inserting the needle or needleless device into the vial and withdrawing it, make sure that it doesn't touch any part of the vial that isn't sterile. Also, make sure that you don't inadvertently contaminate the needleless device with your finger or stick your finger with the needle. To keep your hands steady, brace one against the other while you're inserting and withdrawing the needle or needleless device.
- When drawing up the drug before adding it to the primary solution, make sure to use a syringe that's large enough to hold the entire dose. If you need to use a needle to add the medication to the I.V. bag, make sure the needle is at least 1″ long to penetrate the inner seal of the port on the I.V. bag. In many facilities, practitioners use a 5-micron filter needle for mixing drug powder or withdrawing drugs from glass ampules. This needle is then removed, a sterile 1″ needle or appropriate needleless device is attached to the syringe, and the drug is then admixed. (See *Keep it safe*, page 156.)
- In many facilities, premixed doses are drawn up into a syringe in the pharmacy. A 24-hour supply is delivered to the nursing unit, where the drug is stored in a refrigerator. The nurse then administers the dose using a syringe pump that delivers the medication over a predetermined period.

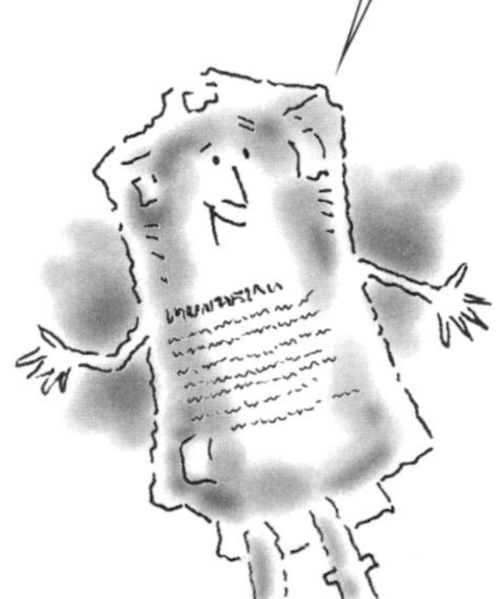

Reconstituting powdered drugs

Many I.V. drugs are supplied in powder form and have to be reconstituted with liquid diluents.

Finding a fluid

Common diluents include:

- normal saline solution
- sterile water for injection
- dextrose 5% in water.

Note the manufacturer's instructions about the appropriate type or amount of diluent. Some drugs should be reconstituted with diluents that contain preservatives. (See *Reconstituting powdered drugs*, page 156.)

Pulling the plug

Some drugs come in double-chambered vials that contain powder in the lower chamber and a diluent in the upper one. To combine the contents, press the rubber stopper on top of the vial to dislodge the rubber plug separating the compartments. The diluent then mixes with the drug in the bottom chamber.

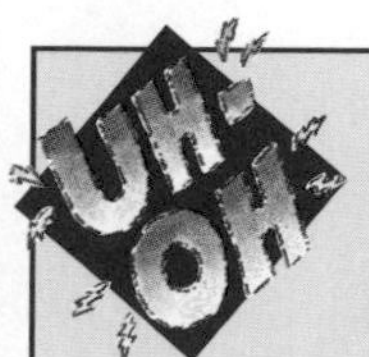

Warning!

Keep it safe

Make sure that you follow a few basic tips to ensure safety when you administer I.V. medications.

Check it out

Check the expiration date on the drug and the diluent, and look for any special diluent requirements. Note whether the drug requires filtration. Also inspect the drug, diluent, and solution for particles and cloudiness. After reconstitution, again check for visible signs of incompatibility in the admixture. Remember, incompatibility is more likely with drugs or I.V. solutions that have a high or low pH. Most drugs are moderately acidic, but some are alkaline, including heparin, aminophylline, ampicillin sodium, and sodium bicarbonate.

Mixing in a minibag

If you're mixing a drug in a minibag or minibottle of normal saline solution or dextrose 5% in water, you may be able to use the solution in the minicontainer as the diluent. However, be sure to inspect it and discard any solution that appears cloudy or contains particles. Some solutions change color after several hours. If you aren't sure whether to use a discolored solution, ask the pharmacist.

Reconstituting powdered drugs

To safely reconstitute powdered drugs, gather your equipment and then follow these step-by-step guidelines.

Draw up and clean

First you need to:
- draw up the amount and type of diluent specified by the manufacturer
- clean the rubber stopper of the drug vial with an alcohol swab, using aseptic technique.

Insert, inject, and mix

When the diluent is drawn up and the stopper is clean, you can insert, inject, and mix:
- Insert the needle or needleless device connected to the syringe of diluent into the stopper at a 45- to 60-degree angle. Angling the needle minimizes coring or breaking off rubber pieces, which would then float inside the vial.
- Inject the diluent.
- Mix thoroughly by gently inverting the vial. If the drug doesn't dissolve within a few seconds, let it stand for 10 to 30 minutes. If necessary, invert the vial several times to dissolve the drug. Don't shake vigorously (unless directed) because some drugs may froth.

Diluting liquid drugs

Liquid medication may be packed in:
- single-dose ampules or vials
- multidose vials
- prefilled syringes
- disposable cartridges.

Liquid drugs don't need reconstitution, but they commonly require further dilution.

Add-ons

There are several methods you can use to add a drug to an I.V. container. Additive vials of a drug can be attached directly to administration tubing. If the vial contains a drug powder, reconstitute it first. Then you can infuse the drug solution directly from the vial, using dedicated vented tubing. (See *Adding a drug to an I.V. container*.)

Labeling solution containers

A container prepared in the pharmacy has a label showing:
- patient's full name
- patient's room number
- date

Best practice

Adding a drug to an I.V. container

To add a drug to an I.V. container, use the following step-by-step techniques for safe mixing.

Adding to an I.V. bottle

To add a drug to an I.V. bottle, first clean the rubber stopper or latex diaphragm with alcohol. Then insert the needle or needleless device of the medication-filled syringe into the center of the stopper or diaphragm and inject the drug. Next, invert the bottle at least twice to ensure thorough mixing. Now remove the latex diaphragm and insert the administration spike.

Adding to an I.V. bag

To add a drug to a plastic I.V. bag, insert the needle or needleless device of the medication-filled syringe into the clean latex medication port and inject the drug. (If you're using a needle, make sure it's at least 1" long; a short needle won't pierce the inner port seal, and a small-volume additive, such as insulin, will remain in the port.) After injecting the drug, grasp the top and bottom of the bag and quickly invert it twice. Don't squeeze or shake the bag.

Adding to an infusing solution

If you have a choice, don't add a drug to an I.V. solution that's already infusing because of the risk of altering the drug concentration. However, if you must add a drug, make sure that the primary solution container has enough solution to provide adequate dilution. To add the drug, clamp the I.V. tubing and take down the container. Then, with the container upright, add the drug.

If you're adding the drug to a bottle, clean the rubber stopper with an alcohol swab, insert the needle or needleless device through the stopper, and inject the drug. If you're adding the drug to an I.V. bag, clean the rubber injection port with an alcohol swab before you inject the drug.

Mix well

After injecting the drug into the container, invert it several times to ensure thorough mixing and prevent a bolus effect.

- name and amount of the I.V. solution and drugs
- other vital information such as the infusion rate.

Becoming label able

If you prepare the drug solution, be sure to label the container with the same information provided by a pharmacy. Also, note the date and time you mixed the drug solution, and sign or initial the label. Make sure that your label doesn't cover the manufacturer's label. If you use a time strip, label it with the patient's name and room number and the infusion rate (in milliliters per hour, drops per minute, or both).

Selecting the equipment

When choosing the equipment you'll use to administer I.V. medications, you need to consider several factors. For example, which drug has been prescribed? What's the ordered drip rate? Is your

Choosing the right equipment

Consider the following questions to help you choose equipment that's appropriate for administering any drug I.V.

Pump

Do you need a pump to deliver a particular drug? Health care facilities usually have policies regarding the use of these devices. Pumps, most of which require specific administration sets, are commonly used when you need a precise or very low infusion rate. They're also used when you're administering fluids or admixtures through a central venous access device.

Drip rate

What's the ordered drip rate and what's your facility's policy on using macrodrip and microdrip tubing? Many policies require microdrip tubing when the infusion rate is less than 63 ml/hour.

Intermittent infusions

Is your patient going to receive intermittent drug infusions as well as the primary drug solution? If so, you may need a primary tubing that has an injection port close to the drip chamber and a backcheck valve that will automatically shut off the primary solution when the secondary solution is infusing.

Simultaneous infusions

Is your patient going to receive a simultaneous infusion of a secondary drug solution? If so, choose tubing that has an injection port close to the venipuncture device so you don't have to stop the primary infusion.

Special tubing

Does the drug solution require special tubing? Tubing without polyvinyl chloride is recommended for certain drugs, such as nitroglycerin or paclitaxel (Taxol).

Glass or plastic

Is the solution container made of glass or plastic? If you're using a glass container, you need vented I.V. tubing. Use nonvented tubing for a collapsible plastic bag.

Infant or small child

Is your patient an infant or a small child? Many facilities have policies that permit only volume-control sets for such patients. These devices limit the volume available to the patient and decrease the risk of inadvertent fluid overload.

Needle-free

Needleless systems are required by The Joint Commission. You can piggyback drugs or additional I.V. solutions into a primary line without using a needle. Instead, a luer-lock system is used that connects the syringe to the port. Luer-locks also help make sure the connection between tubing is secure to decrease the risk of disconnected tubing.

A needleless system can greatly reduce the risk of accidental needle-stick injuries, but it can't eliminate all such injuries because this system can't be used to perform venipunctures. Needleless systems can be used to obtain blood for blood gas analysis and other laboratory tests. Indwelling lines, such as A-lines or central venous access devices, can also be used with the needleless system. It's possible to adapt a line for use with needleless systems with replaceable injection ports.

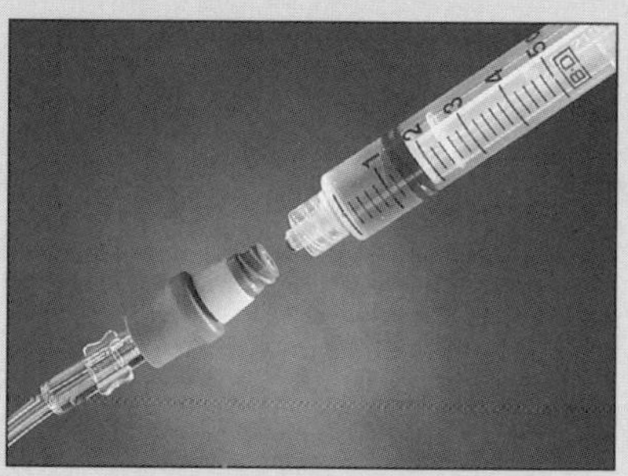

patient an adult or a child? Which equipment options are available? Your selection will depend on the answers to these and many other questions. (See *Choosing the right equipment.*)

Preparing for drug delivery

Before you administer I.V. medication by any method, take time to properly prepare the patient and the medication. Follow these steps:

- Confirm the patient's identity by checking his full name and facility identification number on his wristband. Also, ask him to identify himself, verbally if possible. If the patient can't identify himself, ask another nurse to corroborate his identity. Check his history for allergies and explain the procedure to him. (See *Remember the five rights.*)
- Make sure that you know some key information about the drug you're giving. For instance, you should know the normal dosage, expected effects, adverse reactions, contraindications, and drug interactions. If you're unfamiliar with the drug and don't have access to the drug package insert or a drug reference book, ask your pharmacist any drug-related questions.
- Follow the Centers for Disease Control and Prevention (CDC) guidelines to protect yourself and your patient from blood-borne pathogens and infection. These guidelines require you to wear gloves (and possibly a gown and mask) when exposed to body fluids.

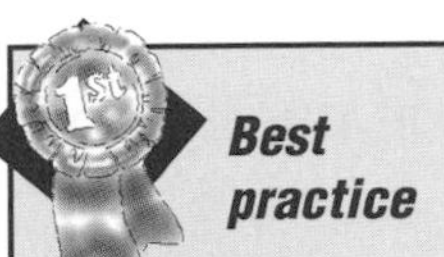

Best practice

Remember the five rights

Before you administer an I.V. drug to a patient, make sure that you check the five rights:

 right drug

 right patient

 right time

right dosage

 right route.

There's actually a sixth right
At the same time, make sure that the patient understands the medication he's to receive and knows he has the right to refuse to take the medication.

Infusion methods

You can give I.V. medications by three methods:

- direct injection
- intermittent infusion
- continuous infusion.

You may also administer an I.V. medication using a specialized device such as a patient-controlled analgesia (PCA) electronic infusion device. (See *Comparing administration methods*, pages 160 and 161.)

Direct injection

Direct injection can be used to deliver a single dose (bolus) or intermittent multiple doses. Commonly called an I.V. push, a direct injection can be administered two ways:

 into an intermittent infusion device

 through an existing infusion line.

Comparing administration methods

This chart gives you the indications, advantages, and disadvantages of common I.V. administration methods.

Methods and indications	Advantages	Disadvantages
Direct injection		
• When a drug is incompatible with the I.V. solution and must be given as bolus injection • When patient has only an intermittent infusion device with no I.V. solution being administered • When a patient requires immediate high blood levels (for example, regular insulin, dextrose 50%, atropine, and antihistamines) • In emergencies, for immediate drug effect	• Doesn't require time or authorization to perform venipuncture because the vein is already accessed • Doesn't require a needle puncture, which can cause patient anxiety • Allows the use of I.V. solution or normal saline solution to test the patency of the venipuncture device before drug administration • Allows continued venous access in case of adverse reactions	• Carries the same inconveniences and risk of complications associated with indwelling venipuncture device (such as infection, infiltration, and pain)
Intermittent infusion		
Piggyback method • Commonly used with drugs given over short periods at varying intervals (for example, antibiotics and gastric-secretion inhibitors)	• Avoids multiple needle injections required by I.M. route • Permits repeated administration of drugs through a single I.V. site • Provides high drug blood levels for short periods without causing drug toxicity	• May cause periods when the drug blood level becomes too low to be clinically effective (for example, when peak and trough times aren't considered in the medication order)
Saline lock • When a patient requires constant venous access but not a continuous infusion	• Provides venous access for patients with fluid restrictions • Provides better patient mobility between doses • Preserves veins by reducing venipunctures • Lowers cost if used with a limited number of drugs	• Requires close monitoring during administration so the device can be flushed on completion

Comparing administration methods *(continued)*

Methods and indications	Advantages	Disadvantages
Intermittent infusion *(continued)*		
Volume-control set • When a patient requires a low volume of fluid	• Requires only one large-volume container • Prevents fluid overload from a runaway infusion • Allows the chamber to be reused	• High cost • Carries a high risk of contamination • If there is no membrane to block air passage when empty, flow clamp must be closed when the set empties
Continuous infusion		
Through primary line • To maintain continuous serum levels, if the infusion isn't likely to be stopped abruptly	• Maintains steady serum levels • Presents less risk of rapid shock and vein irritation because of a large volume of fluid diluting the drug	• Risk of incompatibility increases with drug contact time • Restricts patient mobility • Carries an increased risk of infiltration
Through secondary line • When a patient requires continuous infusion of two or more compatible admixtures administered at different rates • When there's a significant chance of abruptly stopping one admixture without infusing the remaining drug in I.V. tubing	• Allows primary infusion and each secondary infusion to be given at different rates • Allows primary line to be totally shut off and kept on standby to maintain venous access in case secondary line must be abruptly stopped • Short contact time before infusion may allow the administration of incompatible admixtures — something not possible with long contact time	• Can't be used for drugs with immediate incompatibility • Carries an increased risk of vein irritation or phlebitis from an increased number of drugs • Use of multiple I.V. systems (for example, primary lines with secondary lines attached), especially with electronic pumps, can create physical barriers to patient care and limit patient mobility

Local trouble

Direct injection may cause localized site complications. This method exerts more pressure on the vein than other methods, posing a greater risk of infiltration in patients with fragile veins.

Slow down...

Most drugs must be given over a specific period when using direct injection. To avoid speed shock, don't administer a drug in less than 1 minute, unless the order directs you to do so or if the patient is in cardiac or respiratory arrest.

My motto:
Slow down. It helps to avoid speed shock.

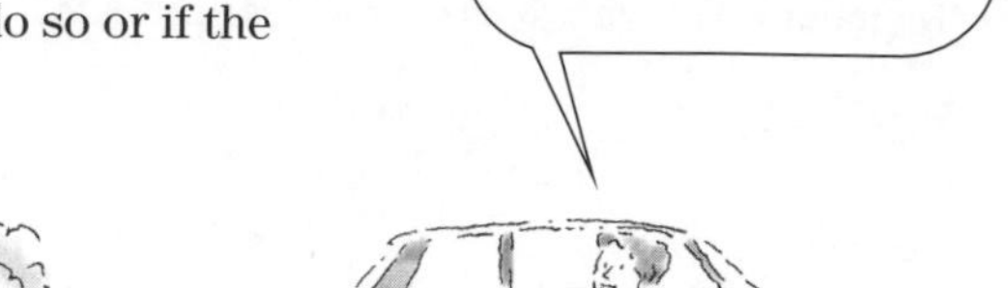

To avoid decreased drug tolerance, slower injection times or greater drug dilution may be required if your patient has:

- systemic edema
- pulmonary congestion
- decreased cardiac output
- reduced urine output, renal flow, or glomerular filtration rate.

...and in some cases speed up!

Certain drugs metabolize quickly and must be administered quickly to achieve the desired effect. One such drug is adenosine, which is used for the treatment of supraventricular tachycardia.

Injection into an intermittent infusion device

To inject a drug into an intermittent infusion device, you need these supplies:

- syringe with medication
- two syringes filled with saline solution
- alcohol swab
- tourniquet
- gloves
- tape. (See *Injecting a drug into an intermittent infusion device.*)

Injecting a drug into an intermittent infusion device

After assembling your equipment, follow the steps outlined here to safely and accurately inject a drug into an intermittent infusion device.

The first steps

Begin with these steps:

- Put on gloves.
- Assess the patient's I.V. site for redness, swelling, or pain. If necessary, remove the intermittent infusion device, and insert a new device in a new location.
- Wipe the injection port of the intermittent infusion device with an alcohol pad, and insert the needleless adapter of the saline-filled syringe.
- Aspirate with the syringe and observe for blood. This verifies the patency of the vein. If none appears, apply a tourniquet slightly above the site and aspirate again. If blood doesn't appear, remove the tourniquet and inject the normal saline solution slowly.
- If you feel any resistance while injecting, stop immediately—the device is occluded and a new device needs to be inserted.
- If blood is aspirated, slowly inject the saline solution and observe for signs of infiltration.
- As you inject the saline, watch for puffiness or pain at the site. If these occur, insert a new intermittent infusion device.
- Remove the saline syringe from the intermittent infusion device.

Injecting a drug into an intermittent infusion device *(continued)*

When patent, proceed
When you're certain the intermittent infusion device is patent, proceed with these steps:
• Insert the needleless adapter and syringe with medication for the direct injection into the injection port of the device.
• Inject the medication at the required rate. Then remove the needleless adapter and syringe from the injection port.
• Insert the needleless adapter of the remaining saline-filled syringe into the injection port, and slowly inject the saline solution.

Following the injection
After the drug is injected, follow-up with these steps:
• Observe your patient for signs of adverse reactions (do this both during and after the injection).
• Dispose of contaminated hazardous equipment where appropriate.
• Document the type and amount of medication administered and the time of administration.

Injection into an existing line

To give an injection directly into the injection port of an existing line, you need these supplies:
- medication
- syringe with a needleless system
- alcohol swab
- saline-filled syringe for flushing. (See *Injecting a drug into an existing line.*)

Injecting a drug into an existing line

After assembling your equipment, follow the step-by-step technique described here to inject a drug safely into an existing line.

Check, flush, invert, clean
Begin with these steps:
• Check the I.V. site for redness, tenderness, edema, or leakage. If you detect any of these signs of complications, change the site before you administer the drug.
• If the new drug and the existing infusate are compatible, keep the infusion running. If the drug isn't compatible with the infusate but is compatible with saline solution, use a saline-filled syringe to flush the line before injecting the drug.
• Invert the syringe and gently push the plunger to remove all air.
• Using an alcohol swab, clean the injection port closest to the venous access device.

Stabilize, inject, observe, withdraw
After completing initial preparations, continue with these steps:
• Stabilize the injection port with one hand and attach the needleless device to the injection port.
• Inject the drug at an even rate, as ordered. Never inject so fast that you stop the primary infusion or allow the drug to flow back into the tubing.
• Observe the patient for signs of a reaction during and after the injection.
• Withdraw the needleless device and reestablish the desired flow rate.

Intermittent infusion

The most common and flexible method of administering I.V. drugs is intermittent infusion. In this method, drugs are administered over a specified period at varying intervals. Doing so helps to maintain and monitor therapeutic blood levels. You may deliver a small volume (1 to 250 ml) over several minutes or a few hours.

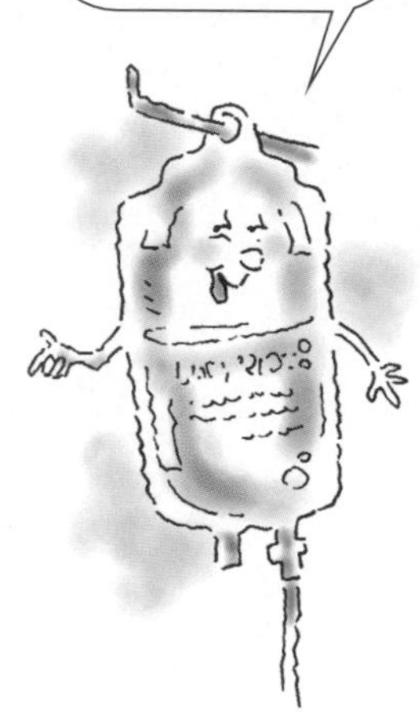

Secondary line

To administer an intermittent infusion through a secondary line, you need these supplies:

- medication in the unit-dose container
- secondary infusion tubing
- alcohol swab
- extension hook for the primary container.

You can deliver an intermittent infusion through a piggyback line that's connected to the primary line with a port, saline lock, or volume-control set.

Check the backcheck

The primary line should have a side Y-port with a backcheck valve that stops the flow from the primary line during drug infusion and resumes the primary flow after infusion. (See *Setting up a piggyback set.*)

Now proceed through the procedure

To perform the procedure, follow these steps:

- Check the I.V. site for infiltration, phlebitis, or infection.
- Check the primary infusion line for patency.
- Ensure that the drug to be piggybacked is compatible with the primary infusion.
- Hang the medication container on the I.V. pole.
- Close the flow clamp on the secondary tubing, remove the covers to the medication container and tubing spike, and insert the spike firmly into the medication container port.
- Using an alcohol swab, clean the injection port on the primary tubing.
- Remove the cover from the secondary tubing. Connect the secondary tubing to the injection port of the primary tubing.
- Lower the primary infusion with the supplied extension hook below the level of the secondary medication container, open the flow clamp of the secondary set, and allow the medication to infuse as prescribed.

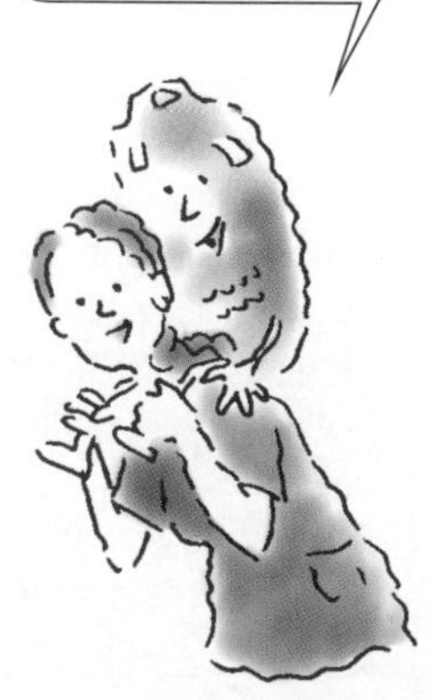

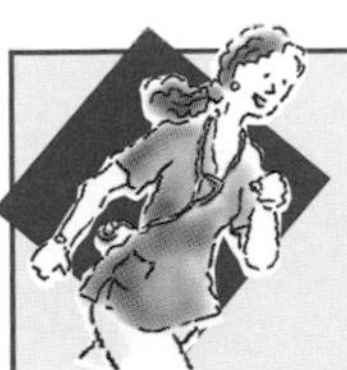

Running smoothly

Setting up a piggyback set

Used only for intermittent drug infusions, a piggyback set includes a secondary container (a small I.V. bag or bottle) and short tubing with a drip chamber. To use it, connect the piggyback set to a primary line with a Y-port (or piggyback port), as shown. You must use an extension hook to position the primary I.V. container below the secondary container.

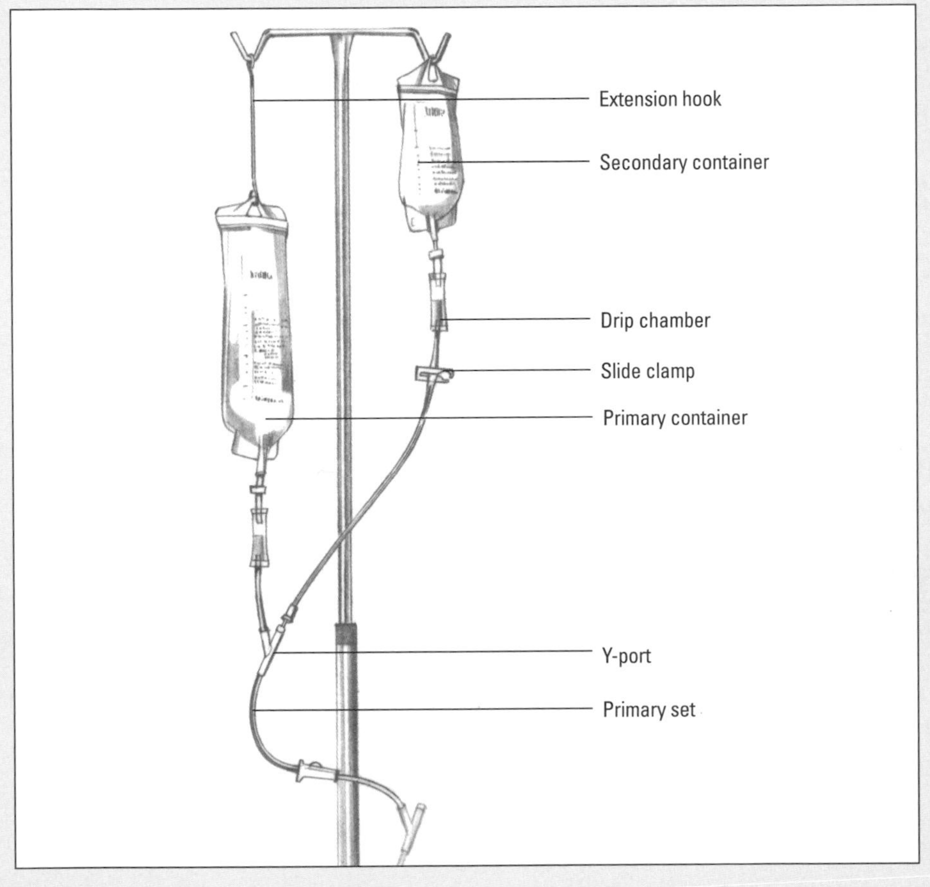

Don't forget to use the extension hook; otherwise, the secondary line won't run.

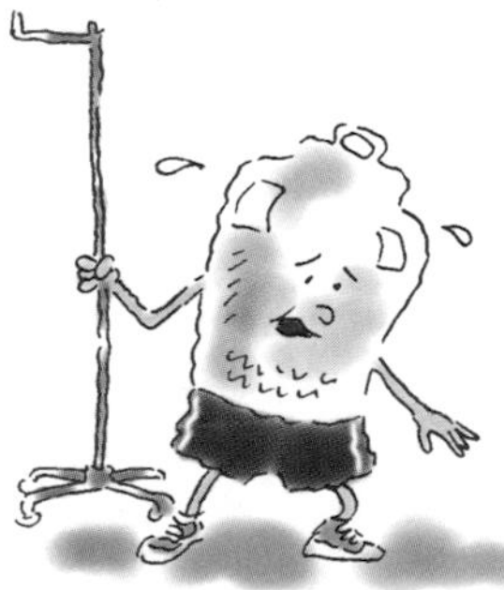

Readjust the primary infusion

Because the secondary container hangs higher than the primary container, fluid flowing from it creates pressure on the backcheck valve and completely shuts off fluid flow from the primary container. After the secondary infusion is completed, the primary fluid automatically flows again. When the primary fluid begins flowing again, close the clamp on the secondary tubing and readjust the flow rate of the primary infusion.

No backcheck valve? Clamp it.

If the primary tubing doesn't have a backcheck valve, you must clamp the primary line; you don't need to lower the primary container. Remember to open the primary clamp when the piggyback infusion is completed. Otherwise, the venous access device may clog and the patient may not receive the volume of I.V. fluid prescribed.

Fight phlebitis

Many drugs pose a high risk of phlebitis. Be sure to check the I.V. site carefully before administering each dose. If necessary, change the site before you administer the medication.

Always check for phlebitis before administering each dose of medication, and change the site when necessary.

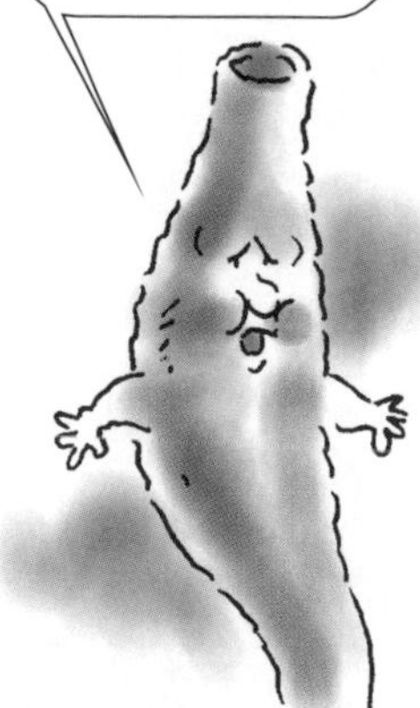

Saline lock

For intermittent I.V. drug infusion with a saline lock or intermittent device, you need these supplies:

- drug solution in its container
- administration set
- needleless device
- alcohol swab.

You also need two syringes filled with saline flush solution each connected to a needleless device. (See *Using a saline lock* and *Hints for handling a saline lock*, page 168.)

Volume-control set

You can use a volume-control set as a primary or secondary line.

Using a saline lock

Use the following step-by-step guidelines to safely administer a medication using a saline lock.

Attach, secure, clean, stabilize

After you have assembled your equipment, begin with these steps:

- Attach the minibag to the administration set and prime the tubing with the drug solution.
- Secure the needleless device to the I.V. tubing device and prime the needleless device with the drug solution.
- Using an alcohol swab, clean the cap on the saline lock.
- Stabilize the saline lock with the thumb and index finger of your nondominant hand.

Insert, flush, secure, infuse

When the saline lock is stabilized, continue with these steps:

- Insert the needleless device of one of the syringes containing flush solution into the injection cap. Pull back on the plunger slightly and watch for a blood return. If blood appears, begin to slowly inject the flush solution. If you feel resistance or if the patient complains of pain or discomfort, stop immediately because the venous access device should be replaced.
- If you don't feel resistance, watch for signs of infiltration as you slowly inject the flush solution. If you note signs of infiltration, remove the venous access device and insert a new device in a new location; if you don't note any signs, you're ready to give the medication.
- Insert the needleless device attached to the administration set into the saline lock.
- Regulate the drip rate, and infuse the medication, as ordered.

Discontinue and clean

To discontinue the infusion:

- Close the I.V. flow clamp and withdraw the needleless device.
- Clean the injection cap and flush the saline lock again.

Primary parts

When using a volume-control set as a primary line, gather these supplies:

- I.V. solution
- medication in a syringe with a needleless device
- alcohol swabs
- a label.

Hints for handling a saline lock

Here are helpful hints for using a saline lock.

Check carefully
Before accessing the lock, check the I.V. site carefully and change it if necessary.

Avoiding movement
When the injection cap serves as a saline lock, stabilize the cap while accessing and removing the I.V. tubing and needleless device to prevent movement at the insertion site. Movement increases the risks of phlebitis and catheter dislodgment.

Be present
You must be present when the infusion runs out so you can disconnect the tubing and flush the device. Otherwise, clots will form in the saline lock.

Every 6 to 24 hours
Flush the device after each use and as needed with the volume of solution recommended by facility policy. The flush solution is typically saline. Flushing may be required every 6 to 24 hours depending on facility policy.

Time for new tubing
Follow your facility's policy for tubing changes. If you have to reconnect used tubing, make sure the end of the tubing hasn't been contaminated. Always use a sterile needleless device.

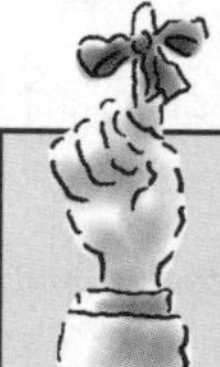

Memory jogger

To remember how to prime the volume-control set, fill the chamber with at least 20 ml of fluid; then use the mnemonic **OSCAR** (after all, you deserve an award):

Open the flow-regulating clamp.

Squeeze and hold the drip chamber.

Close the regulating clamp directly below the drip chamber.

And…

Release the drip chamber.

Secondary supplies

When using a volume-control set as a secondary line, gather these supplies:
- I.V. solution
- medication in a syringe with a needleless device
- alcohol swabs
- a label.

Proceed to the procedure

To perform the procedure, follow these steps:
- Check the I.V. line for patency and the I.V. site for signs of infiltration or phlebitis.
- If you're using the volume-control set as a primary line, prime the tubing with the I.V. solution. Then insert the adapter of the set into the venipuncture device or saline lock.
- If you're using the volume-control set as a secondary line, attach the needleless device to the adapter on the set and prime the tubing with the I.V. solution. Then wipe the injection site on the pri-

mary tubing with an alcohol swab, and insert the needleless device into the injection port.

- To add medication to the chamber, wipe the injection port on the volume-control set with an alcohol swab and inject the medication. (See *Adding to a volume-control set* and *Tips for adding medications.*)
- Place a label on the chamber indicating the drug, dose, time, and date. Don't write directly on the chamber with ink (the plastic can absorb the ink). Also, don't place the label over the numbers of the chamber. Then open the upper clamp; fill the fluid chamber with the prescribed amount of solution to dilute the medication. Close the clamp. Gently rotate the chamber to mix the medication and solution.
- If you're using the volume-control set as a secondary line, either stop the primary infusion or set a low drip rate so the line will be open when the secondary infusion is completed. Then open the lower clamp of the volume-control set, and adjust the drip rate as ordered.
- After the infusion is completed and if the patient can tolerate the extra fluid, open the upper clamp and let 10 ml of I.V. solution flow into the chamber and through the tubing to flush it and complete delivery of the medication to the patient.

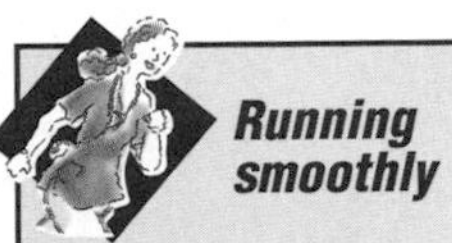

Adding to a volume-control set

After wiping the injection port with an alcohol swab as shown below, inject the medication with a syringe.

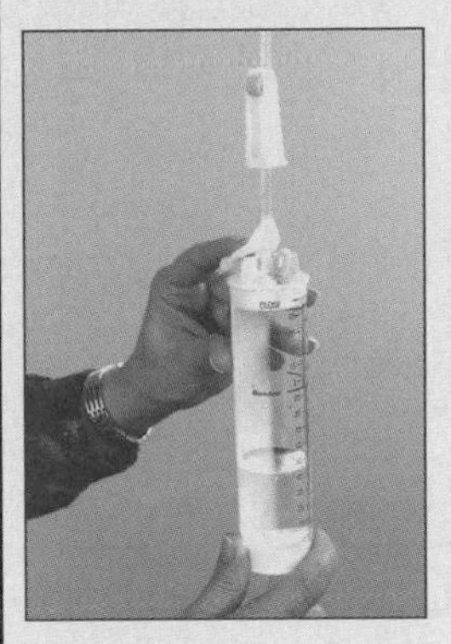

Tips for adding medications

When adding medications to a volume-control set, check for an immediately visible incompatibility—especially if you're using multiple lines. Also, follow these tips.

Tangle-proof

To prevent confusion when using multiple secondary lines, don't let them become tangled. Tag the lines below the drip chamber and at the connection site to the primary line. This clearly identifies the source and tubing connection for each drug.

Pumped up

When possible, use a pump to achieve more accurate dosage control. Put a time strip on the secondary container to help monitor the administration rate.

Secure, patent, and firmly stable

Maintain a secure, patent venous access device. To avoid interrupting drug therapy when you change the I.V. site, establish the new site before disconnecting the old one.

• If you're using the volume-control set as a secondary line, close the lower clamp and reset the flow rate on the primary line. If you're using the set as a primary line, close the lower clamp, refill the chamber to the prescribed amount of primary solution, and restart the infusion.

A novel solution

Instead of using the volume-control set as a primary line, you can mix the medication in the primary solution, then use the volume-control chamber to closely regulate the amount of fluid and the drug dosage the patient receives.

Maintaining the membrane

If you're using a volume-control set with a membrane for intermittent drug administration, fill the chamber with fluid before adding the medication. Filling the chamber prevents the membrane from becoming sticky and difficult to operate. Be sure to read the manufacturer's instructions for priming volume-control sets.

Refill quickly when empty

The infusion stops when the fluid chamber is empty. If the set doesn't have a membrane or shut-off valve, refill the fluid chamber quickly to prevent air from filling the set.

Continuous infusion

A continuous infusion of medication allows you to carefully regulate drug delivery over a prolonged period. A continuous infusion may be given through a peripheral or central venous access device. Sometimes, before you start a continuous infusion, a loading dose is given to achieve peak serum levels quickly.

A continuous infusion enhances the effectiveness of some drugs, such as insulin and heparin. Delivery of these drugs is regulated with an I.V. pump.

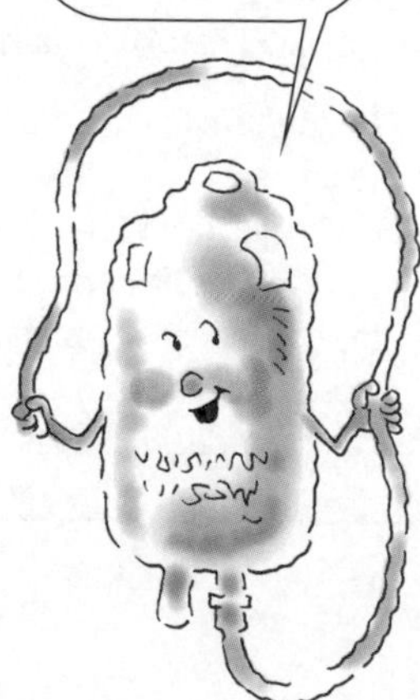

Primary line

To give a continuous infusion through a primary line, you need these supplies:

- prescribed medication in I.V. solution
- administration set
- gloves.

You may also need an infusion pump. If so, make sure that you have the correct administration set for the pump.

A prep talk

Preparations for giving a continuous infusion through a primary line include:

- making sure the I.V. solution container is labeled with the name and dosage of the medication
- attaching the administration set to the solution container and priming the tubing with the I.V. solution
- attaching the administration set to the pump, if appropriate
- performing or assisting with the venipuncture, if necessary.

Begin the performance

To begin the infusion, follow these steps:

- Put on gloves.
- Remove the protective cap at the end of the administration set.
- Attach the set to the venipuncture device.
- Begin the infusion and regulate the flow to the ordered rate. Remember to monitor the patient and the flow rate frequently.
- When the infusion is completed, hang another solution container or change solutions, as ordered.

Eyes on intake, output, and electrolytes

Maintain accurate intake and output records, and be alert for excessive fluid retention and fluid overload. Weigh the patient daily, wearing the same clothes and at the same time of day. When a patient receives small amounts hourly, his total daily volume can be excessive without any obvious signs.

Remember, too, that giving a large volume of fluid can seriously change a patient's electrolyte levels. Make sure that you check the patient's laboratory results to ensure that his electrolyte levels stay within normal limits.

Switching veins

Check the flow rate at regular intervals to ensure that the medication is delivered as ordered. Also, check I.V. sites frequently for signs of complications. If you note tenderness, redness, swelling, or leakage of infusate, discontinue the infusion and treat the site according to facility policy. Restart the infusion in another vein.

Secondary line

To give a continuous infusion through a secondary line, make sure that you have these supplies:

- prescribed medication in I.V. solution
- administration set
- needleless device
- alcohol swabs.

Monitor for fluid retention, fluid overload, and changes in electrolyte levels. And check the I.V. site for signs of complications.

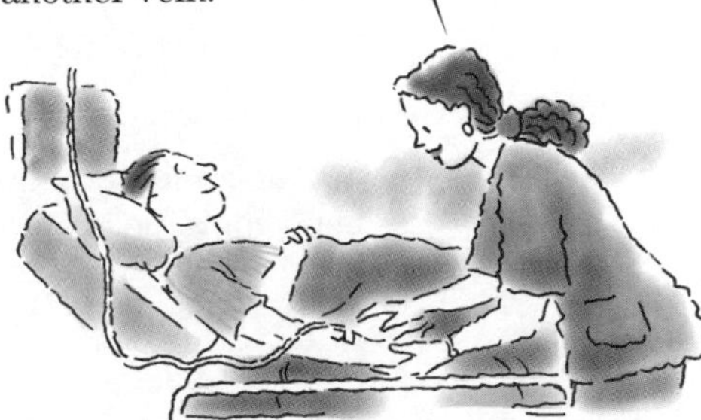

Best practice

Infusing medication through a secondary line

Follow the step-by-step technique here to safely administer medication through a secondary line.

Attach, prime, label, clean

After you have assembled the necessary equipment, begin with these steps:

- Attach the administration set to the solution container and prime the tubing with the I.V. solution. If appropriate, attach the administration set to the pump.
- Place labels with the name of the drug under the drip chamber and at the end of the tubing.
- Clean the injection port on the primary tubing with an alcohol swab.

Insert, adjust, monitor, remove

When you have ensured that the injection port is clean, continue with these steps:

- Connect the needleless adapter to the injection port.
- Regulate the drip rate of the secondary solution and adjust the rate of the primary solution.
- Frequently monitor the patient and the infusion rate.
- When the secondary infusion is finished, remove the needleless device from the injection port. Adjust the flow rate of the primary solution.

You may also need an infusion pump. If so, make sure that you have the correct administration set for the pump. (See *Infusing medication through a secondary line.*)

Patient-controlled analgesia

PCA therapy allows your patient to control I.V. delivery of an analgesic (usually morphine) and maintain therapeutic serum levels of the drug. The computer-controlled PCA pump delivers medication through an I.V. administration set that's attached directly to the patient's I.V. line. The patient can then push a button to receive a dose of analgesic through the I.V. line. Occasionally, a patient may receive PCA therapy through a spinal catheter or subcutaneously.

Locked-out

A timing unit prevents the patient from accidentally overdosing by imposing a lock-out time between doses—usually 6 to 10 minutes. During this interval, the patient won't receive any analgesic despite pushing the button.

Picking patients for PCA therapy

PCA therapy is indicated for patients who require parenteral analgesia. It's commonly used by patients after surgery and those with chronic diseases, particularly patients with terminal cancer or sickle cell anemia.

To receive PCA therapy, a patient must:
- be mentally alert
- be able to understand and comply with instructions and procedures
- have no history of an allergy to the analgesic.

Patients not eligible for therapy include those with:
- limited respiratory reserve
- a history of drug abuse or chronic sedative or tranquilizer use
- a psychiatric disorder.

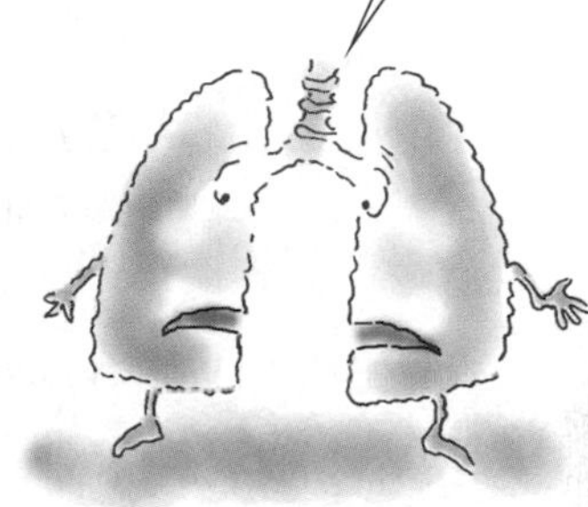

PCA "pluses"

Patients receiving PCA therapy use fewer opioids for pain relief than other patients. Also on the upside, PCA therapy provides these advantages:
- It eliminates the need for I.M. analgesics.
- It provides individualized pain relief; each patient receives the appropriate dosage for his size and pain tolerance.
- It decreases the time between the onset of pain and the administration of the analgesic.
- It gives the patient a sense of control over pain.
- It allows the patient to sleep at night while minimizing daytime drowsiness.

PCA "minuses"

The main adverse effect of opioid analgesics is respiratory depression. Therefore, you must routinely monitor your patient's respiratory rate. In addition to the effects on the respiratory system, opioid analgesics can lower blood pressure. Also, if the opioid analgesic makes your patient nauseated, he may need an antiemetic drug.

When your patient is receiving PCA therapy, be sure to check for infiltration into subcutaneous tissue as well as catheter occlusion, which may cause the drug to back up in the primary I.V. tubing.

Patients who receive PCA therapy use fewer opioids for pain relief and feel a greater sense of control over their pain.

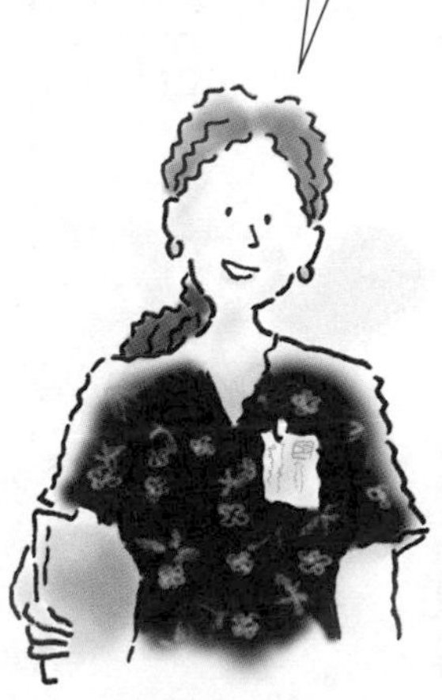

The full story

The practitioner's order for PCA may include the:
- loading dose, which is given by bolus and is programmed by the infusion device

• lock-out interval, during which the PCA device can't be activated (such as every 6 to 10 minutes)
• maintenance dose, if a continuous infusion of opioid analgesia is ordered
• amount the patient will receive when the device is activated (such as 10 mg meperidine or 1 mg morphine)
• maximum amount the patient can receive within a specified time (usually the amount the patient can receive on demand or the maintenance dose over 60 minutes).

Evaluating a PCA pump

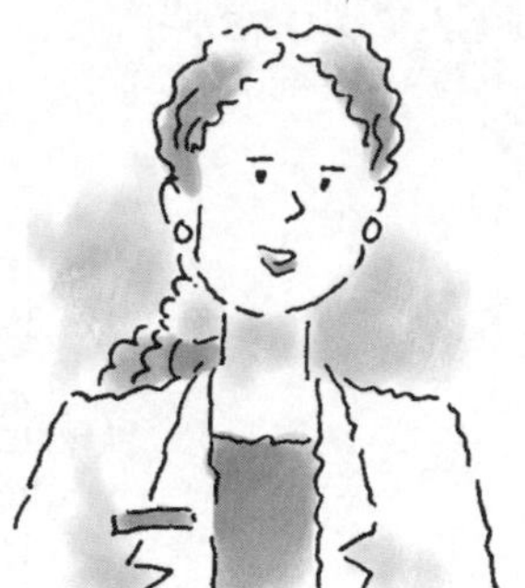

In evaluating a PCA pump, consider cost, complexity, ease of operation, size, and portability.

In evaluating a PCA pump, first consider its cost and the cost of its operation. Ask these questions:
• Does the pump use expensive refill cassettes or less expensive syringes?
• Consider the pump's complexity. How easy is it to operate — for you and the patient?
• What kind of lock-out mechanism is employed by the device? Operating the pump should be a straightforward procedure but not so simple that anyone can manipulate the program.
• Can the pump be used on an I.V pole and carried or worn as well? Evaluate the equipment size and portability. An ambulatory patient should have a small, portable PCA pump.

Focusing on the features

PCA pumps are available with a variety of features:
• Some pumps provide continuous infusion and bolus doses. Others provide only bolus doses.
• PCA pumps that provide continuous infusion and bolus doses may offer several volume settings.
• The pump may have a panel that displays the amount delivered or, if necessary, an alarm message.
• You can program certain pumps to record the concentration in milligrams (mg) or milliliters (ml), allowing greater flexibility in choosing rates.
• With some pumps, you can vary the length of the lock-out interval from 5 to 90 minutes.
• Pumps can be programmed to store and retrieve information such as the total dose allowed in a specified length of time.
• Most pumps can provide the total volume infused to include the opioid analgesia in intake and output measurements.

Managing PCA therapy

With PCA, the patient self-administers drug delivery by pressing a button on a handheld controller that's connected to the pump. Before the device can be used, it must be programmed to deliver specified doses at specified time intervals.

Giving an added boost

If the patient is using a pump that provides continuous infusion and bolus doses, make sure that he understands that he's receiving medication continuously, but that he can give himself intermittent bolus doses for incidental pain (from coughing, for example) using the patient control button.

If you program the pump to deliver a continuous infusion plus bolus doses, remember this rule: The cumulative doses per hour administered by a PCA pump shouldn't exceed the total hourly dose ordered by the practitioner. For example, if the patient needs a total of 6 mg of morphine over 1 hour, the practitioner may begin therapy with a continuous infusion of 3 mg/hour, allowing a bolus dose of 0.5 mg every 10 minutes.

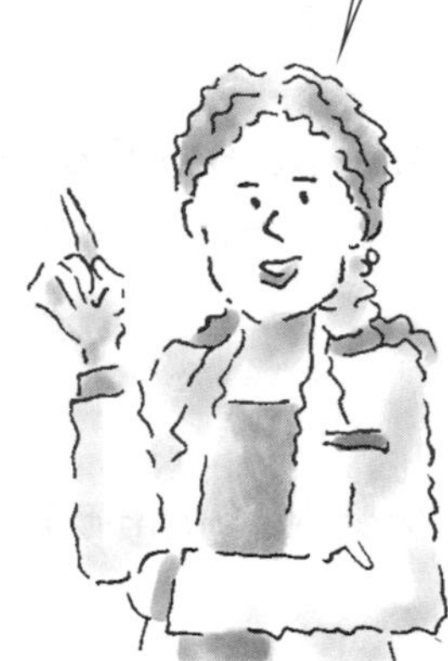

Not the controlling type? That's okay

A PCA pump that provides continuous infusion and bolus doses will provide analgesia regardless of whether the patient uses the control button. This type of PCA is useful for helping patients cope with steady pain that gradually increases or decreases, incidental pain, or pain that's worse at different times. If the patient's pain is intermittent, he may not need continuous infusion.

Check the record first

Before allowing the patient to self-administer opioid analgesics with a PCA pump, review his medication regimen. Concurrent use of two central nervous system (CNS) depressants may cause drowsiness, oversedation, disorientation, and anxiety.

Explain and reassure

Explain to the patient how often he can self-administer the pain medication. Reassure him that the lock-out interval will prevent him from administering medication too frequently.

Determining doses

You and the practitioner may determine the initial trial bolus dose and time interval between boluses, according to the patient's condition and activity level. The practitioner orders ranges of dosing. Then you can enter these prescribed ranges into the PCA pump's program.

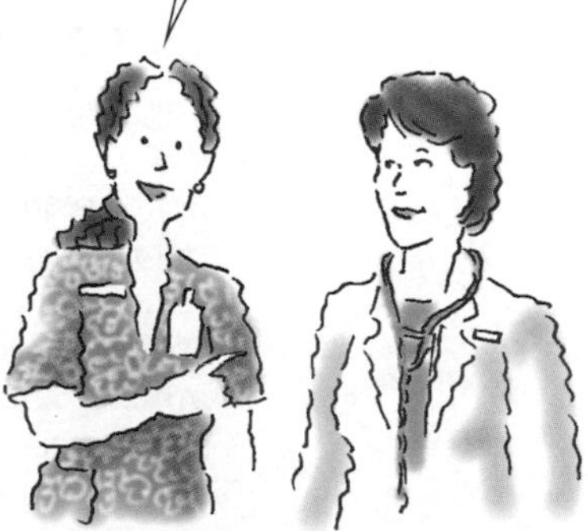

With a push of the button...

When safe limits are set, the patient can push the button to receive a dose when he experiences pain. Explain to him how the PCA device works.

You and the practitioner may decide to change either the dose or the lock-out interval after close monitoring and thorough assessment of the patient.

Looking into the lock-out interval

Here are general guidelines for determining an appropriate lock-out interval. These guidelines apply to pumps that provide bolus doses only and pumps that provide bolus doses plus continuous infusions:

- For I.V. boluses, set the lock-out interval as prescribed by the practitioner. Typically, pain relief after an I.V. opioid bolus takes 6 to 10 minutes.
- For subQ boluses, set the lock-out interval for 30 minutes or more. Typically, pain relief after a subQ bolus takes 30 to 60 minutes.
- For spinal boluses, set the lock-out interval for 60 minutes or more. Typically, pain relief after a spinal bolus takes 30 to 60 minutes.

Until pain subsides

If the patient hasn't been receiving opioids, first program the pump to deliver the drug until his pain is relieved (the loading dose). Then set the pump's hourly infusion rate to equal the total number of milligrams per hour ordered by the practitioner. Check the patient's response every 15 to 30 minutes for 1 to 2 hours.

What to monitor (and be sure to record!)

During therapy, monitor and record:

- amount of analgesic infused
- patient's respiratory rate
- patient's assessment of pain relief using the 0 to 10 scale for pain in which 10 is the most severe pain
- patient's level of consciousness.

If the patient doesn't feel that pain has been sufficiently relieved, notify the practitioner; he may increase the dosage.

Remember to monitor the patient's vital signs, especially when first initializing therapy. Encourage the patient to practice coughing and deep breathing. These exercises promote ventilation and prevent pooling of secretions, which could lead to respiratory difficulty.

PCA complications

The primary complication of PCA administration is respiratory depression. If the patient's respiratory rate declines to 10 or fewer breaths per minute, call his name, touch him, and have him breathe deeply. If he's confused, restless, or can't be roused, stop the infusion, notify the practitioner, and prepare to give oxygen. Administer an opioid antagonist, such as naloxone, if prescribed.

Coughing and deep breathing help prevent respiratory difficulties caused by PCA administration.

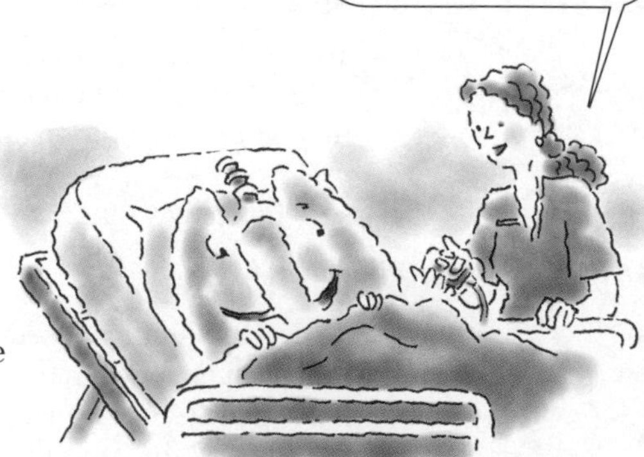

Possible problems with PCA

Infiltration into subcutaneous tissue and catheter occlusion may also occur in PCA therapy. There are other possible complications, including:
- anaphylaxis
- nausea
- vomiting
- constipation
- orthostatic hypotension
- drug tolerance.

A note about nausea

If prescribed, give the patient who experiences nausea an antiemetic such as dolasetron. If the patient has persistent nausea and vomiting during therapy, the practitioner may change the medication.

Patient teaching

Make sure that the patient and caregiver fully understand:
- how the pump works
- when to contact the practitioner
- signs and symptoms of adverse reactions
- signs and symptoms of drug tolerance.

Tell the patient that he'll be able to control his pain and that the pump is safe and effective. Also, remind him that an opioid analgesic relieves pain best when it's taken before the pain becomes intense.

Push the button to receive a dose *before* your pain becomes intense.

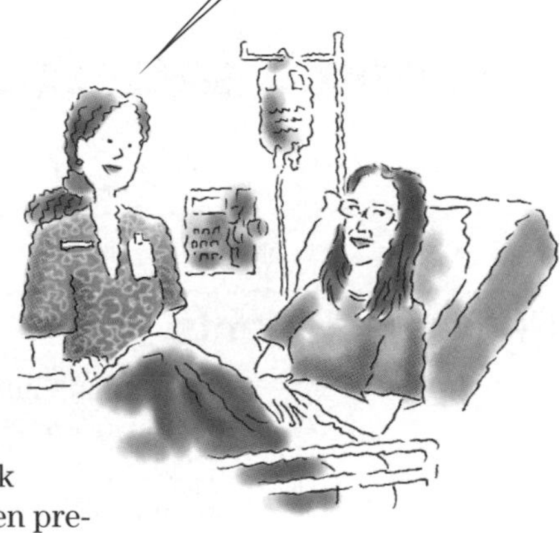

Good advice

Because an opioid analgesic may cause orthostatic hypotension, tell the patient to get up slowly from his bed or a chair. Instruct him to eat a high-fiber diet, drink plenty of fluids, and take a stool softener, if one has been prescribed. Caution him against drinking alcohol because this may enhance CNS depression.

Don't keep it a secret

The patient should notify the practitioner if he fails to achieve adequate pain relief.

The patient's caregiver should report signs of overdose, such as:
- slow or irregular breathing
- pinpoint pupils
- loss of consciousness.

Teach the caregiver how to maintain respiration until help arrives should the need arise.

Did it work?

Evaluate the effectiveness of the drug at regular intervals. Ask these questions:

- Is the patient getting relief?
- Does the dosage need to be increased because of persistent or worsening pain?
- Is the patient developing a tolerance to the drug?
- Is the patient's condition stable?

Documentation

After you administer a drug I.V., always document the procedure, including:

- date and time of each infusion
- drug and dosage
- access site
- duration of administration
- patient's response, including adverse reactions
- your name.

Patients with special needs

When giving I.V. medications to a pediatric or elderly patient, be aware of special considerations.

Pediatric patients

Neonates and infants have precise fluid requirements. Keep these considerations in mind when you give I.V. medications to children:

- Small children can't tolerate the large amount of fluid recommended for diluting many drugs.
- Because the drug dosage is based on the child's weight, each patient has a different normal dosing.
- Because of the small drug volume and slow delivery, you must make sure that no drug remains in the I.V. tubing before you change it.

My dose is different than her dose.
That's because our dosages are based on our weights.

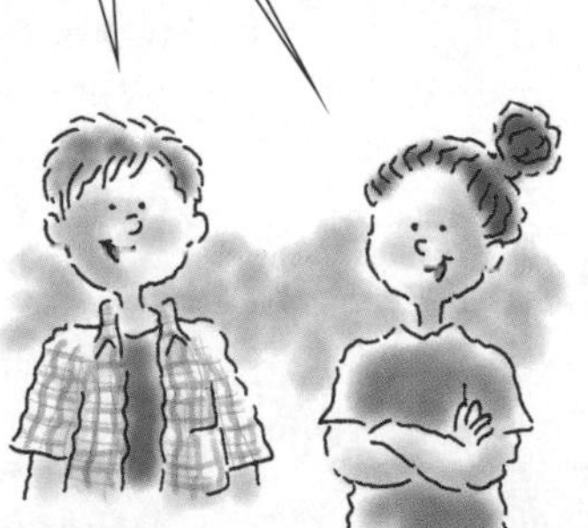

Intermittent infusion

The most common method of giving I.V. drugs to pediatric patients is by intermittent infusion, using a volume-control set.

Out-of-reach, tamper-proof, and anti-free-flow

When setting up the equipment for a pediatric patient, take steps to ensure safety:

- Keep flow-control clamps out of the child's reach.
- Use tamper-proof pumps so the child can't change the rate inadvertently.
- Use an infusion pump with an anti-free-flow device that prevents inadvertent bolus infusions if the pump door is accidentally opened.

Remember, it's safety first when dealing with pediatric patients: Keep clamps out of reach and use tamper-proof pumps with an anti-free-flow device.

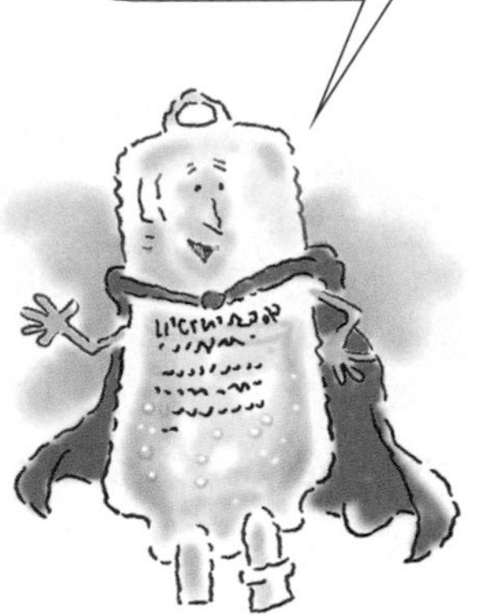

Child care

In many cases, a child's venipuncture device must stay in place longer than an adult's. Be especially careful to protect the I.V. site from accidental dislodgment or contamination. Also, use aseptic technique whenever you're administering I.V. medications.

Retrograde administration

Retrograde administration offers one method for dealing with infants' precise fluid requirements. This method uses a coiled, low-volume tubing and a displacement syringe to prevent fluid overload.

Advantages

Retrograde administration allows you to administer an I.V. antibiotic over a 30-minute period without increasing the volume of fluid delivered to the patient. This method requires only one tubing to administer all I.V. fluids and medications. Also, you don't have to change the primary flow rate to administer I.V. drugs.

Disadvantages

One downside of retrograde administration is that drug delivery is unpredictable, particularly with flow rates of less than 5 ml/hour. Also, the low-volume tubing must be able to hold the entire diluted drug volume. If any is displaced into the syringe, it must be discarded.

The drug must be diluted in a volume equal to half that used at the milliliter-per-hour rate of the primary infusion to allow for a 30-minute drug infusion. Therefore, if the primary rate is changed, the diluted drug volume must be changed as well.

Syringe pump

A syringe pump is especially useful for giving intermittent I.V. medications to pediatric patients. It provides the greatest control for small-volume infusions.

Syringe pump safeguards

Make sure that the pump you use is tamper-proof, has a built-in guard against uncontrolled flow rates, and has an alarm sensitive to low-pressure occlusion. It should operate accurately with syringe sizes from 1 to 60 ml using low-volume tubing.

Intraosseous infusion

When venous access can't be established in an emergency, intraosseous infusion may be administered. This type of administration is the infusion of I.V. medication into a bone.

In cases of emergency

Intraosseous infusion is usually performed by emergency personnel. It's a simple, quick, and relatively safe method for short-term emergency administration of lifesaving I.V. fluids and medications.

Fast, effective, and temporary

Drugs used in intraosseous infusion may be given by continuous or intermittent infusion or by direct injection. Intraosseous infusion is as quick and effective as the I.V. route. However, intraosseous infusion should be used only until venous access can be established.

Elderly patients

When administering an I.V. analgesic to an elderly patient, watch closely for signs of respiratory depression or CNS depression, including confusion. Also, when giving a drug that can cause renal toxicity, monitor the patient closely for this complication. Remember, the aging process alone means many elderly patients have decreased functioning in several of their biological systems.

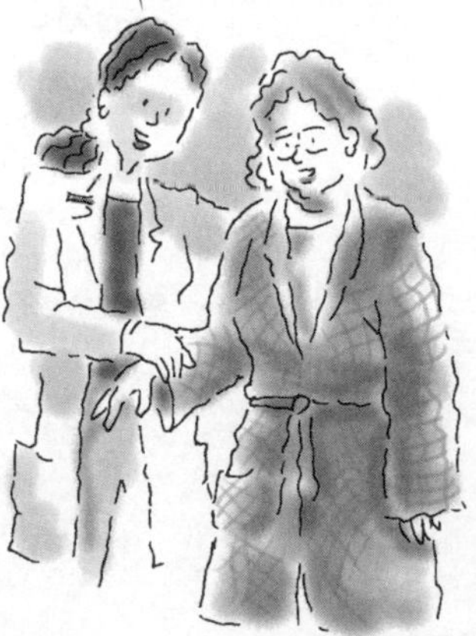

Fragile veins and fluid overload

Because many elderly patients have fragile veins, they're prone to infiltration and phlebitis. Carefully assess the I.V. site for signs and symptoms of these complications. If necessary, restart the infusion before you give a medication I.V.

Many I.V. drugs are particularly irritating to fragile veins, so you may have to dilute a drug in a larger volume than you normally would. Remember, though, that elderly patients are prone to fluid overload. Keep accurate intake and output records, and include all fluids given for I.V. drug administration.

Managing complications

To protect a patient receiving I.V. medication therapy, watch for signs and symptoms of these serious complications:
- hypersensitivity
- infiltration
- extravasation
- phlebitis
- infection. (See *Managing complications of I.V. drug therapy*, pages 182 and 183.)

Hypersensitivity

Before you administer a drug, take steps to find out if your patient may be prone to hypersensitivity:
- Ask the patient if he has any allergies, including allergies to food or pollen.
- Ask if he has a family history of allergies. Patients with a personal or family history of allergies are more likely to develop a drug hypersensitivity.
- If your patient is an infant less than 3 months old, be sure to ask about the mother's allergy history because maternal antibodies may still be present.

Following through with care

After giving an I.V. medication, follow through with these precautions:
- Stay with the patient for 5 to 10 minutes to detect early signs and symptoms of hypersensitivity, such as sudden fever, joint swelling, rash, urticaria, bronchospasm, and wheezing.
- If the patient is receiving a drug for the first time, check him every 5 to 10 minutes or according to your facility's policy. Otherwise, check every 30 minutes for a few hours.

Immediate response

At the first sign of hypersensitivity, discontinue the infusion and notify the practitioner immediately. Remember, immediate severe reactions are life-threatening. If necessary, assist with emergency treatment or resuscitation.

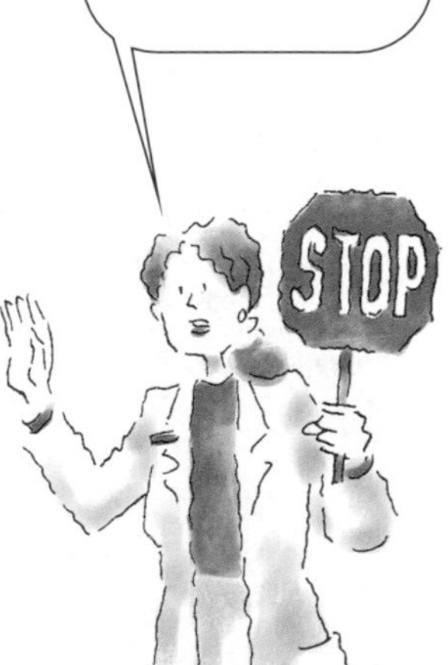

Infiltration

Infiltration occurs when I.V. fluid leaks into surrounding tissue. It commonly stems from improper placement or dislodgment of the catheter. In elderly patients, this complication may occur because the veins are thin and fragile.

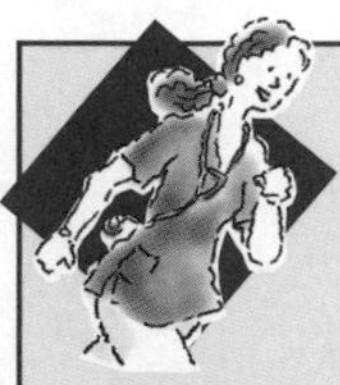

Running smoothly

Managing complications of I.V. drug therapy

Use this chart to correct possible complications of I.V. drug administration.

Complications	Signs and symptoms	Nursing interventions
Circulatory overload	• Neck vein distention or engorgement • Respiratory distress • Increased blood pressure • Crackles • Positive fluid balance	• Stop the infusion, and place the patient in semi-Fowler's position, as tolerated. • Reduce the patient's anxiety. • Administer oxygen as ordered. • Notify the practitioner. • Administer diuretics as ordered.
Hypersensitivity	• Itching, urticarial rash • Tearing eyes, runny nose • Bronchospasm • Wheezing • Anaphylactic reaction	• Stop the infusion immediately. • Maintain a patent airway. • Administer an antihistaminic steroid, an anti-inflammatory, and antipyretic medications as ordered. • Give 0.2 to 0.5 ml of 1:1,000 aqueous epinephrine subQ; repeat at 3-minute intervals and as needed. • Monitor the patient's vital signs.
Infiltration (peripheral I.V.)	• Swelling • Discomfort • Burning • Tightness • Cool skin • Blanching	• Stop the infusion and remove the device (unless medication is a vesicant; in such cases, consult the pharmacy). • Elevate the limb. • Check the patient's pulse and capillary refill. • Restart the I.V. and infusion. • Document the patient's condition and interventions. • Check the site frequently.
Phlebitis (peripheral I.V.)	• Redness or tenderness at the tip of the device • Puffy area over the vein • Elevated temperature	• Stop the infusion and remove the device. • Apply a warm pack. • Document the patient's condition and interventions. • Insert a new I.V. catheter using a larger vein or a smaller device and restart the infusion.
Systemic infection	• Elevated temperature • Malaise	• Stop the infusion. • Notify the practitioner. • Remove the device. • Culture the site and device as ordered. • Administer medications as prescribed. • Monitor the patient's vital signs.

Managing complications of I.V. drug therapy *(continued)*

Complications	Signs and symptoms	Nursing interventions
Venous spasm	• Pain along the vein • Sluggish flow rate when clamp is completely open • Blanched skin over the vein	• Apply warm soaks over the vein and surrounding tissue. • Slow the flow rate.
Speed shock	• Headache • Syncope • Flushed face • Tightness in chest • Irregular pulse • Shock • Cardiac arrest	• Stop the infusion. • Call the practitioner. • Give dextrose 5% in water at keep-vein-open rate.

Raising the risk

The risk of infiltration increases when the tip is positioned near a flexion area. In this case, patient movement may cause the device to telescope within the vein or slip out or through the lumen of the vessel.

If only a small amount of an isotonic solution or nonirritating drug infiltrates, the patient usually experiences only mild discomfort. Routine comfort measures in this case include elevating the extremity. Document your infiltration findings using the infiltration scale (see *The infiltration scale*, page 184).

Extravasation

Extravasation, leaking of vesicant drugs such as various antineoplastic drugs and sympathomimetics into surrounding tissue, can produce severe local tissue damage, which may:

- cause discomfort
- delay healing
- produce infection, tissue necrosis, and disfigurement
- lead to loss of function and possibly amputation.

For prevention tips, see *Preventing extravasation*, page 185.

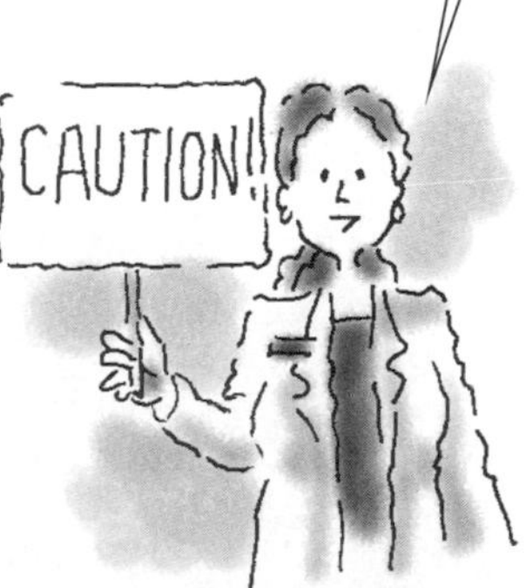

Extra! Extra! Case of extravasation suspected!

If you suspect extravasation, follow your facility's protocol. Essential steps are as follows:

- Stop the I.V. flow and remove the I.V. line, unless you need the catheter in place to infiltrate the antidote.

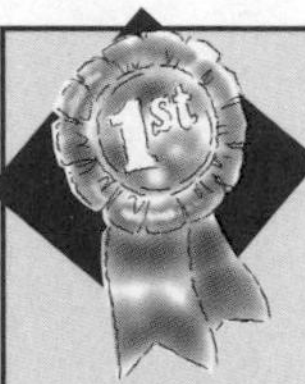

Best practice

The infiltration scale

The 2006 Infusion Nurses Society Revised Standards of Practice have classified the degrees of infiltration. Use these classifications, outlined in the chart below, when documenting instances of infiltration.

Degree	Description
0	• No symptoms
1+	• Skin blanched • Edema less than 1″ in any direction • Cool to touch • With or without pain
2+	• Skin blanched • Edema 1″ to 6″ in any direction • Cool to touch • With or without pain
3+	• Skin blanched, translucent • Gross edema more than 6″ in any direction • Cool to touch • Mild to moderate pain • Possible numbness
4+	• Skin blanched, translucent, tight, leaking, discolored, bruised, swollen • Gross edema more than 6″ in any direction • Deep, pitting tissue edema • Circulatory impairment • Moderate to severe pain • Infiltration of any amount of blood product, irritant, or vesicant

- Estimate the amount of extravasated solution and notify the practitioner.
- Instill the appropriate antidote according to facility protocol.
- Elevate the extremity.
- Record the extravasation site, the patient's symptoms, the estimated amount of infiltrated solution, and the treatment. Also record the time you notified the practitioner and his name. Continue documenting the appearance of the site and associated symptoms.
- Following manufacturer's recommendations, apply either ice packs or warm compresses to the affected area.

Preventing extravasation

Extravasation—the leaking of vesicant (blistering) drugs or fluids into the surrounding tissue—can occur when a vein is punctured or when there's leakage around an I.V. site. If extravasation occurs, severe local tissue damage may result. To prevent extravasation when you're giving vesicants, adhere strictly to proper administration techniques and follow the guidelines described here.

Site selection, venipuncture, and infusion

When preparing the patient for drug administration, keep these guidelines in mind:

- Don't use an existing I.V. catheter unless its patency is assured. Perform a new venipuncture to ensure correct catheter placement and vein patency.
- Select the site carefully. Use a distal vein that allows successive venipunctures. To avoid tendon and nerve damage from possible extravasation, avoid using the back of the hand. Also avoid the wrist and fingers (which are hard to immobilize) and areas previously damaged or that have poor circulation.
- Probing for a vein may cause trauma. Stop and begin again at another site.
- Always start the infusion with dextrose 5% in water (D_5W) or normal saline solution.

Check it out

Check for infiltration before giving the medication. Apply a tourniquet above the catheter to occlude the vein, then see if the flow continues. If the flow stops, the solution isn't infiltrating. Alternatively, simply lower the I.V. container and watch for blood backflow. The latter method is less reliable because the needle may have punctured the opposite vein wall though the catheter is still resting partially in the vein. Flush the catheter to ensure patency. If swelling occurs at the I.V. site, the solution is infiltrating.

During and after administration

When you're ready to administer the drugs, follow these guidelines:

- Give the drugs by slow I.V. push through a free-flowing I.V. line or by small-volume infusion (50 to 100 ml).
- Give vesicants last when multiple drugs are ordered. Use a low-flow electronic infusion device to administer vesicants. A high-pressure pump will continue the infusion if infiltration occurs.
- During administration, observe the infusion site for erythema or infiltration. Tell your patient to report any burning, stinging, pain, or sensation of sudden "heat" at the site.
- Use a transparent semipermeable dressing to allow frequent inspection of the I.V. site.
- After drug administration, instill several milliliters of D_5W or normal saline solution to flush the drug from the vein and prevent drug leakage when the catheter is removed.

Extravasation extra credit

Nurses commonly test for blood return to determine if extravasation is occurring. However, the absence of blood return doesn't always indicate extravasation. Blood return may not be possible if:

- you're using a small catheter in a small vein or in one with low venous pressure
- the tip of the venous access device is lodged against the vein wall.

Here's the truth about other common misconceptions:

- Extravasation doesn't always cause a hard lump. When the catheter tip is completely out of the vein wall, a lump may form. However, if fluid leaks out of the vein slowly (as it may when the catheter tip partially punctures the vein wall), extravasation may produce only a flat, diffuse swelling.
- The patient may not always experience coldness or discomfort with extravasation. He may feel cold if extravasation occurs during rapid administration of a medication. Rarely will a patient feel cold, however, from extravasation during a slow infusion.

Phlebitis

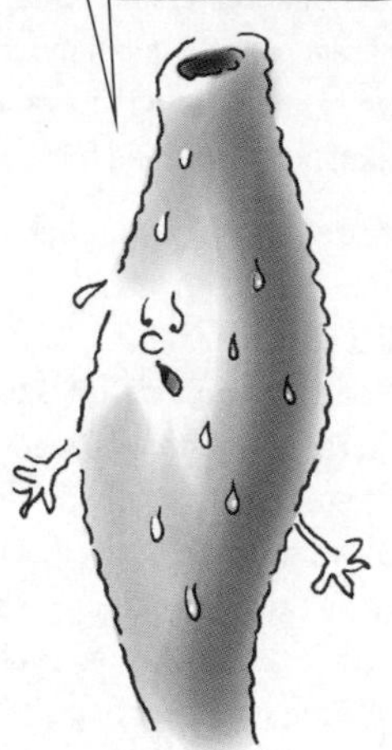

Phlebitis, inflammation of a vein, is a common complication of I.V. therapy. It may be associated with drugs or solutions that:

- are acidic
- are alkaline
- have high osmolarity.

Other contributing factors include:

- vein trauma during insertion
- using a vein that's too small
- using a vascular access device that's too large
- prolonged use of the same I.V. site.

Ph-ollowing phlebitis' development

Phlebitis can follow any infusion — or even an injection of a single drug — but it's more common after continuous infusions. Typically, phlebitis develops 2 to 3 days after the vein is exposed to the drug or solution. Phlebitis develops more rapidly in distal veins than in the larger veins close to the heart.

The direct route

Drugs given by direct injection generally don't cause phlebitis when administered at the correct dilution and rate. However, phenytoin and diazepam, which are frequently given by direct injection, can produce phlebitis after one or more injections at the same I.V. site.

The usual suspects

When piggybacked, certain irritating I.V. drugs are likely to cause phlebitis, such as:

- erythromycin
- tetracycline
- nafcillin sodium
- vancomycin
- amphotericin B.

Large doses of potassium chloride (40 mEq/L or more), amino acids, dextrose solutions (10% or more), and multivitamins can also cause phlebitis.

Reducing the risk

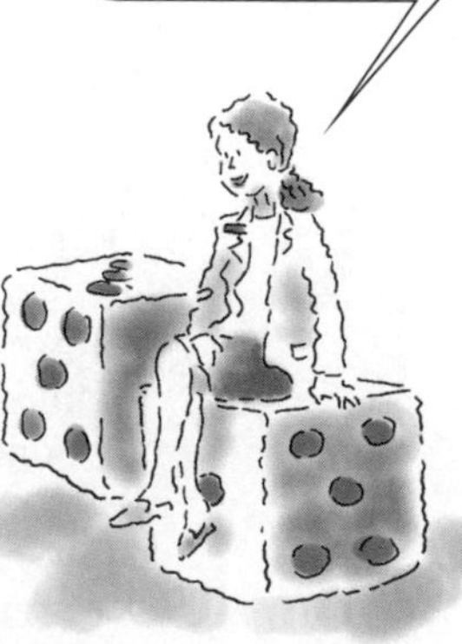

If ordered and if the patient's condition can tolerate it, add 250 to 1,000 ml of diluent to irritating drugs to help reduce the risk of irritation. You still should change the I.V. site every 72 hours or more frequently if necessary. If peripheral access is limited, suggest the placement of a central venous access device to reduce the number of needle sticks, especially for long-term therapy.

Phlebitis can also result from motion and pressure of the venous access device. Also, particles in drugs and I.V. solutions can produce phlebitis, but you can reduce this risk by using filter needles.

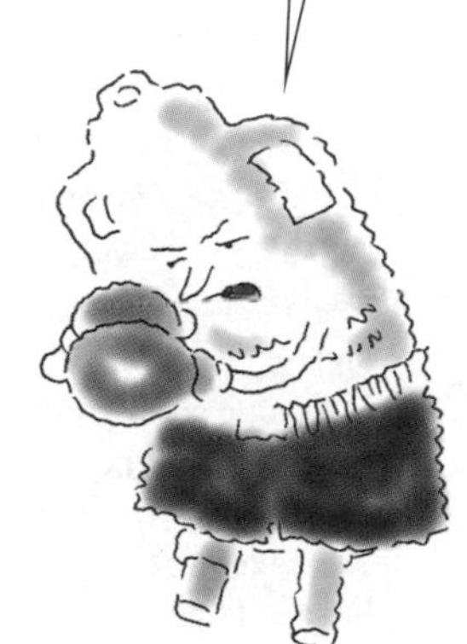

Reducing the risk even further...

To help prevent phlebitis, the pharmacist can alter drug osmolarity and pH without affecting the primary medication. Additional measures you can take include:

- using proper venipuncture technique
- diluting drugs correctly
- monitoring administration rates
- observing the I.V. site frequently
- changing the infusion site regularly.

Site inspection

To detect phlebitis, inspect the I.V. site several times per day. Use a transparent semipermeable dressing so you can see the skin distal to the tip of the access device as well as the insertion site. (See *Detecting and classifying phlebitis*, page 188.)

Fighting phlebitis

If you suspect phlebitis, follow these steps to care for your patient:

- At the first sign of redness or tenderness, move the venipuncture device to another site, preferably on the opposite arm.
- To ease your patient's discomfort, apply warm packs, or soak the arm in warm water.
- Notify the practitioner and document the assessment of the I.V. site and your interventions.

Infection

A patient receiving I.V. medication therapy may develop a local infection at the I.V. site. Monitor your patient for signs and symptoms of infection, such as redness and discharge at the site.

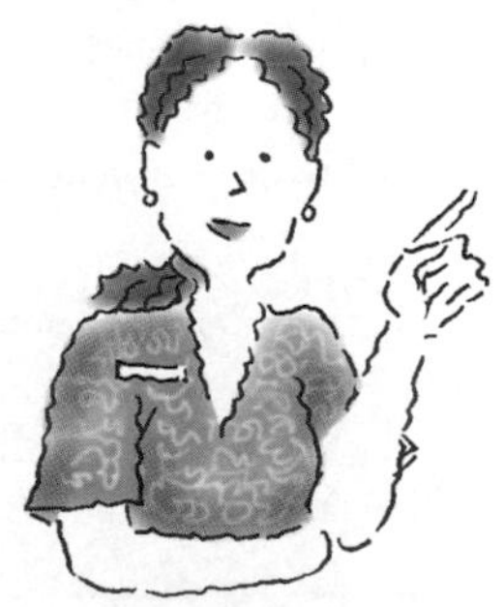

Protection begins with you

Keep in mind that you're at risk for exposure to serious infection. If your patient has the hepatitis B virus, human immunodeficiency virus, or another blood-borne pathogen, it can be transmitted to caregivers through poor technique or failure to use standard precautions.

To protect yourself, follow the precautions for handling blood and body fluids recommended by the CDC. Remember to treat all patients as potentially infected and take appropriate precautions. Also, if you administer I.V. drugs and solutions, you should receive the hepatitis B vaccine (if you don't already have hepatitis B antibodies).

Best practice

Detecting and classifying phlebitis

If you detect phlebitis early, it can be treated effectively. If undetected, however, phlebitis can cause local infection, severe discomfort and, possibly, sepsis.

A brief explanation

Here's a brief explanation of how the signs and symptoms of phlebitis develop. As platelets aggregate at the damage site, a clot begins to form and histamine, bradykinin, and serotonin are released. Increased blood flow to the injury site and clot formation at the vein wall cause redness, tenderness, and slight swelling.

If you don't remove the venous access device at this stage, the vein wall becomes hard and tender and may develop a red streak 2″ to 6″ (5 to 15 cm) long. Left untreated, phlebitis may produce exudate at the I.V. site, accompanied by an elevated white blood cell count and fever. It can also produce pain at the I.V. site, but a lack of pain doesn't eliminate the possibility of phlebitis.

How to classify it

According to the 2006 Infusion Nurses Society Revised Standards of Practice, the degrees of phlebitis are classified as follows:

0 = no clinical symptoms

1+ = erythema with or without pain

2+ = erythema with pain, edema may or may not be present

3+ = erythema with pain, edema may or may not be present, streak formation, palpable cord

4+ = erythema with pain, edema may or may not be present, streak formation, palpable cord longer than 1″, purulent drainage.

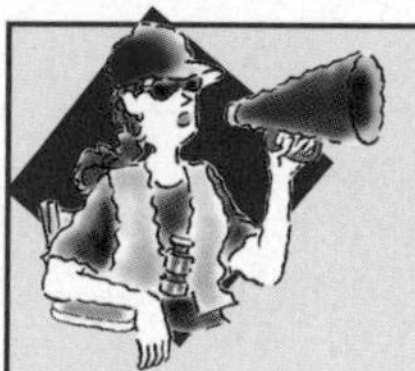

That's a wrap!

I.V. medications review

Benefits

- Achieve rapid therapeutic drug levels
- Are absorbed more effectively than drugs given by other routes
- Permit accurate titration
- Produce less discomfort

Risks

- May cause solution and drug incompatibilities
- May lead to poor vascular access
- Can produce immediate adverse reactions

I.V. administration methods

Direct injection

- Drug injected directly into an intermittent infusion device or through an existing I.V. line
- Drug injected slowly (unless specified) to prevent adverse reactions and vein trauma

Intermittent infusion

- Drug administered over a specified interval
- Drug delivered through a piggyback line, saline lock, or volume-control set

I.V. medications review *(continued)*

Continuous infusion
- Drug delivery regulated over an extended time
- Drug delivered through a primary or secondary line

PCA therapy
- Analgesic delivery controlled by the patient
- Overdose prevented by lock-out interval
- Patient uses fewer opioids for pain relief

Monitoring
- Patient monitored for respiratory depression
- Patient monitored for decreased blood pressure

Assessment
- Pain relief (frequently)
- Infiltration into surrounding tissues

Potential complications
- Hypersensitivity
- Infiltration
- Extravasation
- Phlebitis
- Infection

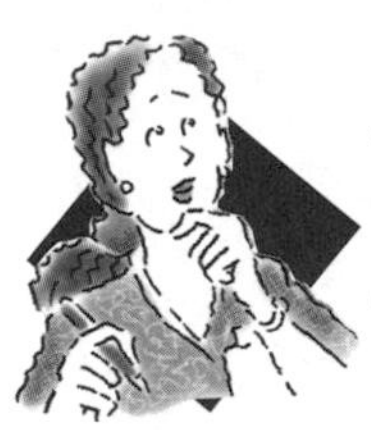

Quick quiz

1. I.V. medication may be indicated when:
A. the patient needs a slower therapeutic effect.
B. the medication can't be absorbed by the GI tract.
C. the medication given orally is stable in gastric juices.
D. the medication isn't irritating to muscle tissues.

Answer: B. I.V. medication has a rapid effect and may be indicated if the medication can't be absorbed by the GI tract, is unstable in gastric juices, or causes pain or tissue damage when given I.M. or subQ.

2. What's the preferred route of medication in emergencies?
A. I.V.
B. SubQ
C. I.M.
D. Oral

Answer: A. The I.V. route allows therapeutic levels to be achieved rapidly.

3. Loading dose, lock-out interval, and maintenance doses are basic to:
A. I.V. therapy.
B. PCA therapy.
C. continuous I.V. morphine drips.
D. TPN.

Answer: B. These concepts are basic to PCA therapy.

4. A patient receiving I.V. therapy has redness at the I.V. site. The patient denies feeling pain at the area. These findings suggest what degree of phlebitis?

A. 4+
B. 3+
C. 2+
D. 1+

Answer: D. According to the Intravenous Nurses Society Revised Standards of Practice, phlebitis that involves erythema with or without pain is classified as 1+.

5. Elderly patients are more prone to which complications of I.V. therapy?

A. Hypersensitivity
B. Phlebitis
C. Infection
D. Extravasation

Answer: B. Because many elderly patients have fragile veins, they're more prone to phlebitis and infiltration.

6. The one way to prevent extravasation is by:

A. using a high-pressure pump to infuse vesicants.
B. using a small vein to insert the access device.
C. using a gauze dressing over the insertion site.
D. using an existing I.V. catheter only after patency has been assured.

Answer: D. An existing I.V. catheter should only be used after its patency has been assessed. If the catheter isn't patent, perform a new venipuncture to ensure correct catheter placement and vein patency.

Scoring

☆☆☆ If you answered all six questions correctly, wow! Whether you used a direct, intermittent, or continuous approach, you caught the essence of this chapter.

☆☆ If you answered four or five questions correctly, great! You're right in line — no significant absorption problems.

☆ If you answered fewer than four questions correctly, don't panic! There are five more quick quizzes to go.

Transfusions

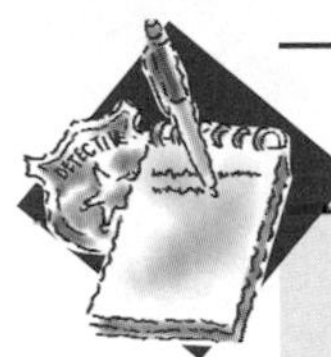

Just the facts

In this chapter, you'll learn:

- blood composition and physiology
- two ways to administer whole blood, blood components, plasma, and plasma fractions
- special considerations for pediatric and geriatric patients
- signs of common transfusion complications and appropriate responses to them.

Understanding transfusion therapy

The circulatory system is the body's main mover of blood and its components. The bloodstream carries oxygen, nutrients, hormones, and other vital substances to all other tissues and organs of the body. When illness or injury decreases the volume, oxygen-carrying capacity, or vital components of blood, transfusion therapy may be the only solution.

Purpose of transfusion therapy

Transfusion therapy is the introduction of whole blood or blood components directly into the bloodstream. It's used mainly to:

- restore and maintain blood volume
- improve the oxygen-carrying capacity of blood
- replace deficient blood components and improve coagulation.

Pump up the volume

The average adult body contains about 5 L of blood. However, hemorrhage, trauma, or burns can send blood

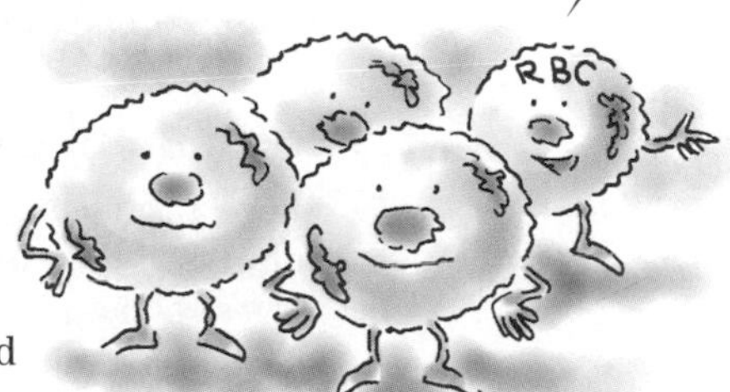

volume plunging. Restoring and maintaining the volume of blood in the body is important because blood helps maintain fluid balance. When blood transfusion is contraindicated in a patient, fluid infusions can restore circulatory volume. Unlike blood, however, fluid infusions can't improve oxygen-carrying capacity or replace deficient components.

Blood carries on

When a person breathes in, air surges into the lungs. Blood then harvests oxygen from the air mixture and carries it throughout the body. The oxygen-carrying capacity of blood may be depleted from respiratory disorders, sepsis, carbon monoxide poisoning, acute anemia due to blood loss, or sickle cell disease or other chronic diseases. I.V. transfusion of red blood cell (RBC) components can help restore the role of blood in oxygen delivery.

Getting it back together

The coagulation capacity of blood can be depleted by hemorrhage, liver failure, bone marrow suppression, platelet depletion (thrombocytopenia), medication- and disease-induced coagulopathies, or vitamin K deficiency. I.V. transfusion may be used to replace the missing coagulation components of blood.

Transfusing blood products

The two ways to administer blood and blood products are:

- through a peripheral I.V. catheter
- through a central venous (CV) access device.

A license to transfuse

Most states allow licensed registered nurses (but not licensed practical nurses [LPNs] or licensed vocational nurses) to administer blood and blood components. In some states, LPNs may regulate transfusion flow rates, observe patients for reactions, discontinue transfusions, and document procedures. Know your state practice act before performing a transfusion or transfusion-related procedure.

Administering blood and blood components is the registered nurse's responsibility in most states. Know your state practice act *before* you perform or participate in a blood transfusion.

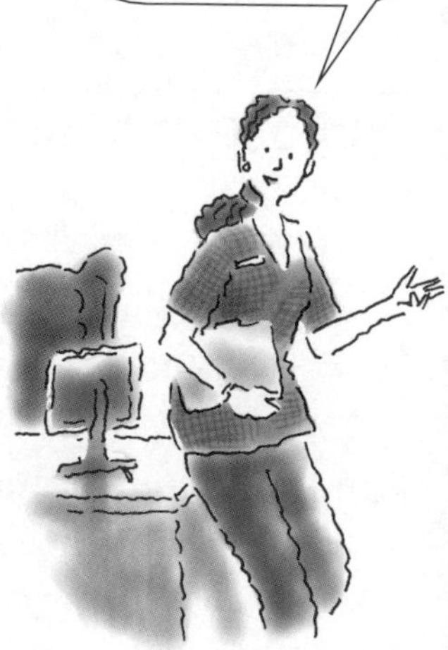

Peripheral I.V. catheter

Blood products can be transfused through a peripheral I.V. catheter, but it isn't the best idea if large volumes must be transfused quickly. It's recommended that a 20G or larger peripheral I.V. catheter be used for rapid transfusions in acute situations. Peripheral veins are commonly used in nonacute transfusion situations. The small diameter of the vein and peripheral resistance (resistance to blood flow in the vein) can slow the transfusion.

CV access device

Large volumes of blood products can be delivered quickly through a CV access device because of the large size of the blood vessels and their decreased resistance to infusion.

1st

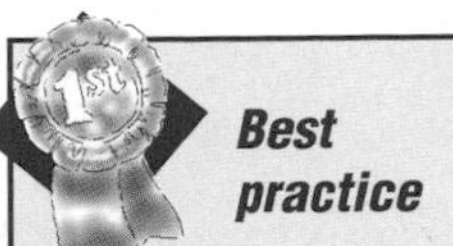

Best practice

Protect yourself

When transfusing blood, remember to protect yourself from exposure to transmissible diseases, such as viral hepatitis and human immunodeficiency virus. The Centers for Disease Control and Prevention guidelines recommend wearing gloves, a mask, goggles, and a gown when transfusing blood, in case of blood spills or sprays.

Transfusion risks

Because of careful screening and testing, the supply of blood is safer today than it has ever been. Even so, a patient who receives a transfusion is still at risk for life-threatening complications, such as a hemolytic reaction (which destroys RBCs), and exposure to infectious diseases, such as human immunodeficiency virus (HIV) and hepatitis. Therefore, the practitioner, the nurse, and the patient (when able) must weigh the benefits of a transfusion against the risks. The patient must be informed of the risks of a transfusion. Many facilities have special consent forms for transfusions. (See *Protect yourself.*)

Blood composition

Blood contains two basic components:

 cellular elements

 plasma.

It's elementary!

The cellular (or formed) elements make up about 45% of the blood volume. They include:
- erythrocytes, or RBCs
- leukocytes, or white blood cells (WBCs)
- thrombocytes (platelets).

Plasma — part by part

Plasma, the liquid component of blood, makes up about 55% of blood volume. The two most significant components of plasma are:
- water (serum)
- protein (albumin, globulin, and fibrinogen).

Other elements in plasma include:
- lipids
- electrolytes

About 55% of the total blood volume is plasma, the liquid component of blood. The remaining 45% consists of formed, cellular elements—RBCs, WBCs, and platelets.

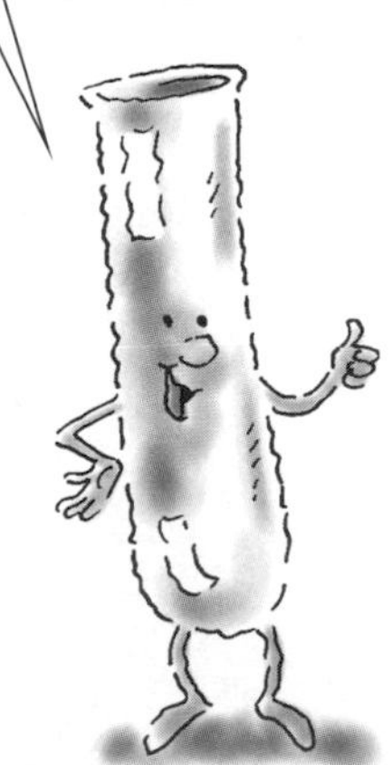

- vitamins
- carbohydrates
- nonprotein nitrogen compounds
- bilirubin
- gases.

Blood products

Generally, only a patient who has lost a massive amount of blood in a short time requires a whole blood transfusion. Usually, a patient can be treated with individual blood products — the separate components that make up whole blood.

The order's for two units of RBCs. Let's get to work… it's transfusion time!

Singled out

Current technology allows freshly donated whole blood to be separated into its component parts:

- RBCs
- plasma
- platelets
- leukocytes
- plasma proteins, such as immune globulin, albumin, and clotting factors.

Partial components but full solutions

Individual blood components can be used to correct specific blood deficiencies. The availability of blood components usually makes it unnecessary to transfuse whole blood.

Compatibility

Recipient blood is choosy about donor blood. Any incompatibility can cause serious adverse reactions. The most severe is a hemolytic reaction, which destroys RBCs and may become life-threatening. Before a transfusion, testing helps to detect incompatibilities between recipient and donor blood.

Typing and crossmatching blood ensures compatibility and minimizes the risk of a hemolytic reaction.

Making a match

Typing and crossmatching establish the compatibility of donor and recipient blood. This precaution minimizes the risk of a hemolytic reaction. The most important tests include:

- ABO blood typing
- Rh typing
- crossmatching
- direct antiglobulin test

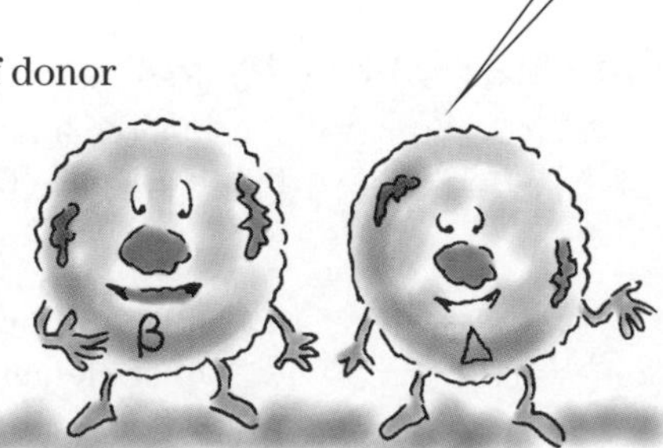

• antibody screening test
• screening for such diseases as hepatitis B and C, HIV, human T-cell lymphotrophic virus type I (HTLV-1) and type II (HTLV-2, or hairy cell leukemia), syphilis and, for certain patients, cytomegalovirus (CMV).

ABO blood type

The four blood types in the ABO system are:

 A

 B

 AB

 O.

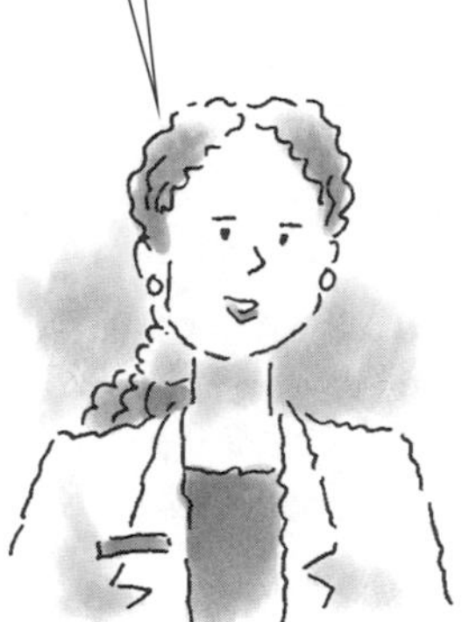

Antigens and antibodies: A stimulating discussion

An antigen is a substance that can stimulate the formation of an antibody. Each blood group in the ABO system is named for antigens—A, B, both of these, or neither—that are carried on a person's RBCs. An antigen may induce the formation of a corresponding antibody if given to a person who doesn't normally carry the antigen.

An antibody is an immunoglobulin molecule synthesized in response to a specific antigen. The ABO system includes two naturally occurring antibodies: anti-A and anti-B. One, both, or neither of these antibodies may be found in the plasma. The interaction of corresponding antigens and antibodies of the ABO system can cause agglutination (clumping together). (See *Blood type compatibility*, page 196.)

The major antigens, such as those in the ABO system, are inherited. Blood transfusions can introduce other antigens and antibodies into the body. Most are harmless, but any could cause a transfusion reaction.

A mismatch is a hemolytic hazard

A hemolytic reaction occurs when donor and recipient blood types are mismatched. It could happen, for example, if blood containing anti-A antibodies is transfused to a recipient who has blood with A antigens.

A hemolytic reaction can be life-threatening. With as little as 10 ml infused, symptoms can occur quickly—including chest pain, dyspnea, facial flushing, fever, chills, hypotension, flank pain, a burning sensation along the vein receiving blood, shock, and renal failure. Because this reaction is so fast, always adhere

Blood type compatibility

Precise typing and crossmatching of donor and recipient blood helps avoid transfusing incompatible blood, which can be fatal. The chart below shows ABO compatibility for both recipient and donor.

Blood group	Antibodies present in plasma	Compatible red blood cells	Compatible plasma
Recipient			
O	Anti-A and anti-B	O	O, A, B, AB
A	Anti-B	A, O	A, AB
B	Anti-A	B, O	B, AB
AB	Neither anti-A nor anti-B	AB, A, B, O	AB
Donor			
O	Anti-A and anti-B	O, A, B, AB	O
A	Anti-B	A, AB	A, O
B	Anti-A	B, AB	B, O
AB	Neither anti-A nor anti-B	AB	AB, A, B, O

strictly to your facility's policy and procedures for assessing vital signs during transfusions.

Blood feud

When mismatching occurs, antigens and antibodies of the ABO system do battle. Antibodies attach to the surfaces of the recipient's RBCs, causing the cells to clump together.

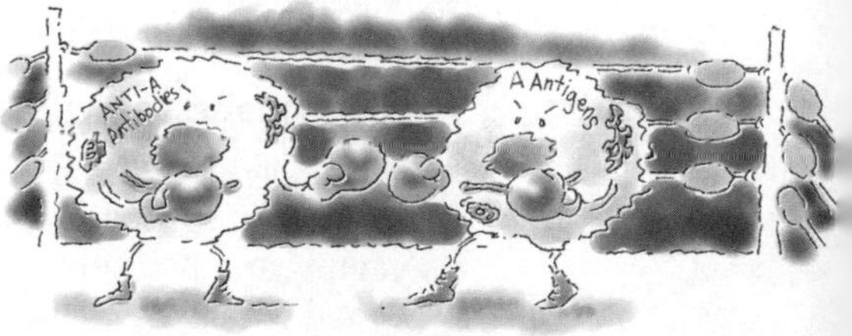

Eventually, the clumped cells can plug small blood vessels. This antibody-antigen reaction activates the body's complement system, a group of enzymatic proteins that cause RBC destruction (hemolysis). RBC hemolysis releases free hemoglobin (an RBC component) into the bloodstream, which can damage renal tubules and lead to kidney failure.

O, you're everybody's type

Because group O blood lacks both A and B antigens, it can be transfused in limited amounts in an emergency to any patient—regardless of the recipient's blood type—with little risk of adverse reaction. That's why people with group O blood are called *universal donors.*

Any donor will do

A person with AB blood type has neither anti-A nor anti-B antibodies. This person may receive A, B, AB, or O blood, making him a *universal recipient.*

Rh blood group

Another major blood antigen system, the Rhesus (Rh) system, has two groups:

 Rh-positive

 Rh-negative.

The Rh system consists of different inherited antigens—D, C, E, c, or e. These antigens are highly immunogenic—they have a high capacity for initiating the body's immune response.

D is the difference

D, or D factor, is the most important Rh antigen. The presence or absence of D is one of the factors that determines whether a person has Rh-positive or Rh-negative blood.

Rh-positive blood contains a variant of the D antigen or D factor; Rh-negative blood doesn't have this antigen. A person with Rh-negative blood who receives Rh-positive blood will gradually develop anti-Rh antibodies. The first exposure won't cause a reaction because anti-Rh antibodies are slow to form. Subsequent exposures, however, may pose a risk of hemolysis and agglutination.

A person with Rh-positive blood doesn't carry anti-Rh antibodies because they would destroy his own RBCs.

Nearly 95% of Blacks, Native Americans, and Asians have Rh-positive blood; about 85% of Whites have Rh-positive blood. The rest of the population has Rh-negative blood.

A pregnant pause

There are two ways Rh-positive blood can get into Rh-negative blood: by transfusion or during a pregnancy in which the fetus has Rh-positive blood.

Rh factor incompatibility can cause a problem in pregnancy if a mother has Rh-negative blood and her fetus inherits Rh-positive blood from the father. During her first pregnancy, the woman becomes sensitized to Rh-positive fetal blood factors, but her antibodies usually aren't sufficient to harm the fetus. Sensitization may occur after a miscarriage or an abortion.

In a subsequent pregnancy with an Rh-positive fetus, increasing amounts of the mother's anti-Rh antibodies attack the fetus, destroying RBCs. As the fetus's body produces new RBCs, cell destruction escalates, releasing bilirubin (a red cell component). The fetal liver's inability to properly process and excrete bilirubin can cause jaundice (soon after birth), other liver problems and, possibly, brain damage. Severely affected infants may develop life-threatening hemolytic disease.

Giving Rh immune globulin by I.M. injection within 72 hours of delivery prevents the formation of anti-Rh antibodies, thereby preventing the development of hemolytic disease in neonates.

Rh incompatibility rarely affects a first child, but it could pose a risk for subsequent pregnancies if left untreated.

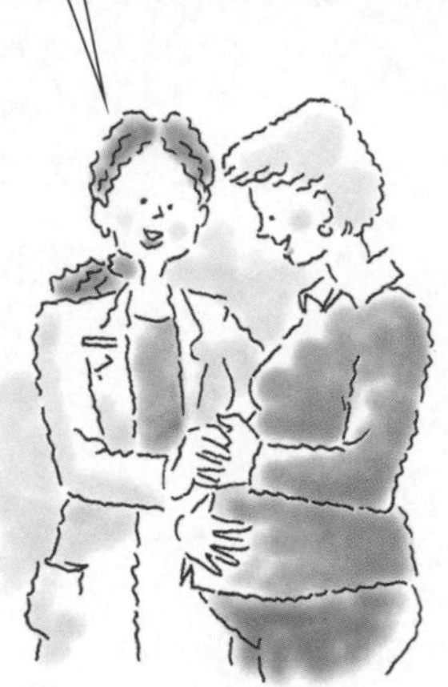

HLA blood group

Human leukocyte antigens (HLAs) are essential to immunity. HLA is part of the histocompatibility system. This system controls compatibility between transplant or transfusion recipients and donors.

The HLA system:
- is responsible for graft success or rejection
- may be involved with host defense against cancer
- may be involved when WBCs or platelets fail to multiply after being transfused. (If this happens, the HLA system could trigger a fatal immune reaction in the patient.)

Make me a match

Generally, the closer the HLA match between donor and recipient, the less likely the tissue or organ will be rejected.

HLA testing benefits patients receiving massive, multiple, or frequent transfusions. HLA evaluation is also conducted for patients who:
- will receive platelet and WBC transfusions
- will undergo organ or tissue transplant
- have severe or refractory febrile transfusion reactions.

Administering transfusions

There are two kinds of transfused blood:

 autologous (from the recipient himself)

 homologous (from a donor).

Who can and can't give blood

Donors must be screened to reduce the risks associated with transfusions.

Eligible

Eligible donors must:
- be at least 17 years old
- weigh at least 110 lb (50 kg)
- be free from active infection
- not have donated in the last 56 days
- have a hemoglobin level of at least 12.5 g/dl and a hematocrit of at least 38%.

Ineligible

Ineligible donors include those:
- who have human immunodeficiency virus or acquired immunodeficiency syndrome
- who are male and have had sex with other men since 1977
- who have taken illegal drugs I.V.
- who have had sex with prostitutes in the last 12 months
- who have had sex with anyone in the above categories
- who have had viral hepatitis
- with certain types of cancer
- with hemophilia
- who have received a blood transfusion in the last 12 months
- who spent a total of 3 months in the United Kingdom between January 1, 1980 and December 31, 1996
- who have been treated for syphilis or gonorrhea in the past 12 months
- who have received an organ transplant from another person in the last 12 months.

Autologous blood reduces the risks normally associated with transfusions, but it may not be available. Homologous blood undergoes rigorous screening and testing to ensure its quality. Part of this screening involves the donors themselves. (See *Who can and can't give blood.*)

Your primary responsibility

Whatever the source of the blood or blood products, your primary responsibility is to prevent a potentially fatal hemolytic reaction by making sure the patient receives the correct product. Whether you transfuse whole blood, cellular products, or plasma, you'll follow the same basic procedure. Always begin by checking, verifying, and inspecting. (See *Check, verify, and inspect*, page 200.)

Whole blood and cellular products

Before a transfusion, you need to send for the blood or cellular products ordered. Then gather and set up the appropriate equipment.

Cellular products

The patient's condition dictates which type of cellular product is needed in transfusion therapy. (See *Guide to whole blood and cellular products*, pages 201 and 202.)

Transfused cellular products include:
- whole blood
- packed RBCs

Check, verify, and inspect

The most common cause of a severe transfusion reaction is receiving the wrong blood. Before administering any blood or blood product, take the steps described here.

Check

Check to make sure an informed consent form was signed. Then double-check the patient's name, medical record number, ABO and Rh status (and other compatibility factors), and blood bank identification number against the label on the blood bag. Also check the expiration date on the bag.

Verify

Ask another nurse or practitioner to verify all information, according to facility policy. (Some facilities routinely require double identification.) Make sure that you and the nurse or practitioner who checked the blood or blood product have signed the blood confirmation slip. If even a slight discrepancy exists, don't administer the blood or blood product. Instead, immediately notify the blood bank and return the blood or blood product.

Inspect

Inspect the blood or blood product to detect abnormalities. Then confirm the patient's identity by checking the name, room number, and bed number on his wristband and, if possible, with the patient himself.

- leukocyte-poor RBCs
- WBCs
- platelets.

Would you like that whole or packed?

To replenish decreased blood volume or to boost the oxygen-carrying capacity of blood, the practitioner orders a transfusion of whole blood or packed RBCs (blood from which 80% of the plasma has been removed).

If your patient is receiving whole blood or packed RBCs, don't send for the blood until just before you gather the equipment; RBCs deteriorate after 4 hours at room temperature.

Whole blood transfusions are used to increase blood volume. They're usually needed because of massive hemorrhage (loss of more than 25% of total blood) resulting from trauma or vascular or cardiac surgery. Whole blood transfusions may also be used for exchange transfusions in sickle cell disease.

Packed RBCs are transfused to maintain or restore oxygen-carrying capability. They can also replace RBCs lost because of GI bleeding, dysmenorrhea, surgery, trauma, or chemotherapy. Packed RBCs are also used occasionally for red cell exchange.

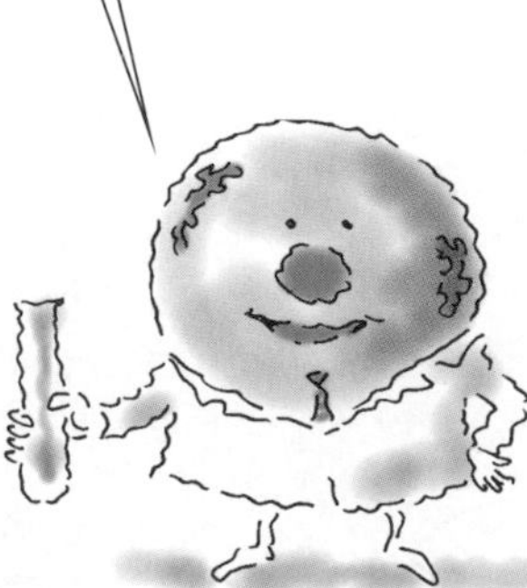

Leaving out the leukocytes

Leukocyte-poor RBCs are transfused when a patient has had a febrile, nonhemolytic transfusion reaction, caused by WBC antigens reacting with the patient's WBC antibodies or platelets.

Guide to whole blood and cellular products

This chart outlines various blood components and their indications for transfusion, along with relevant nursing considerations for each.

Blood component	Indications	Compatibility	Nursing considerations
Whole blood Complete (pure) blood	• To restore blood volume lost from hemorrhaging, trauma, or burns • Exchange transfusion in sickle cell disease	• ABO identical: Group A receives A; group B receives B; group AB receives AB; group O receives O • Rh type must match	• Remember that whole blood is seldom administered. • Use blood administration tubing to infuse within 4 hours. • Closely monitor patient volume status for volume overload. • Warm blood if giving a large quantity. • Use only with normal saline solution.
Packed red blood cells (RBCs) Same RBC mass as whole blood but with 80% of the plasma removed	• To restore or maintain oxygen-carrying capacity • To correct anemia and surgical blood loss • To increase RBC mass • Red cell exchange	• Group A receives A or O • Group B receives B or O • Group AB receives AB, A, B, or O • Group O receives O • Rh type must match • Same as packed RBCs • Rh type must match	• Use blood administration tubing to infuse over more than 4 hours. • Use only with normal saline solution. • Avoid administering packed RBCs for anemic conditions correctable by nutritional or drug therapy.
Leukocyte-poor RBCs Same as packed RBCs with about 70% of the leukocytes removed	• Same as packed RBCs • To prevent febrile reactions from leukocyte antibodies • To treat immunocompromised patients • To restore RBCs to patients who have had two or more nonhemolytic febrile reactions	• Same as packed RBCs • Rh type must match	• Use blood administration tubing. • May require a 40-micron filter suitable for hard-spun, leukocyte-poor RBCs. • Other considerations are same as those for packed RBCs. Cells expire 24 hours after washing.

(continued)

Guide to whole blood and cellular products *(continued)*

Blood component	Indications	Compatibility	Nursing considerations
White blood cells (leukocytes)			
Whole blood with all the RBCs and about 80% of the plasma removed	• To treat sepsis that's unresponsive to antibiotics (especially if patient has positive blood cultures or a persistent fever exceeding 101° F [38.3° C]) and life-threatening granulocytopenia (granulocyte count less than 500/µl)	• Same as packed RBCs • Compatibility with human leukocyte antigen (HLA) preferable but not necessary unless patient is sensitized to HLA from previous transfusion • Rh type must match	• Use a blood administration set. Give 1 unit daily for 4 to 6 days or until infection resolves. • As prescribed, premedicate with antihistamines, acetaminophen (Tylenol), or steroids. • If fever occurs, administer an antipyretic, don't discontinue transfusion; instead, reduce flow rate, as ordered, for patient comfort. • Because reactions are common, administer slowly over 2 to 4 hours. Check patient's vital signs and assess him every 15 minutes throughout transfusion. • Give transfusion with antibiotics to treat infection.
Platelets			
Platelet sediment from RBCs or plasma platelets	• To treat bleeding caused by decreased circulating platelets or functionally abnormal platelets • To improve platelet count preoperatively in a patient whose count is 50,000/µl or less	• ABO compatibility identical; Rh-negative recipients should receive Rh-negative platelets	• Use a blood filter or leukocyte-reduction filter. • As prescribed, premedicate with antipyretics and antihistamines if patient's history includes a platelet transfusion reaction or to reduce chills, fever, and allergic reactions. • Use single donor platelets if patient has a need for repeated transfusions. • Platelets aren't used to treat autoimmune thrombocytopenia or thrombocytopenic purpura unless patient has a life-threatening hemorrhage.

Several methods are used to remove leukocytes from blood, including:

- centrifugal force along with filtration and the addition of sedimentary agents, such as dextran and hydroxyethyl starch
- leukocyte removal filters

- washing the cells in a special solution (the most expensive and the least effective method; it also removes about 99% of the plasma).

Granulocytes to go

Transfusion of granulocytes (leukocytes containing granules) may be ordered to fight antibiotic-resistant septicemia and other life-threatening infections or when the granulocyte supply is severely low (granulocytopenia). This therapy is repeated for 4 to 5 days or longer, as ordered, unless the bone marrow recovers or severe reactions occur.

Because some RBCs normally remain in WBC concentrates, granulocytes are tested for compatibility (ABO, Rh, and HLA).

Platelets step to the plate

Platelets can be transfused to:

- treat bleeding caused by decreased platelets or platelets that have abnormal function, such as in patients receiving chemotherapy or who have aplastic anemia
- increase preoperative platelet counts in patients who have a platelet count of less than 50,000/µl.

Only normal saline solution should be given with blood.
Other isotonic solutions may cause cells to clump.

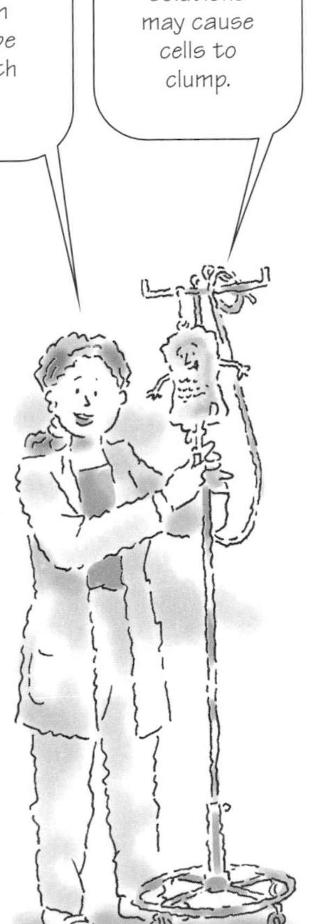

Selecting equipment

Before beginning a transfusion, gather the following equipment:

- gloves, gown, mask, and goggles to wear when handling blood products
- in-line or add-on filters as specified by the practitioner's order or as appropriate for the product being infused
- I.V. pole
- transfusion component, exactly as ordered
- venipuncture equipment, if necessary.

Normal saline solution only

No I.V. solution other than normal saline (0.9% sodium chloride) should be given with blood. If a primary line has been used to deliver a solution other than normal saline, a blood administration set shouldn't be affixed or "piggybacked" to it without first flushing the line.

Ready to filter through some advice?

Always use blood filters on blood products to avoid infusing fibrin clots or cellular debris that forms in the blood bag. There are many types of filters, each with unique features and indications. A standard blood administration set comes with a 170-micron filter, which traps particles that are 170 microns or larger. This filter doesn't remove smaller particles, called microaggregates, which form after only a few days of blood storage.

Microaggregates form from degenerating platelets and fibrin strands and may contribute to the formation of microemboli (small clots that obstruct circulation) in the lungs. To remove microaggregates, the practitioner may order a 20- to 40-micron filter, called a microaggregate filter. This filter removes smaller particles but is costly and may slow the infusion rate — a particular problem when seeking to deliver a massive, rapid transfusion.

Filters may be used to screen out leukocytes during the transfusion of RBCs or platelets. Use new tubing and a new filter for every unit of blood you transfuse. Never use a microaggregate filter to transfuse WBC concentrates or platelets; the filter will trap them. Instead, use a leukocyte reduction filter made specifically for the component.

Heat it up

A blood warmer may be ordered to prevent:
- hypothermia (for example, from large volumes of blood administered quickly)
- arrhythmias from hypothermia (86° F [30° C]).

Let's jump to a pump

In some facilities, an infusion pump is used to regulate the administration of blood and blood products. Always check the manufacturer's instructions to find out whether a particular pump can be used to administer blood or blood products. Also check to see if special blood tubing is needed if you're using an infusion pump with blood products.

Starting the transfusion

So far, you have identified the patient, inspected and verified the blood product, obtained baseline vital signs, and assembled the necessary equipment and supplies. Now you're ready to begin the transfusion. (See *Transfusing blood.*)

After you begin the transfusion, assess the patient and monitor his vital signs according to his transfusion history and your facility's policy — usually every 15 minutes for the first hour.

I'll need to monitor your status throughout the entire transfusion.

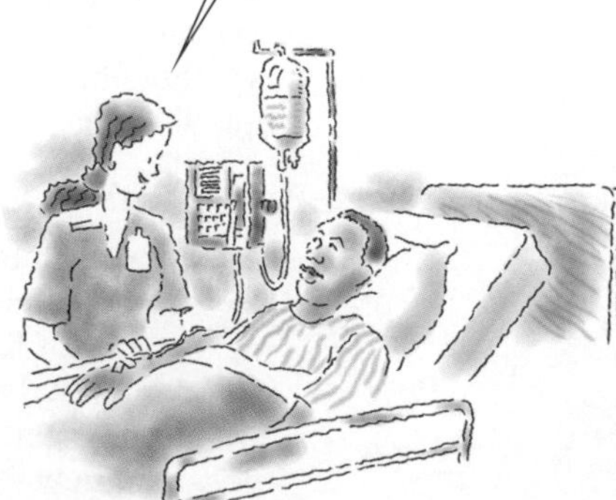

Stop the transfusion!

Watch for these signs or symptoms of a transfusion reaction:
- fever
- chills
- rigors
- headache
- nausea
- facial flushing.

Transfusing blood

To begin transfusing blood, follow the steps described here.

Let's begin

- Explain the procedure to the patient, including possible signs and symptoms of a transfusion reaction (chills, rash, fever, back pain, or dizziness), and obtain his consent according to your facility policy.
- Wash your hands and put on gloves, a gown, goggles, and a mask.
- If the patient doesn't have an I.V. catheter in place, perform a venipuncture using a 20G or larger-diameter catheter.
- Obtain the ordered blood or blood product from the blood bank.

Check, recheck, and verify

When you're ready to start the transfusion, proceed with the following steps:

- Check, recheck, and verify the type, Rh, and expiration date of the blood or cellular component. Also, double-check that you're giving the right blood or cellular component to the right patient, as shown below.
- Observe the blood or cellular component for abnormal color, clumping of red blood cells (RBCs), gas bubbles, and extraneous material that might indicate bacterial contamination. If you see any of these signs, return the bag to the blood bank.

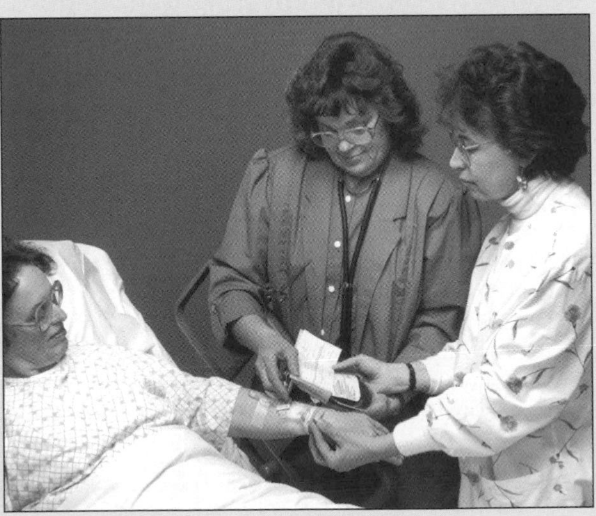

Ready to start

- Using a blood administration set, begin by closing all the clamps on the set. Then insert the spike of the line you're using for the normal saline solution into the bag of normal saline solution. Next, open the port on the blood bag and insert the spike of the line you're using to administer the blood or cellular component into the port. Hang the bag of normal saline solution and blood or cellular component on the I.V. pole, as shown in the left photograph on page 206.
- Open the clamp on the line of normal saline solution, and squeeze the drip chamber until it's half full of normal saline solution. Then remove the adapter cover at the tip of the blood administration set, open the main flow clamp, and prime the tubing with normal saline solution. Close the clamp and recap the adapter.

The transfusion itself

To transfuse the blood or cellular component, follow these steps:

- Take the patient's vital signs to serve as baseline values. Recheck vital signs after 15 minutes (or according to facility policy).
- Attach the prepared blood administration set to the venous access device using a needleless connection and flush it with normal saline solution.
- When administering whole blood or white blood cells, gently invert the bag several times during the procedure to mix the cells. (During the transfusion, gently agitate the bag to prevent the viscous cells from settling.)
- After you've flushed the venous access device, begin to transfuse the blood.
- Adjust the flow clamp closest to the patient to deliver a flow rate no greater than 5 ml/minute for the first 15 minutes of the transfusion, as shown on the next page. The type of blood product given and the patient's clinical condition determine the rate of transfusion. A unit of RBCs may be given over a period of 1 to 4 hours; platelets and coagulation factors may be given more quickly than RBCs and granulocytes.

(continued)

Transfusing blood *(continued)*

- A transfusion shouldn't take longer than 4 hours because the risk of contamination and sepsis increases after that. Discard or return to the blood bank any blood or blood products not given within this time, as facility policy directs.
- If the patient can't tolerate an infusion of 1 unit of blood within 4 hours, it may be appropriate to have the blood bank divide the unit and keep one portion refrigerated until it can be administered.

Hanging the bag

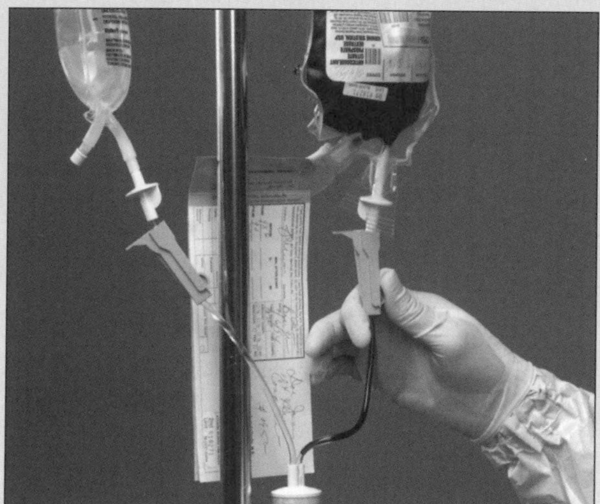

Adjusting the clamp

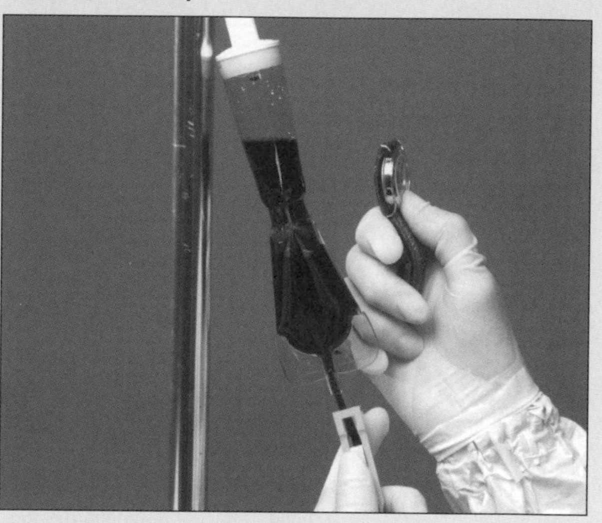

If you detect any of these signs or symptoms, quickly stop the transfusion and reestablish the normal saline solution infusion. *Note:* If you're using a Y-set, don't restart the infusion by opening the clamp; you'll just deliver more of the blood that's causing the problem. Instead, use a new bag and tubing to restart the infusion. (See *Monitoring a blood transfusion.*)

Next, check and record the patient's vital signs. Notify the practitioner immediately and don't dispose of the blood. If no signs of a reaction appear within 15 minutes, adjust the flow clamp to achieve the ordered infusion rate. Monitor the patient throughout the entire transfusion according to your facility's policy and procedures. (See *Transfusion don'ts*, page 208.)

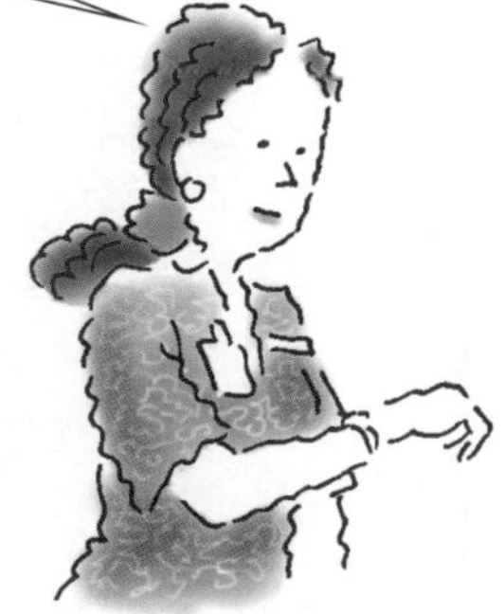

Monitoring a blood transfusion

To help avoid transfusion reactions and safeguard your patient, follow these guidelines:

- Record the patient's vital signs before the transfusion, 15 minutes after the start of the transfusion, and just after the transfusion is complete, and more frequently if warranted by the patient's condition and transfusion history or the facility's policy. Most acute hemolytic reactions occur during the first 30 minutes of the transfusion, so watch your patient carefully during the first 30 minutes.
- Always have sterile normal saline solution, an isotonic solution, set up as a primary line along with the transfusion.
- Act promptly if your patient develops wheezing and bronchospasm. These signs may indicate an allergic reaction or anaphylaxis. If, after a few milliliters of blood are transfused, the patient becomes dyspneic and shows generalized flushing and chest pain (with or without vomiting and diarrhea), he could be having an anaphylactic reaction. Stop the blood transfusion immediately, start the normal saline solution, check and document the patient's vital signs, and call the practitioner and initiate anaphylaxis procedure.
- If the patient develops a transfusion reaction, return the remaining blood together with a posttransfusion blood sample and any other required specimens to the blood bank.

Pressure points (or cuff stuff)

A pressure cuff on the blood container can increase the flow rate. If you use one, make sure that it's equipped with a pressure gauge and it exerts uniform compression against all parts of the container. Check the manufacturer's guidelines before using these devices to administer blood or blood components. (See *The pressure is on*, page 209.)

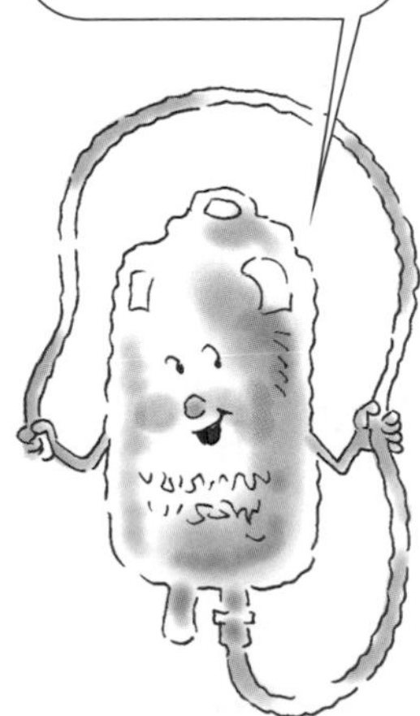

Terminating the transfusion

After a transfusion is complete, follow these steps:

- Flush the blood tubing with an adequate amount of normal saline solution according to the patient's condition.
- On a Y-type set, close the clamp on the blood line and open the clamp on the saline solution line.

Transfusion don'ts

A blood transfusion requires extreme care. Here are some tips on what not to do when administering a transfusion:

- Don't add medications to the blood bag.
- Never give blood products without checking the order against the blood bag label—the only way to tell if the request form has been stamped with the wrong name. Most life-threatening reactions occur when this step is omitted.
- Don't transfuse the blood product if you discover a discrepancy in the blood number, blood slip type, or patient identification number.
- Don't piggyback blood into the port of an existing infusion set. Most solutions, including dextrose in water, are incompatible with blood. Administer blood only with normal saline solution.
- Don't hesitate to stop the transfusion if your patient shows changes in vital signs, is dyspneic or restless, or develops chills, hematuria, or pain in the flank, chest, or back. Your patient could go into shock, so don't remove the I.V. device that's in place. Keep it open with a slow infusion of normal saline solution; call the practitioner and the laboratory.

- Discard the tubing, filter, and blood bag according to your facility's policy.
- Reassess the patient's condition and vital signs.

Don't forget to document

Make sure that you record:

- date and time of the transfusion
- identification number on the blood bag
- type and amount of blood transfused
- volume of normal saline solution infused
- status of the venous access device
- patient's vital signs
- signs or symptoms of a reaction (or the absence of signs or symptoms)
- how the patient tolerated the procedure.

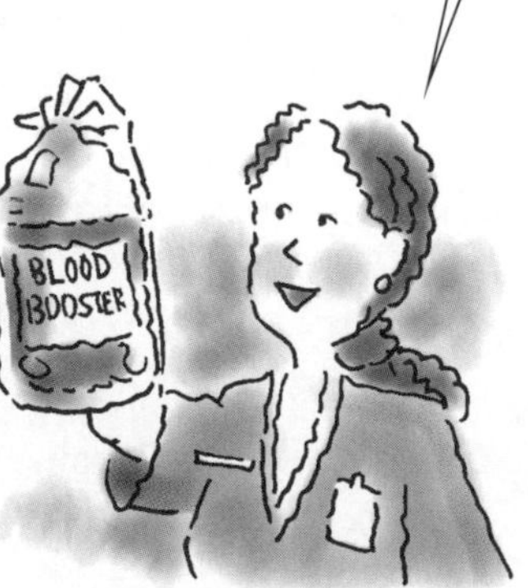

Plasma and plasma fractions give a boost to the circulating blood volume.
BLOOD BOOSTER

Plasma and plasma fractions

Plasma and plasma fractions are the anticoagulated clear portion of blood that has been run through a centrifuge. They make up about 55% of blood and are used in transfusion therapy to:

(Text continues on page 210.)

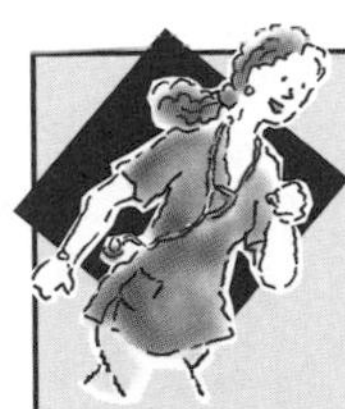

Running smoothly

The pressure is on

Rapid blood replacement requires transfusing blood under pressure. A pressure cuff is placed over the blood bag like a sleeve and inflated, as shown below. The pressure gauge, attached to the cuff, is calibrated in millimeters of mercury (mm Hg).

Prepare, prime, correct

To use this device, prepare the patient and set up the equipment as you would with a straight-line blood administration set. Prime the filter and tubing with normal saline solution to remove all air from the administration set. Connect the tubing to the catheter hub.

Note: By increasing the pressure, you also increase the speed at which complications, such as infiltration, can occur. Therefore, watch the patient closely.

Using a pressure cuff

To use a pressure cuff:

- Insert your hand into the top of the pressure cuff sleeve and pull the blood bag up through the center opening. Then hang the blood bag loop on the hook provided with the sleeve.
- Hang the pressure cuff and blood bag on the I.V. pole. Open the flow clamp on the tubing.
- To set the flow rate, turn the screw clamp on the pressure cuff counterclockwise. Compress the pressure bulb of the cuff to inflate the bag until you achieve the desired flow rate. Then turn the screw clamp clockwise to maintain this constant flow rate.
- As the blood bag empties, the pressure decreases, so check the flow rate regularly and adjust the pressure in the pressure cuff as necessary to maintain a consistent rate. Don't allow the cuff needle to exceed 300 mm Hg; excessively high pressure can cause hemolysis and damage the component container or rupture the blood bag.

Pressure cuff

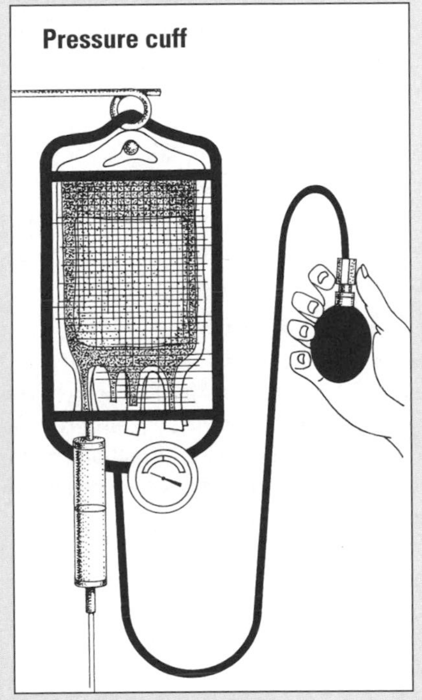

- correct blood deficiencies such as a low platelet count
- control bleeding tendencies that result from clotting factor deficiencies
- increase the patient's circulating blood volume.

Perusing plasma products

Before a transfusion, obtain the plasma or plasma fractions ordered. Commonly transfused plasma products include:
- fresh frozen plasma
- albumin
- cryoprecipitate
- factor VIII concentrate.

The patient's condition dictates which plasma product is needed. (See *Guide to plasma products.*)

Plasma proxies

Plasma substitutes may be used to maintain blood volume in an emergency, such as acute hemorrhage and shock. Plasma substitutes lack oxygen-carrying and coagulation properties, but using them allows time to get the patient's blood typed and crossmatched.

Depending on the circumstances, you may give:
- synthetic volume expander such as dextran in saline solution
- natural volume expander, such as plasma protein fraction and albumin.

Faced with an emergency? Plasma substitutes can buy valuable time.
EMERGENCY
RESCUE

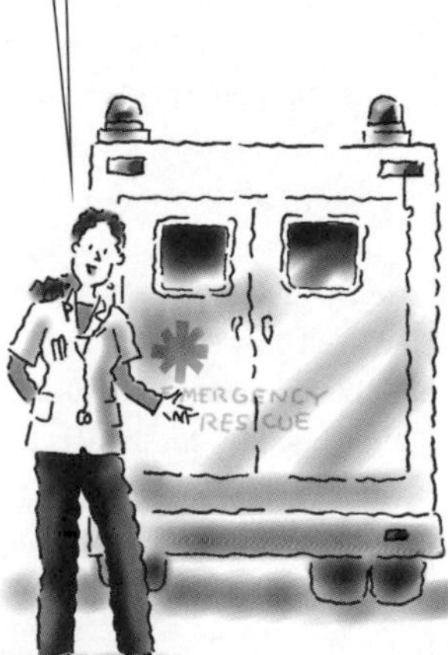

Selecting equipment

Gather the following infusion equipment:
- in-line or add-on filters or a filter system designated for the ordered component (usually a 170-micron filter) (*Note:* Never use a microaggregate filter to infuse platelets or plasma; it could remove essential components from the transfusion.)
- normal saline solution
- I.V. pole
- clean gloves, gown, mask, and goggles
- ordered plasma or plasma fractions
- venipuncture equipment, if necessary.

Starting the transfusion

Before you begin a transfusion, review the procedure. (See *Transfusing plasma or plasma fractions*, page 213.)

Guide to plasma products

The chart below lists various plasma products and their indications for transfusion along with relevant nursing considerations for each.

Blood component	Indications	Compatibility	Nursing considerations
Fresh frozen plasma (FFP)			
Uncoagulated plasma separated from RBCs and rich in coagulation factors V, VIII, and IX	• To treat postoperative hemorrhage • To correct an undetermined coagulation factor deficiency • To replace a specific factor when that factor isn't available • Warfarin reversal	• ABO compatibility required • Rh match not required	• Use a blood administration set, and administer infusion rapidly. • Keep in mind that large-volume transfusions of FFP may require correction for hypocalcemia because citric acid in FFP binds calcium. • Infuse within 24 hours of being thawed.
Albumin 5% (buffered saline); albumin 25% (salt-poor)			
A small plasma protein prepared by fractionating pooled plasma	• To replace volume lost because of shock from burns, trauma, surgery, or infections • To treat hypoproteinemia (with or without edema)	• Not required	• Use administration set supplied by manufacturer and set rate based on patient's condition and response. • Keep in mind that albumin is contraindicated in severe anemia. • Administer cautiously in cardiac and pulmonary disease because heart failure may result from circulatory overload.
Factor VIII concentrate (antihemophilic factor)			
Cold insoluble portion of plasma recovered from FFP	• To treat a patient with hemophilia A • To treat a patient with von Willebrand's disease	• ABO compatibility not required	• Administer by I.V. injection using a filter needle, or use administration set supplied by manufacturer.
Cryoprecipitate			
Insoluble plasma portion of FFP containing fibrinogen, factor VIIIc, factor VIIvWF, factor XIII and fibronectin	• To treat factor VIII deficiency and fibrinogen disorders • To treat significant factor XIII deficiency	• ABO compatibility required • Rh match not required	• Administer with a blood administration set. • Add normal saline solution to each bag of cryoprecipitate, as necessary, to facilitate infusion. • Keep in mind that cryoprecipitate must be administered within 6 hours of thawing. • Before administration, check laboratory studies to confirm a deficiency of one of specific clotting factors present in cryoprecipitate. • Be aware that patients with hemophilia A or von Willebrand's disease should only be treated with cryoprecipitate when appropriate factor VIII concentrates aren't available.

When you're ready to begin the transfusion, follow these steps:

- Make sure that the patient has a functional venous access device (20G or greater), or insert one as needed.
- Put on clean gloves and other protective equipment that your facility requires.
- Verify that you have the correct blood product and that it matches the number designated for the patient.
- Check the expiration date of the plasma or plasma fraction.
- Double-check that you're giving the right plasma or plasma fraction.
- Inspect the plasma or plasma fraction for cloudiness and turbidity, which could indicate possible contamination.
- Spike the bag with component-specific tubing (if the blood bank provided it) or with the blood tubing specified by your facility's policy and procedures.
- Prime the tubing.
- Explain the procedure to the patient.
- Obtain the patient's baseline vital signs, and continue to check vital signs frequently according to your facility's policy.
- Attach the plasma, fresh frozen plasma, albumin, factor VIII concentrate, platelets, or cryoprecipitate to the patient's flushed venous access device.
- Begin the transfusion, and adjust the flow rate as ordered.
- Take the patient's vital signs, and assess him frequently for signs or symptoms of a transfusion reaction, such as fever, chills, or nausea. If a reaction occurs, quickly stop the infusion and start a normal saline solution infusion at a keep-vein-open rate. Check and record the patient's vital signs. Notify the practitioner.
- After the infusion, flush the line with saline solution, according to your facility's policy. Then disconnect the I.V. tubing. If therapy will continue, hang the original I.V. solution and adjust the flow rate as ordered.
- Record the type and amount of plasma or plasma fraction administered, duration of transfusion, baseline vital signs, adverse reactions, and how the patient tolerated the procedure.

If you suspect a transfusion reaction, stop the infusion quickly and start a normal saline solution at a keep-vein-open rate. Document your patient's vital signs, and notify the practitioner right away.

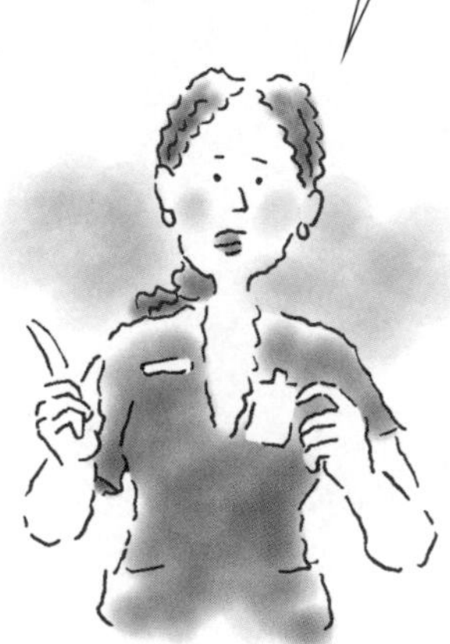

Transfusing plasma or plasma fractions

To transfuse plasma or plasma fractions, follow these steps:
- Obtain baseline vital signs.
- Flush the patient's venous access device with normal saline solution.
- Attach the plasma, fresh frozen plasma, albumin, factor VIII concentrate, platelets, or cryoprecipitate to the patient's venous access device.
- Begin the transfusion, and adjust the flow rate as ordered.
- Take the patient's vital signs, and assess him frequently for signs or symptoms of a transfusion reaction, such as fever, chills, and nausea.
- After the infusion, flush the line with 20 to 30 ml of normal saline solution. Then disconnect the I.V. tubing. If therapy is to continue, resume the prescribed infusate and adjust the flow rate, as ordered.
- Record the type and amount of plasma or plasma fraction administered, duration of transfusion, baseline vital signs, and any adverse reactions.

Specialized transfusion methods

Specialized methods for administering blood include:
- autotransfusion, the process of collecting, filtering, and reinfusing the patient's own blood
- hemapheresis, the process of collecting and removing specific blood components and then returning the remaining components to the donor.

A self-help movement

Many patients prefer autotransfusion because it eliminates the risk of infectious disease. They can begin giving blood 4 to 6 weeks before surgery; the units are collected, labeled, and stored until needed.

Blood can also be collected during surgery. It's treated with an anticoagulant and collected in a sterile container that's fitted with a filter. The blood is reinfused as whole blood or processed before infusion. Salvaged blood can't be stored because the filtering and processing can't remove bacteria completely.

Autotransfusion uses the patient's own blood, eliminating the risk of infectious disease.

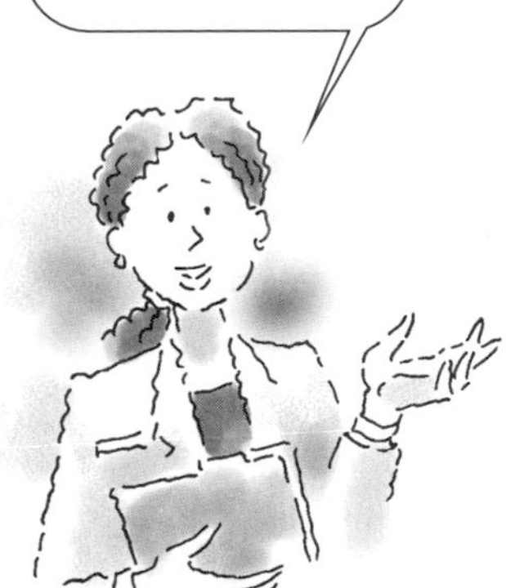

Seeking skilled nurses

Hemapheresis and autotransfusion must be performed by skilled personnel. Only nurses who are familiar with the procedures should monitor and evaluate a patient's condition throughout the transfusion.

Patients with special needs

Pediatric and elderly patients require special care during transfusion therapy. For instance, transfusing blood into a neonate requires specialized skills because the neonate's physiologic requirements differ vastly from those of an older infant, child, adolescent, or adult.

There are significant differences — such as equipment, amount, and rate, to name a few — in transfusions for children.

Pediatric patients

Transfusions in children differ significantly from transfusions in adults.

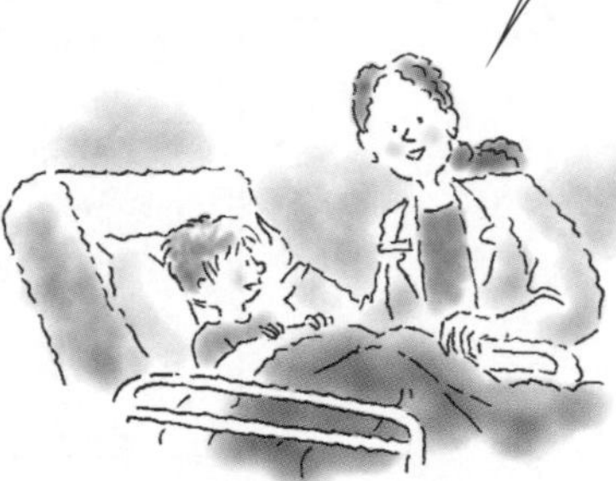

Half-unit for half-pints

Blood units for pediatric patients are prepared in half-unit packs, and a 24G catheter is used to administer the blood.

Rating children differently

The rate of the infusion also differs. Usually, a child receives 5% to 10% of the total transfusion in the first 15 minutes of therapy. To maintain the correct flow rate, be sure to use an electronic infusion device.

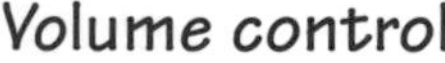

Volume control

A child's normal circulating blood volume determines the amount of blood transfused. The average blood volume for children and infants older than 1 month is 75 ml/kg. The proportion of blood volume to body weight decreases with age.

Good communication

Whenever you transfuse blood in an infant or child, explain the procedure, its purpose, and the possible complications to the parents or legal guardian. If appropriate, also include the child in the explanation. Ask the parents for the child's transfusion history, and obtain their consent.

A watchful eye

Closely monitor the child, particularly during the first 15 minutes, to detect early signs of a reaction. Use a blood warmer, if indicated, to prevent hypothermia and cardiac arrhythmias, especially if you're administering blood through a central venous access device.

A child's problem with grown-up indications

In massive hemorrhage and shock, the indications for blood component transfusion in children remain similar to those for adults, although accurate assessment is difficult. Draw blood from a central vein to get more accurate hemoglobin and hematocrit measurements, or use blood pressure readings to assess blood volume.

Aging slows the immune system, placing elderly patients at higher risk for delayed transfusion reactions.

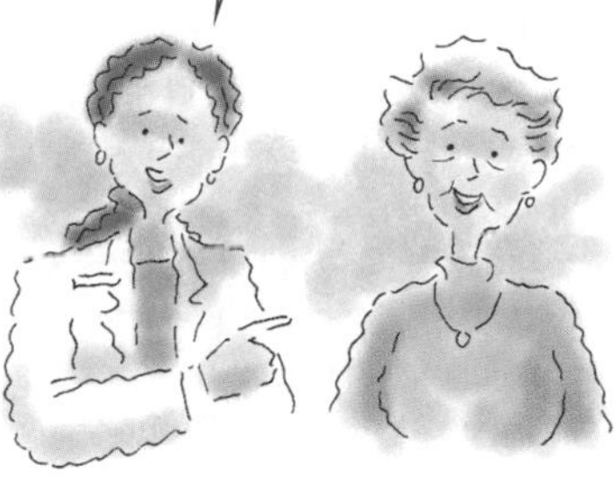

Elderly patients

An elderly patient with preexisting heart disease may be unable to tolerate rapid transfusion of an entire unit of blood without exhibiting shortness of breath or other signs of heart failure. The patient may be better able to tolerate half-unit blood transfusions.

Delayed reaction

Age-related slowing of the immune system puts an older adult at risk for delayed transfusion reactions. Because greater quantities of blood products transfuse before signs or symptoms appear, the patient may experience a more severe reaction. Also, an elderly patient tends to be less resistant to infection.

Complications

Always take steps to prevent transfusion complications, and know how to manage them when they arise. (See *Correcting transfusion problems*, page 216.)

Transfusion reactions

Usually attributed to major antigen-antibody reactions, transfusion reactions may occur up to 96 hours after the transfusion begins. Transfusion reactions occur more commonly with the administration of platelets, WBCs, and cryoprecipitate than with whole blood, RBCs, or plasma.

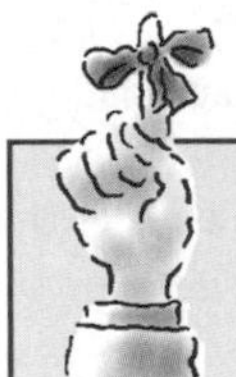

Memory jogger

To remember what to do in the event of a transfusion reaction, think of the acronym **SPIN:**

Stop the infusion.

Pulse and other vital signs (check 'em).

Infuse normal saline solution.

Notify the practitioner.

Stop immediately!

Whenever you detect signs or symptoms of an acute transfusion reaction, immediately stop the transfusion. Then follow these steps:

- Change the I.V. tubing to prevent infusing more blood. Save the blood tubing and bag for analysis.
- Administer normal saline solution to keep the vein patent (open).
- Take and record the patient's vital signs.
- Notify the practitioner.

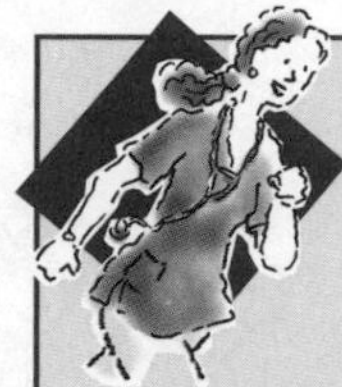

Running smoothly

Correcting transfusion problems

A patient who receives excellent care can still encounter problems during a transfusion. Here's how to proceed when common transfusion problems occur.

It stopped!

If the transfusion stops, follow these steps:

- Check that the I.V. container is at least 3′ (1 m) above the level of the I.V. site.
- Make sure that the flow clamp is open.
- Make sure that the blood completely covers the filter. If it doesn't, squeeze the drip chamber until it does.
- Gently rock the bag back and forth, agitating blood cells that may have settled on the bottom.
- If using a Y-type blood administration set, close the flow clamp to the patient and lower the blood bag. Next, open the normal saline solution line clamp and allow the solution to flow into the blood bag. Rehang the blood bag, open the flow clamp to the patient, and reset the flow rate.

Hematoma

If a hematoma develops at the I.V. site, follow these steps:

- Immediately stop the infusion.
- Remove the catheter. Cap the tubing with a new needleless connection.
- Notify the practitioner and expect to place ice on the site for 24 hours; after that, apply warm compresses.
- Promote reabsorption of the hematoma by having the patient gently exercise the affected limb.
- Document your observations and actions.

An empty bag

If the blood bag empties before the next one arrives when using a Y-type set, close the blood line clamp, open the normal saline solution line clamp, and let the normal saline solution run slowly until the new blood arrives. Make sure that you decrease the flow rate or clamp the line before attaching the new unit of blood.

If you encounter a transfusion stoppage, check the I.V. container and flow clamp.
STOP

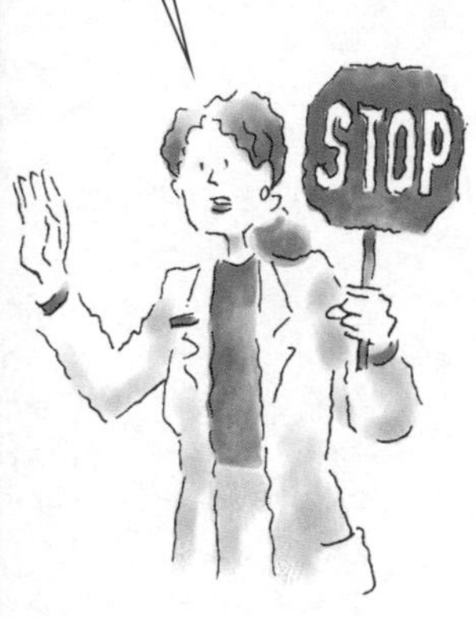

- Obtain a urine specimen and blood sample and send them to the laboratory.
- Prepare for further treatment.
- Complete a transfusion reaction report and an incident report according to your facility's policies and procedures.

The practitioner or blood bank may eliminate some of these steps if a patient has a history of frequent mild reactions.

The rundown on reactions

Transfusion of blood products that have been processed and preserved increases the patient's risk of complications, especially if the patient receives frequent transfusions of large amounts. Hemolytic, febrile, and allergic reactions can follow any transfusion. (See *Managing transfusion reactions*, pages 218 and 219.)

Hemolytic reactions

An acute hemolytic reaction is life-threatening. It occurs as a result of incompatible blood. It also can occur as a result of improper storage of blood.

Clean up clerical errors

A hemolytic reaction almost always results from a clerical error, such as mislabeling or failing to identify the patient properly. It may progress to shock and renal failure.

Febrile reactions

Nonhemolytic febrile reactions are characterized by a temperature increase of 1.8° F (1° C). Such reactions are related to a transfusion and aren't caused by disease.

Antibodies battling antigens

Febrile reactions usually result from the patient's anti-HLA antibodies reacting against antigens on the donor's WBCs or platelets. Febrile reactions may occur in approximately 1% of transfusions. They can occur immediately or within 2 hours after completion of a transfusion.

Signs and symptoms of febrile reactions include:

- fever
- chills
- headache
- nausea and vomiting
- hypotension
- chest pain
- dyspnea
- nonproductive cough
- malaise.

Keep a watchful eye for these signs of a febrile reaction.

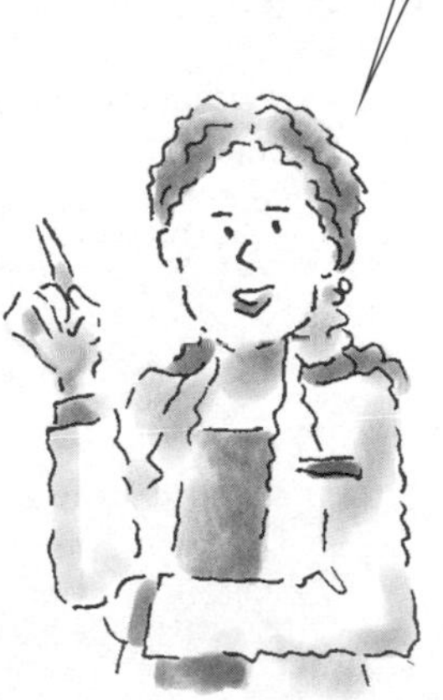

(Text continues on page 220.)

Managing transfusion reactions

If your patient experiences a transfusion reaction, stop the infusion and consult this chart for further steps and tips for preventing future reactions.

Reaction	Nursing interventions	Prevention
Reactions from any transfusion		
Hemolytic	• Monitor blood pressure. • Treat shock as indicated by the patient's condition, using I.V. fluids, oxygen, epinephrine, a diuretic, and a vasopressor. • Obtain posttransfusion reaction blood and urine samples for evaluation. • Observe for signs of hemorrhage resulting from disseminated intravascular coagulation.	• Before the transfusion, check donor and recipient blood types to ensure blood compatibility; also identify the patient with another nurse or practitioner present. • Transfuse blood slowly for the first 15 to 20 minutes; closely observe the patient for the first 30 minutes of the transfusion.
Febrile	• Relieve symptoms with an antipyretic or antihistamine.	• Premedicate with an antipyretic, an antihistamine and, possibly, a steroid. • Use leukocyte-poor or washed red blood cells (RBCs). Use a leukocyte removal filter specific to the component.
Allergic	• Administer antihistamines. • Monitor for anaphylactic reaction and administer epinephrine and steroids, if indicated.	• Premedicate with an antihistamine if the patient has a history of allergic reactions. • Observe the patient closely for the first 30 minutes of the transfusion.
Plasma protein incompatibility	• Treat for shock by administering oxygen, fluids, epinephrine and, possibly, a steroid as ordered.	• Transfuse only immunoglobulin A-deficient blood or well-washed RBCs.
Bacterial contamination	• Treat with a broad-spectrum antibiotic and a steroid.	• Inspect blood before the transfusion for gas, clots, and dark purple color. • Use air-free, touch-free methods to draw and deliver blood. • Maintain strict storage control. • Change the blood tubing and filter every 4 hours. • Infuse each unit of blood over 2 to 4 hours; terminate the infusion if the period exceeds 4 hours. • Maintain sterile technique when administering blood products.

Managing transfusion reactions *(continued)*

Reaction	Nursing interventions	Prevention
Reactions from any transfusion *(continued)*		
Circulation overload	• Stop the transfusion. • Maintain the I.V. with normal saline solution. • Administer oxygen. • Elevate the patient's head. • Administer diuretics as ordered by the practitioner.	• Transfuse blood slowly. • Don't exceed 2 units in 4 hours; fewer for elderly patients, infants, or patients with cardiac conditions.
Reactions from multiple transfusions		
Hemosiderosis	• Perform a phlebotomy to remove excess iron.	• Administer blood only when absolutely necessary.
Bleeding tendencies	• Administer platelets. • Monitor the platelet count.	• Use only fresh blood (less than 7 days old) when possible.
Elevated blood ammonia level	• Monitor the ammonia level. • Decrease the amount of protein in the diet. • If indicated, give neomycin sulfate or lactulose.	• Use only RBCs, fresh frozen plasma, or fresh blood, especially if the patient has hepatic disease.
Increased oxygen affinity for hemoglobin	• Monitor arterial blood gas levels and give respiratory support as needed.	• Use only RBCs or fresh blood if possible.
Hypothermia	• Stop the transfusion. • Warm the patient with blankets. • Obtain an electrocardiogram (ECG).	• Warm the blood to 95° to 98° F (35° to 37° C), especially before massive transfusions.
Hypocalcemia	• Monitor potassium and calcium levels. • Use blood less than 2 days old if administering multiple units. • Slow or stop the transfusion, depending on the reaction. Expect a worse reaction in hypothermic patients or patients with elevated potassium levels. • Slowly administer calcium gluconate I.V.	• Infuse blood slowly.
Potassium intoxication	• Obtain an ECG. • Administer sodium polystyrene sulfonate (Kayexalate) orally or by enema. • Administer I.V. insulin and glucose.	• Use fresh blood when administering massive transfusions.

Allergic reactions

An allergic reaction is the second most common transfusion reaction. It occurs because of an allergen in the transfused blood. Signs of an allergic reaction may include:

- itching
- hives
- fever
- chills
- facial swelling
- wheezing
- throat swelling.

An anaphylactic advance

An allergic reaction may progress to an anaphylactic reaction. This reaction can occur immediately or within 1 hour after infusion. Severe anaphylactic reactions produce bronchospasm, dyspnea, pulmonary edema, and hypotension. Treatment includes immediate administration of epinephrine, corticosteroids, and antihistamines.

Plasma protein incompatibility

Plasma protein incompatibility usually results from blood that contains immunoglobulin A (IgA) proteins being infused into an IgA-deficient recipient who has developed anti-IgA antibodies. The reaction can be life-threatening and usually resembles anaphylaxis. Signs and symptoms include:

- flushing and urticaria
- abdominal pain
- chills
- fever
- dyspnea and wheezing
- hypotension
- shock
- cardiac arrest.

As storage time and temperature increase, growth of microorganisms also increases.

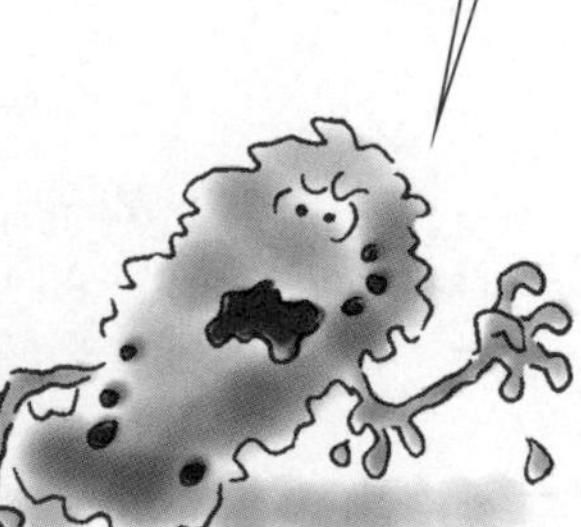

Bacterial contamination

Blood and blood products may be contaminated during the collection process. As storage times and temperature increase, growth of microorganisms also increases. The resulting transfusion reaction is most commonly related to the endotoxins produced by gram-negative bacteria. Signs and symptoms of bacterial contamination include:

- chills
- fever
- vomiting

- abdominal cramping
- diarrhea
- shock
- kidney failure.

Reactions from multiple transfusions

Reactions from multiple transfusions include:

- hemosiderosis
- bleeding tendencies
- elevated blood ammonia levels
- increased oxygen affinity for hemoglobin
- hypothermia
- hypocalcemia
- potassium intoxication.

Hemosiderosis

Accumulation of an iron-containing pigment (hemosiderin) may be associated with RBC destruction in patients who receive many transfusions. In hemosiderosis, the patient's iron plasma level is greater than 200 mg/dl.

Bleeding tendencies

A low platelet count — which can develop in stored blood — can cause bleeding tendencies. Signs and symptoms may include abnormal bleeding, oozing from a cut or break in the skin surface, and abnormal clotting values.

Elevated blood ammonia level

Blood ammonia levels can increase in patients receiving transfusions of stored blood. Signs and symptoms of high blood ammonia levels include forgetfulness and confusion. The patient may also have a sweet mouth odor. High ammonia levels can cause behaviors that range from stuporlike to combative.

Does your patient seem to be in a stupor? Or, at the other extreme, combative? Check ammonia levels.

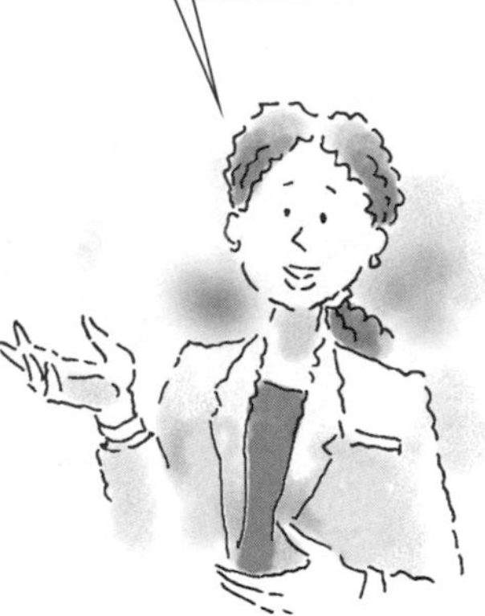

Increased oxygen affinity for hemoglobin

A blood transfusion can cause a decreased level of 2,3-diphosphoglycerate (2,3-DPG). Found on RBCs but scarce in stored blood, 2,3-DPG affects the oxyhemoglobin dissociation curve. This curve represents hemoglobin saturation and desaturation in graph form. Levels of 2,3-DPG (as well as other factors) cause the curve to shift either to the right (causing a decrease in oxygen affinity) or to the left (causing an increase in oxygen affinity).

A shift to the left

When 2,3-DPG levels are low, they produce a shift to the left. This shift causes an increase in oxygen affinity for hemoglobin, so the oxygen stays in the patient's bloodstream and isn't released into other tissues. Signs of this reaction include a depressed respiratory rate, especially in patients with chronic lung disease.

Hypothermia

A rapid infusion of large amounts of cold blood can cause hypothermia. The patient may experience shaking chills, hypotension, and cardiac arrhythmias, which may become life-threatening. Cardiac arrest can occur if core temperature falls below 86° F (30° C).

Infusing large amounts of cold blood rapidly can cause hypothermia. Aah... now that's better!

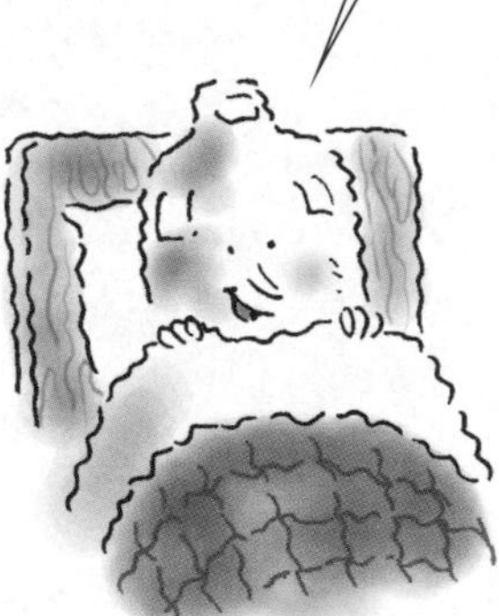

Hypocalcemia

If blood is infused too rapidly, citrate toxicity can occur. (Citrate is used to preserve blood.) Because citrate binds with calcium, calcium deficiency results. Hypocalcemia can also occur if normal citrate metabolism is hindered by a liver disorder.

Signs and symptoms of calcium deficiency include:

- tingling in the fingers
- muscle cramps
- nausea
- vomiting
- hypotension
- cardiac arrhythmias
- seizures.

Potassium intoxication

Some cells in stored RBCs may leak potassium into the plasma. Intoxication usually doesn't occur with transfusions of 1 to 2 units of blood; larger volumes, however, may cause potassium toxicity.

Signs and symptoms of potassium toxicity may include:

- irritability
- intestinal colic
- diarrhea
- muscle weakness
- oliguria
- renal failure
- electrocardiogram changes with tall, peaked T waves
- bradycardia that may proceed to cardiac arrest.

Transmission of disease

Unlike a transfusion reaction, an infectious disease transmitted during a transfusion may go undetected until days, weeks, or months later, when signs and symptoms appear. Remember, all blood products are potential carriers of infectious disease, including:

- hepatitis
- HIV
- CMV.

Steps to prevent disease transmission include laboratory testing of blood products and careful screening of potential donors. Neither of these precautions is foolproof.

Hepatitis in hiding?

Hepatitis C (non-A, non-B) accounts for most posttransfusion hepatitis cases. However, the test that detects hepatitis C can produce false-negative results and may allow some contamination to go undetected. Until the specific hepatitis C antibody is detected, diagnosis is principally established by obtaining negative test results for hepatitis A, B, and D.

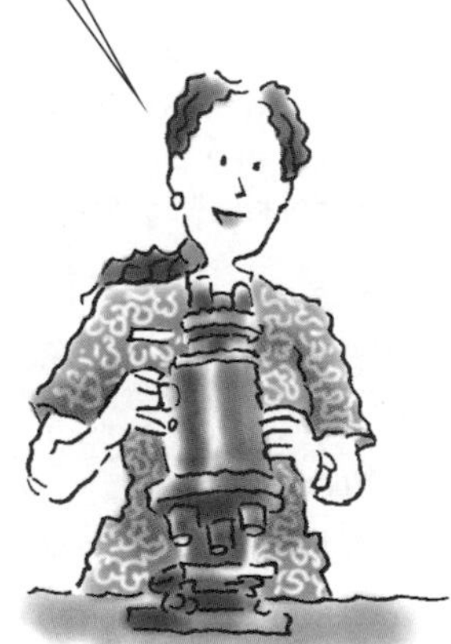

HIV watch

HIV screening determines the presence of antibodies and antigens to HIV. The Food and Drug Administration requires that the antigen test be used in conjunction with the antibody test to reduce the risk of exposure from blood transfusions. False-negative results can occur, particularly during the incubation period of about 6 to 12 weeks after exposure. The Centers for Disease Control and Prevention estimates that undetected infection occurs in 1 out of every 1,000,000 donations per year.

See any CMV?

Many facilities screen blood for CMV. Blood with CMV is especially dangerous for an immunosuppressed, seronegative patient.

Scanning for syphilis (just in case)

Facilities also test blood for the presence of syphilis, although the routine practice of refrigerating blood kills the syphilis organism. These measures have virtually eliminated the risk of transfusion-related syphilis.

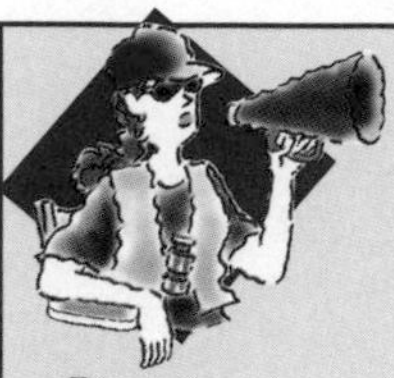

That's a wrap!

Transfusions review

Purpose

- To restore and maintain blood volume
- To improve the oxygen-carrying capacity of blood
- To replace deficient blood components

Compatibility

- ABO blood type: A, B, AB, O
- Rh blood group: Rh-positive, Rh-negative
- HLA blood group: controls compatibility between transfusion recipients and donors

Transfusion products

Whole blood

- Used to increase blood volume after massive hemorrhage

Packed RBCs

- Used to maintain or restore oxygen-carrying capability and capacity

Leukocyte-poor RBCs

- Used for patients who need RBCs but who have had a febrile or nonhemolytic reaction in the past

Granulocytes

- Used when granulocytes are low or to fight overwhelming infection

Platelets

- Used to control or prevent bleeding

Plasma and plasma fractions

- Used to correct blood deficiencies, control bleeding tendencies caused by clotting factor deficiencies, and increase circulating blood volume

Transfusion reactions

Hemolytic

- Caused by incompatible blood
- May result in renal failure and shock
- May be life-threatening

Febrile

- Occurs when the patient's anti-HLA antibodies react against the donor's WBCs or platelets
- Causes flulike symptoms, chest pain, and hypotension

Allergic

- Caused by an allergen present in the transfused blood
- Causes hives, itching, fever, chills, facial swelling, wheezing, and sore throat

Plasma protein incompatibility

- Occurs when blood that contains immunoglobulin A (IgA) proteins is infused into an IgA-deficient recipient who has developed anti-IgA antibodies
- Causes flushing, abdominal pain, chills, fever, hypotension, shock, and cardiac arrest

Bacterial contamination

- Caused by contamination during the collection process
- Causes chills, fever, vomiting, abdominal cramping, diarrhea, shock, and kidney failure

Multiple transfusion reactions

- Hemosiderosis
- Bleeding tendencies
- Increased blood ammonia levels
- Increased oxygen affinity for hemoglobin
- Hypothermia
- Hypocalcemia
- Potassium intoxication

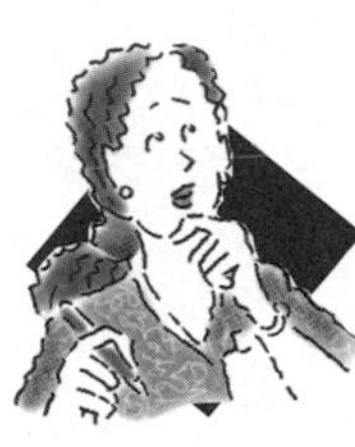

Quick quiz

1. What's the size of the micron filters that come with standard blood transfusion sets?

A. 60 microns
B. 170 microns
C. 100 microns
D. 120 microns

Answer: B. The standard blood administration set comes with a 170-micron filter.

2. Which type of transfusion involves collecting, filtering, and reinfusing the patient's own blood?

A. Autotransfusion
B. Hemapheresis
C. Plasmapheresis
D. Homologous

Answer: A. Autotransfusion involves collecting, filtering, and reinfusing the patient's own blood.

3. Fresh frozen plasma must be transfused within:

A. 6 hours.
B. 5 hours.
C. 4 hours.
D. 8 hours.

Answer: C. Plasma must be transfused within 4 hours because it doesn't contain preservatives.

4. If you detect signs or symptoms of a transfusion reaction, the first thing you should do is:

A. slow down the infusion rate.
B. notify the blood bank.
C. notify the practitioner.
D. stop the infusion.

Answer: D. If you detect signs or symptoms of a transfusion reaction, stop the transfusion and quickly take and record the patient's vital signs. Then start infusing normal saline solution at a slow rate and notify the practitioner.

5. You should start a blood transfusion at a slow rate to:

A. maintain blood volume.
B. observe for the effects of a transfusion reaction.
C. prevent clot formation at the tip of the venipuncture device.
D. prevent hypothermia.

Answer: B. Always start the transfusion at a slow rate to observe for the effects of a transfusion reaction.

6. The plasma product albumin is administered to:
A. correct an undetermined coagulation factor deficiency.
B. treat hypoproteinemia.
C. treat a patient with hemophilia A.
D. treat a congenital factor deficiency.

Answer: B. Albumin is a protein that's used to treat hypoproteinemia as well as to replace volume in shock and burns.

Scoring

☆☆☆ If you answered all six questions correctly, congrats! The information recipient (you) and the information donor (this chapter) are clearly compatible.

☆☆ If you answered four or five questions correctly, good going! The micron filter of your mind has allowed the key particles of information to successfully transfuse.

☆ If you answered fewer than four questions correctly, don't fret. Perhaps the flow rate on your information infusion device was set too low.

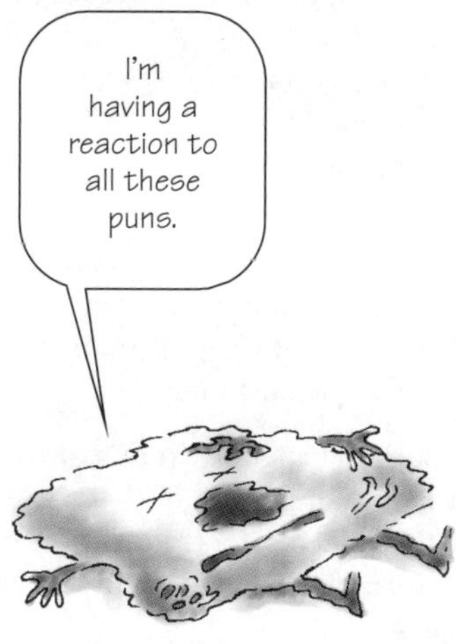

Chemotherapy infusions

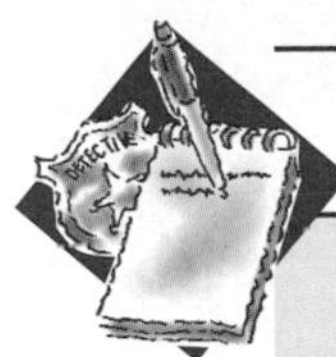

Just the facts

In this chapter, you'll learn:

- the way in which chemotherapy treats cancer
- types of chemotherapeutic drugs
- techniques for administering chemotherapy
- adverse effects of chemotherapy
- complications of chemotherapeutic drugs and how to avoid them.

Understanding I.V. chemotherapy

Chemotherapy, surgery, and radiation are the mainstays of cancer treatment. Chemotherapy is most commonly administered I.V., using peripheral or central veins—although it's also administered by the oral, subcutaneous (subQ), intrathecal, I.M., intra-arterial, and intracavitary routes.

Chemotherapeutic drugs may be administered in the practitioner's office, in an outpatient clinic, in the patient's home, or in a long-term care facility or hospital. Wherever treatments take place, the same basic principles of I.V. therapy apply. Because of rapid changes in health care delivery leading to a rise in chemotherapy administration outside the hospital setting, emphasis on patient teaching has also increased.

Once again, my ability to deliver an exact dose recommends me for the job.

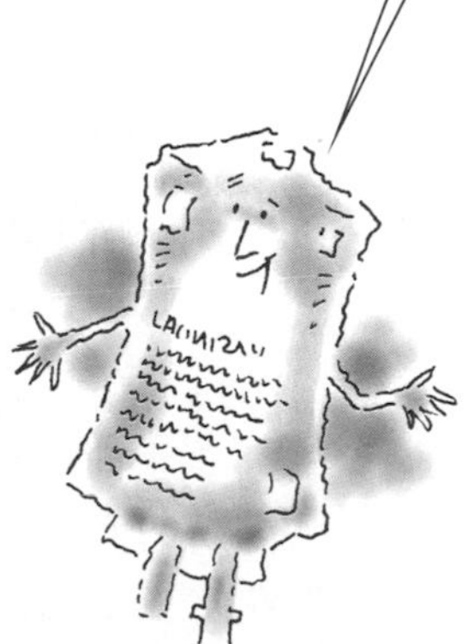

Precision is part of the decision

Suppressing rapidly dividing cancer cells with chemotherapy requires effective delivery of an exact dose of these toxic drugs. I.V. chemotherapy achieves this effective dosing. Additional benefits include complete absorption and systemic distribution.

Which cell is well?

Although chemotherapy is intended to control or eliminate cancer cells, it can also damage healthy cells. Healthy cells are attacked because the chemotherapy can't differentiate between healthy cells and cancerous ones. Chemotherapy attacks all rapidly growing cells. Because hair and nail follicles are rapidly growing cells, patients undergoing chemotherapy typically lose their hair and their nails become brittle.

Long-term I.V. chemotherapy, which involves frequent venipunctures, can make veins sclerotic. Patients can also be at risk for phlebitis or tissue necrosis caused by certain chemotherapeutic drugs.

Cycle-specific drugs are effective only during a specific phase of my life cycle…

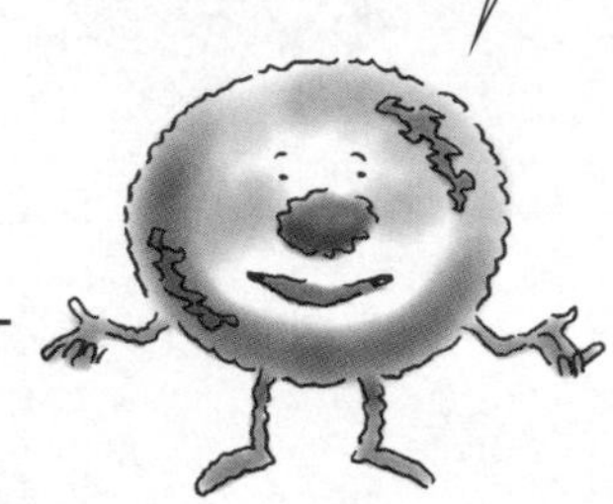

How chemotherapy works

Healthy and cancerous cells pass through similar life cycles and are similarly vulnerable to chemotherapeutic drugs. Some of these drugs are cycle-specific — designed to disrupt a specific biochemical process, making them effective only during specific phases of the cell cycle. Other drugs are cycle-nonspecific, meaning that their prolonged action is independent of the cell cycle, allowing them to act on both reproducing and resting cells.

Covering all the bases

Because tumor cells are active in various phases of the cell cycle, chemotherapy typically employs more than one drug. This way, each drug can target a different site or take action during a different phase of the cell cycle.

Let's get specific…as well as nonspecific

During a single administration of a cycle-nonspecific chemotherapeutic drug, a fixed percentage of normal and malignant cells die, while a percentage of normal and malignant cells survive.

When cycle-specific chemotherapy is administered, cells in the resting phase survive. (See *The cell cycle and chemotherapeutic drugs.*)

…whereas cycle-nonspecific drugs act independently of the cell cycle.

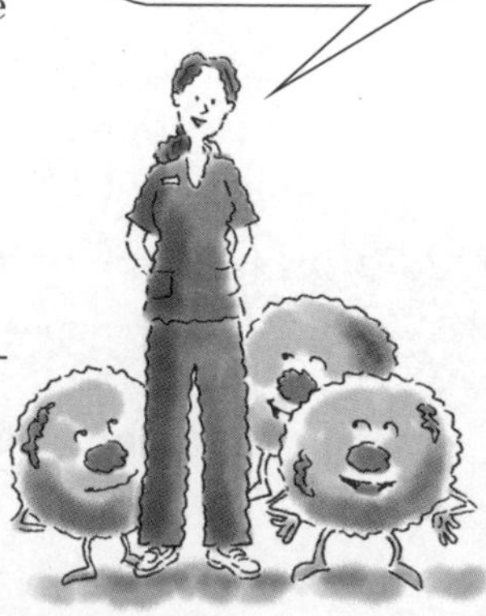

Calculating collateral cost

The challenge is to provide a drug dose large enough to kill the greatest number of cancer cells but small enough to avoid irreversibly damaging normal tissue or causing toxicity. Given in combination, chemotherapeutic drugs potentiate each other, and the tumor responds as it would to a larger dose of a single drug.

In addition, because different drugs work at different stages of the cell cycle or employ different mechanisms to kill cancer cells, using several drugs decreases the likelihood that the tumor will develop resistance to the chemotherapy.

The cell cycle and chemotherapeutic drugs

All cells cycle through five phases. Chemotherapeutic drugs that are active on cells during one or more of these phases are called cycle-specific. The illustration below tells what happens at each phase of the cell cycle and gives examples of cycle-specific drugs that are active during each phase.

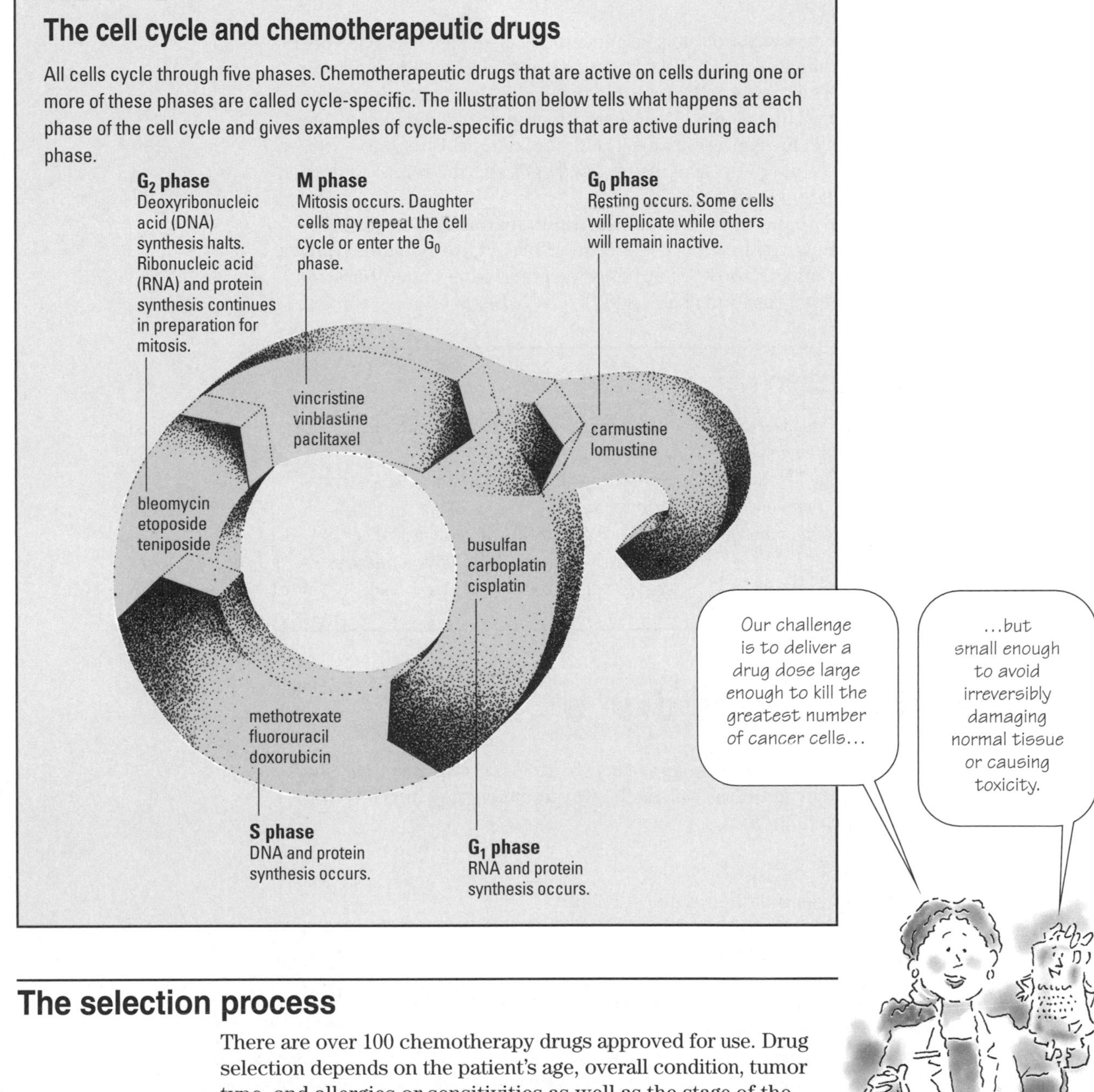

The selection process

There are over 100 chemotherapy drugs approved for use. Drug selection depends on the patient's age, overall condition, tumor type, and allergies or sensitivities as well as the stage of the cancer. Practitioners strive to select the most effective drugs for the first round of chemotherapy because this is when cancer cells respond best. Second- or third-line chemotherapeutic drugs may be used depending on the patient's hypersensitivity reaction or the tumor's resistance to the drugs.

Going in cycles

Eradicating a tumor calls for repeated drug doses, which is considered a single course of chemotherapy and is repeated on a cyclic basis. The cycle can be repeated daily, weekly, every other week, or every 3 to 4 weeks. Treatment cycles are carefully planned so normal cells can regenerate. The timing of repeat treatment cycles depends on the cycle of the targeted cells and the return of normal blood counts.

Most patients require at least three treatment cycles before they show any beneficial response. However, every patient differs. Some patients show faster tumor response time than others and some don't respond at all. (See *Determining tumor response.*)

Determining tumor response

The following scale is recommended by the World Health Organization to determine how a tumor responds to chemotherapy. The tumor size is measured 1 month after treatment begins and is compared to the size of the tumor at the beginning of treatment.

Complete response (CR)—complete disappearance of the tumor
Partial response (PR)—at least a 50% decrease in tumor size
Stable disease (SD)—no change in tumor size
Progressive disease (PD)—25% increase in tumor size or appearance of a new tumor

Chemotherapeutic drugs

Chemotherapeutic drugs are categorized according to their pharmacologic action as well as the way in which they interfere with cell production.

Dividing up the drugs

Cycle-specific drugs are divided into:
- antimetabolites
- plant alkaloids
- enzymes.

Cycle-nonspecific drugs are divided into:
- alkylating agents
- nitrosureas
- antineoplastics
- antibiotic antineoplastics
- miscellaneous drugs.

Other drugs used to inhibit tumor cell growth include steroids, hormones, and antihormones. These drugs work in the intracellular environment. Steroids, which normally act as anti-inflammatory agents, make malignant cells vulnerable to damage from cell-specific drugs. Hormones alter the environment of cells by affecting the permeability of their membranes. Antihormones affect hormone-dependent tumors by inheriting the production of those hormones or neutralizing their effects. (See *Selected chemotherapeutic drugs.*)

Steroids, hormones, and antihormones work within tumor cells to inhibit growth.

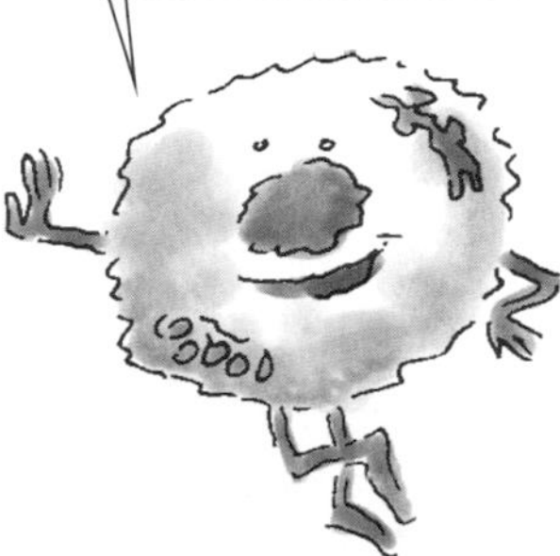

Multitasking drugs

Practitioners order chemotherapeutic drugs to control cancer, to cure cancer, to prevent metastasis, or for palliation. Drugs may be given alone or in combinations called *protocols.* (See *Sample chemotherapy protocols.*)

Selected chemotherapeutic drugs

Compare the characteristics and toxic effects of these chemotherapeutic drugs.

Category	Characteristics	Toxic effects
Cycle-specific		
Antimetabolites cytarabine, floxuridine, fluorouracil, gemcitabine, methotrexate, thioguanine	• Interfere with nucleic acid synthesis • Attack during S phase of cell cycle	• Effects on bone marrow (myelosuppression), central nervous system (CNS), and GI system
Vinca alkaloids vinblastine, vincristine	• Prevent mitotic spindle formation • Cycle-specific to M phase	• Effects on CNS, GI system • Myelosuppression • Tissue damage
Enzymes asparaginase, pegaspargase	• Useful only in leukemias • Cycle-specific to G_1 phase	• Hypersensitivity reactions
Cycle-nonspecific		
Alkylating agents busulfan, carmustine, cyclophosphamide, ifosfamide, thiotepa	• Disrupt deoxyribonucleic acid (DNA) replication	• Infertility • Secondary carcinoma • Effects on renal system
Antibiotic antineoplastics bleomycin, dactinomycin, doxorubicin, idarubicin, mitomycin, mitoxantrone	• Bind with DNA to inhibit synthesis of DNA and ribonucleic acid	• Effects on GI, renal, and hepatic systems • Effects on bone marrow

(continued)

Selected chemotherapeutic drugs *(continued)*

Category	Characteristics	Toxic effects
Hormones and hormone inhibitors		
androgens (testolactone), antiandrogens (flutamide), antiestrogens (tamoxifen), estrogens (estramustine), gonadotropin (leuprolide), progestins (megestrol)	• Interfere with binding of normal hormones to receptor proteins, manipulate hormone levels, and alter hormone environment • Mechanism of action not always clear • Usually palliative, not curative	• No known toxic effect
Folic acid analogs		
leucovorin	• Antidote for methotrexate toxicity	• Hypersensitivity reaction possible
Cytoprotective agents		
dexrazoxane, mesna	• Protect normal tissue by binding with metabolites of other cytotoxic drugs	• None

Sample chemotherapy protocols

Chemotherapeutic drugs are commonly given in combinations called protocols. Here are some protocols typically given for common cancers.

Specific cancers	Protocols	Drugs
Bladder cancer	M-VAC	• methotrexate • vinblastine • Adriamycin (doxorubicin) • cisplatin
Breast cancer	ACT	• Adriamycin (doxorubicin) • cyclophosphamide • Taxol (paclitaxel) or Taxotere (docetaxel)
Cervical cancer	CF	• cisplatin • fluorouracil

Both generic and trade names may be used in protocol abbreviations.

Sample chemotherapy protocols *(continued)*

Specific cancers	Protocols	Drugs
Prostate cancer	CE	• cisplatin • etoposide
Gastric cancer	ECF	• epirubicin • cisplatin • fluorouracil
Laryngeal cancer	CF	• cisplatin • fluorouracil (5-Fu)
Acute lymphocytic leukemia, induction	DVPA	• daunorubicin • vincristine • prednisone • asparaginase
Melanoma	CVD	• cisplatin • vinblastine • dacarbazine
Acute myelocytic leukemia	POMP	• prednisone • Oncovin (vincristine) • methotrexate • Purinethol (mercaptopurine)
Lymphoma (non-Hodgkin's)	CHOP	• cyclophosphamide • doxorubicin/ hydroxydoxorubicin • Oncovin (vincristine) • prednisone
Lung cancer, small-cell	CE	• cisplatin • etoposide
Lung cancer, non-small-cell	PC	• paclitaxel • cisplatin

(continued)

When a trade name is used, you'll find the generic name in parentheses.

Sample chemotherapy protocols *(continued)*

Specific cancers	Protocols	Drugs
Lymphoma (Hodgkin's disease)	ABVD	• Adriamycin (doxorubicin) • bleomycin • vinblastine • dacarbazine
Lymphoma, malignant	BEACOPP	• bleomycin • etoposide • Adriamycin (doxorubicin) • cyclophosphamide • Oncovin (vincristine) • procarbazine • prednisone • filgrastim
Multiple myeloma	VAD	• vincristine • Adriamycin (doxorubicin) • dexamethasone
Testicular cancer	BEP	• bleomycin • etoposide • Platinol (cisplatin)

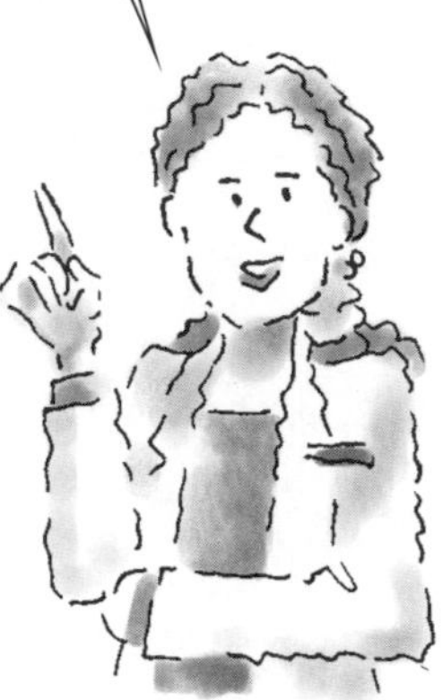

Still hard at work

The search for new cancer treatments is ongoing. Each year, the National Cancer Institute screens about 15,000 potential new compounds for chemotherapeutic action.

Immunotherapy

In cancer immunotherapy, drugs known as *biological response modifiers* are used to enhance the body's ability to destroy cancer cells.

Bringing up strong, healthy cells

Cancer immunotherapy seeks to evoke effective immune response to human tumors by altering the way cells grow, mature, and respond to cancer cells. This approach is unique because it manipu-

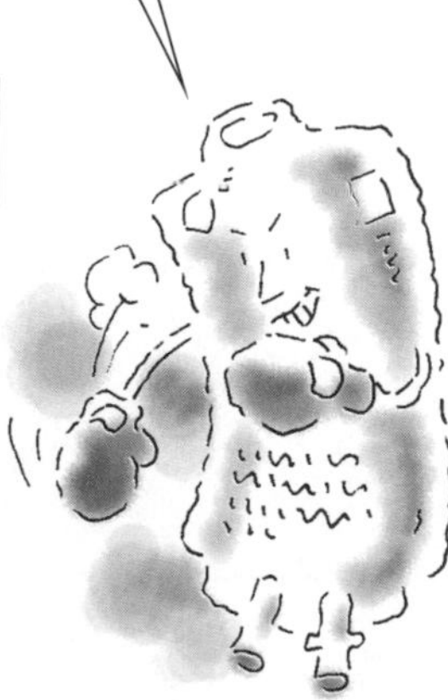

lates the body's natural resources instead of introducing toxic substances that aren't selective and can't differentiate between normal and abnormal processes or cells. Immunotherapy may include the administration of monoclonal antibodies and immunomodulatory cytokines.

Monoclonal antibodies

Monoclonal antibodies, which specifically target tumor cells, are a form of immunotherapy.

All about antibodies

Antibodies are immunoglobulins produced by mature B cells or plasma cells in response to antigens—proteins found on the surface of normal and abnormal cells. Antibodies recognize specific antigens and bind exclusively to them; this process is referred to as a lock-and-key mechanism. When these antibodies attach to antigens, they can cause tumor-cell inactivation or destruction. A monoclonal antibody recognizes only a single unique antigen.

One-shot wonders

Several monoclonal antibodies have been approved by the Food and Drug Administration for cancer therapy. Examples of monoclonal antibodies include:

- rituximab (Rituxan)
- trastuzumab (Herceptin)
- bevacizumab (Avastin).

Rituximab is specifically indicated for relapsed or refractory low-grade Hodgkin's disease and non-Hodgkin's lymphoma.

Trastuzumab is effective against metastatic breast cancer. This monoclonal antibody may be used as a first-line treatment in combination with chemotherapy or as a second-line single agent.

Bevacizumab is used in patients with metastatic colon cancer. It prevents the formation of new blood vessels so that tumor cells don't receive blood, oxygen, and other nutrients needed for growth.

Immunomodulatory cytokines

Immunomodulatory cytokines are intracellular messenger proteins (proteins that deliver messages within cells that can affect immune response). These proteins include:

- interferon alpha
- interleukins

- tumor necrosis factor (TNF)
- colony-stimulating factors (CSFs).

Immunomodulatory cytokines are proteins that deliver messages within cells.

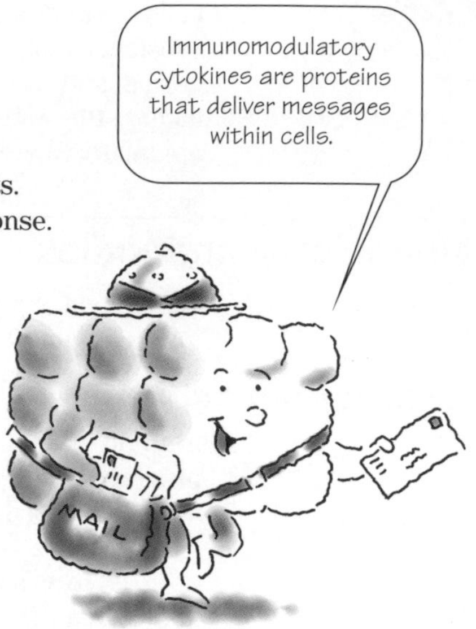

Interferon alpha

Interferon alpha has antiviral and antitumorigenic effects. It slows cell replication and stimulates an immune response. Interferon alpha is approved for treating chronic myeloid leukemia, hairy cell leukemia, and acquired immunodeficiency syndrome–related Kaposi's sarcoma. It's also used with low-grade malignant lymphoma, multiple myeloma, and renal cell carcinoma.

Interleukins

Interleukins are cytokines that primarily function to deliver messages to leukocytes. Interleukin-2 (IL-2) is an approved anticancer agent. IL-2 stimulates the proliferation and cytolytic activity of T cells and natural killer cells. High doses of IL-2 have been effective in a few patients with metastatic renal cell carcinoma and melanoma. The other interleukins remain under investigation for cancer therapy.

Tumor necrosis factor

TNF plays a role in the inflammatory response to tumors and cancer cells. In animal studies, TNF has sometimes produced impressive antitumor responses. This drug is considered investigational.

Colony-stimulating factors

CSFs are substances that are naturally produced by the body. They stimulate the growth of different types of cells found in the blood and the immune system. CSFs have been helpful in the clinical care of patients receiving myelosuppressive therapy. Examples of CSFs include:

- Erythropoietin (Epogen, Procrit) induces erythroid maturation (maturation of red blood cells [RBCs]) and increases the release of reticulocytes from the bone marrow, which stimulates production and might reduce the number of blood transfusions needed by the patient. Darbopoetin (Aranesp) is a long-acting form of erythropoietin.

• Granulocyte CSF (Neupogen) stimulates proliferation, differentiation, and functional activity of neutrophils, causing a rapid rise in the white blood cell count. Granulocyte CSF is given to reduce the incidence of infection in patients receiving chemotherapy drugs. Pegfilgrastim (Neulasta) is a long-acting granulocyte CSF.
• Granulocyte-macrophage CSF (Leukine) is indicated for patients receiving chemotherapy for acute myelogenous leukemia, for patients undergoing bone marrow transplants, and for peripheral blood progenitor collection.

Drug preparation

Many health care facilities use existing guidelines as a basis for their policies and procedures regarding chemotherapeutic drugs. The major sources for these guidelines include these agencies and associations:

- The American Society of Health-System Pharmacists has published guidelines for the preparation of chemotherapeutic drugs since 1990.
- The Occupational Safety and Health Administration (OSHA) published its revised standards for controlling exposure to chemotherapeutic drugs in 1995, and needle-stick protection in 2001.
- The Oncology Nursing Society published guidelines for nursing education, practice, and administration of chemotherapeutic drugs in 2005.
- The Infusion Nurses Society published revised standards of practice for safe delivery of chemotherapeutic drugs in 2000.

Certification required

At the local level, most health care facilities require nurses and pharmacists involved in the preparation and delivery of chemotherapeutic drugs to complete a certification program, covering the safe delivery of chemotherapeutic drugs and care of the patient with cancer.

Make sure you're up-to-date on guidelines and certified, if necessary, to administer chemotherapeutic drugs in your facility.

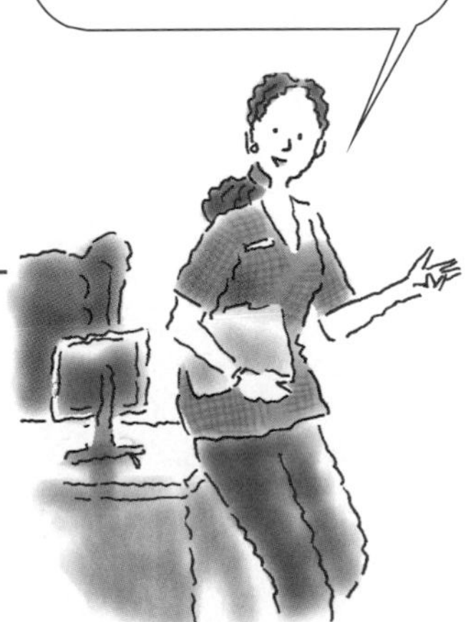

Protective measures

Preparation of chemotherapeutic drugs requires adherence to guidelines regarding:

- drug preparation areas and equipment
- protective clothing
- specific safety measures.

Area and equipment

Drug preparation may be performed by a trained nurse, a pharmacist or, in states that allow it, a supervised pharmacy technician.

Protect the air when you prepare

Prepare chemotherapeutic drugs in a well-ventilated workspace. Perform all drug admixing or compounding within a Class II Biological Safety Cabinet or a "vertical" laminar airflow hood with a high-efficiency particulate air filter, which is vented to the outside. The hood pulls the aerosolized chemotherapeutic drug particles away from the compounder. If a Class II Biological Safety Cabinet isn't available, OSHA recommends that you wear a special respirator.

Close to you

Have close access to a sink, alcohol sponges, and gauze pads as well as OSHA-required chemotherapy hazardous waste containers, sharps containers, and chemotherapy spill kits. (See *Equipment for preparing chemotherapeutic drugs.*)

Hazardous waste!

Hazardous waste containers should be made of puncture-proof, shatter-proof, leakproof plastic. Chemotherapy waste is usually identified with yellow biohazard labels. Use them to dispose of all chemotherapy-contaminated I.V. bags, tubing, filters, and syringes. Red sharps containers are used to dispose of all contaminated sharps such as needles.

Best practice

Equipment for preparing chemotherapeutic drugs

The Occupational Safety and Health Administration recommends having these items available in your work area when preparing chemotherapeutic drugs:

- patient's medication order or record
- prescribed drugs
- appropriate diluent (if necessary)
- medication labels
- long-sleeved gown
- chemotherapy gloves
- face shield or goggles and face mask
- 20G needles
- hydrophobic filter or dispensing pin
- syringes with luer-lock fittings and needles of various sizes
- I.V. tubing with luer-lock fittings
- 70% alcohol
- sterile gauze pads
- plastic bags with "hazardous drug" labels
- sharps disposal container
- hazardous waste container
- chemotherapy spill kit.

Clothing

Essential protective clothing includes:
- cuffed gown
- gloves
- goggles or face shield.

> **Memory jogger**
> To remember the clothing you should wear when preparing chemotherapeutic drugs, think of the three ***G's:***
> **G**own
> **G**loves
> **G**oggles.

The lowdown on gowns and gloves

Gowns should be disposable, water resistant, and lint free with long sleeves, knitted cuffs, and a closed front.

Gloves designed for use with chemotherapeutic drugs should be disposable and made of thick latex or thick non-latex material. They should also be powder-free because powder can carry contamination from the drugs into the surrounding air. Double gloving is an option when the gloves aren't of the best quality. Change gloves whenever a tear or puncture occurs. Wash your hands before putting on the gloves and after removing them.

Safety measures

Take care to protect staff, patients, and the environment from unnecessary exposure to chemotherapeutic drugs. Don't leave the drug preparation area while wearing the protective gear you wore during drug preparation. Eating, drinking, smoking, or applying cosmetics in the drug preparation area violates OSHA guidelines.

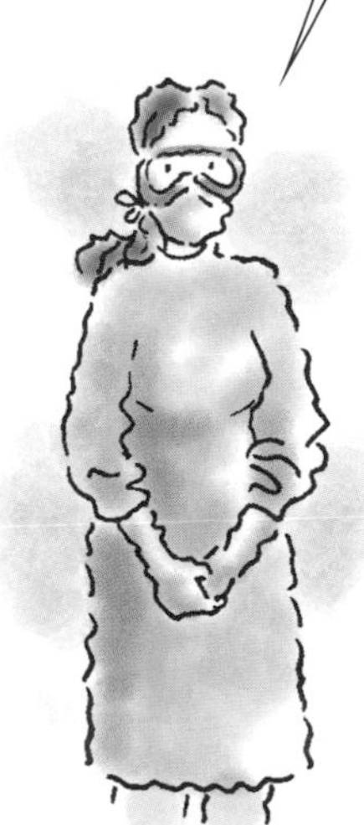

Laying the groundwork for safety

Put on protective gear before you begin to compound the chemotherapeutic drugs. Before preparing the drugs, clean the work area inside the cabinet with 70% alcohol and a disposable towel; do the same after you're finished and after a spill. Discard the towel into the yellow leakproof chemotherapy waste container.

Feeling exposed

If a chemotherapeutic drug comes in contact with your skin, wash the skin thoroughly with soap and water. This will prevent drug absorption into the skin. If the drug comes in contact with your eye, immediately flood the eye with water or isotonic eyewash for at least 5 minutes, while holding the eyelid open.

After an accidental exposure, notify your supervisor immediately. Your supervisor may send you to employee health, where the exposure event will be documented in your employee health record.

Better safe than sorry

Here are some other safety precautions to keep in mind:
- Use aseptic technique when preparing all drugs.
- Use a needle-free system whenever possible.

- Use needles with a hydrophobic filter to remove solutions from vials.
- Vent vials with a hydrophobic filter or use the negative pressure technique to reduce the amount of aerosolized drugs released.
- When you break ampules, wrap a gauze pad around the neck of the vial to decrease the chances of droplet contamination and glove puncture.
- Wear a face mask and goggles to protect yourself against splashes and aerosolized drugs.
- Place all contaminated needles in the sharps container, and don't recap needles.
- Use only syringes and I.V. sets that have a luer-lock fitting.
- Label all chemotherapeutic drugs with a yellow biohazard label.

Transport tactics

Transport the prepared chemotherapy drugs in a sealable plastic bag that's prominently labeled with a yellow chemotherapy biohazard label.

The spiel on spills

Make sure that your facility's protocols for spills are available in all areas where chemotherapeutic drugs are handled, including patient care areas. Chemotherapy spill kits should be readily available. (See *Inside a chemotherapy spill kit.*)

If a spill occurs, follow your facility's protocol, which is probably based on OSHA guidelines. This protocol will likely instruct you to follow these steps:

- Put on protective garments, if you aren't already wearing them.
- Isolate the area and contain the spill with absorbent materials from the spill kit.
- Use the disposable dustpan and scraper to collect broken glass or desiccant absorbing powder. Carefully place the dustpan, scraper, and collected spill in a leakproof, puncture-proof, chemotherapy designated hazardous waste container.
- Prevent the aerosolization of the drug at all times.
- Clean the spill area with a detergent or bleach solution.

Best practice

Inside a chemotherapy spill kit

Based on Occupational Safety and Health Administration guidelines and your facility's protocols, a chemotherapy spill kit should contain:

- long-sleeved gown that's water-resistant and nonpermeable, with cuffs and back closure
- shoe covers
- two pairs of powder-free surgical gloves (for double gloving)
- respirator mask
- chemical splash goggles
- disposable dustpan and plastic scraper (for collecting broken glass)
- plastic-backed absorbent towels, or spill-control pillows
- desiccant powder or granules (for absorbing wet contents)
- disposable sponges
- two large cytotoxic waste disposal bags.

Drug administration

Because dosage, route, and timing must be exact to avoid possibly fatal complications, only chemotherapy certified nurses should be involved in administering these drugs. If you have the skill and educational background, follow these four steps:

 Perform a preadministration check.

Obtain I.V. access.

 Give drugs.

 Conclude treatment.

Performing a preadministration check

Before administering a chemotherapeutic drug, double-check the order with another chemotherapy certified nurse.

Count on doing this

The patient's blood count should be checked before beginning the chemotherapy infusion. Many facilities have nursing policies that require the nurse to notify the practitioner for approval to administer the chemotherapeutic drug if the patient's blood count drops below a predetermined value.

Chemotherapeutic drugs that are excreted through the kidneys, such as cisplatin and carboplatin, require checking serum creatinine levels.

Which drugs? Which route?

Make sure that you understand clearly which drugs are to be given and by which route. Check whether the drug is classified as a vesicant, nonvesicant, or irritant. (See *Risks of tissue damage.*)

Check serum creatinine levels before giving drugs that excrete through me!

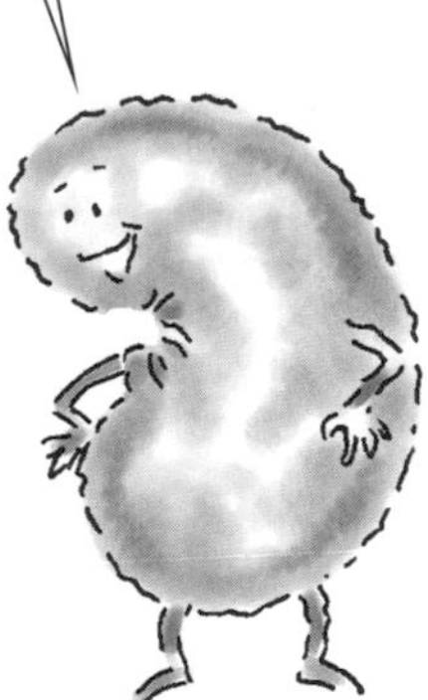

Who's on first?

Should the irritant or vesicant be administered first or last? The answer to this question is controversial and is related to the comfort level of the nurse infusing the chemotherapeutic drugs. Document the sequence of the infused drugs.

Confirm and verify

Confirm any written orders for needed antiemetics, fluids, diuretics, or electrolyte supplements to be given before, during, or after chemotherapy administration. Verify the patient's level of understanding of the treatment and adverse effects. Make sure that either the patient or a legally authorized person has signed an informed consent form for each specific chemotherapy drug they're to receive and for the insertion of the I.V. device, if required. (See *Preventing errors*, page 243.)

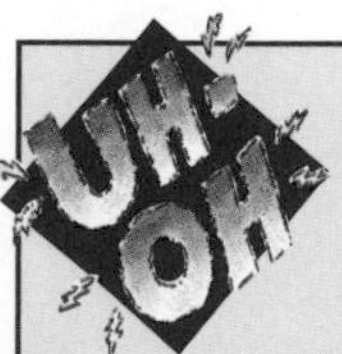

Warning!

Risks of tissue damage

To administer chemotherapy safely, you need to know each drug's potential for damaging tissue. In this regard, chemotherapeutic drugs are classified as vesicants, nonvesicants, or irritants.

Vesicants

Vesicants cause a reaction so severe that blisters form and tissue is damaged or destroyed. Chemotherapeutic vesicants include:

- cisplatin
- dactinomycin
- daunorubicin
- doxorubicin
- epirubicin
- idarubicin
- mechlorethamine
- mitomycin
- mitoxantrone
- nitrogen mustard
- vinblastine
- vincristine
- vinorelbine.

Nonvesicants

Nonvesicants don't cause irritation or damage. Chemotherapeutic nonvesicants include:

- asparaginase
- bleomycin
- cyclophosphamide
- cytarabine
- floxuridine
- fluorouracil.

Irritants

Irritants can cause a local venous response, with or without a skin reaction. Chemotherapeutic irritants include:

- carboplatin
- carmustine
- dacarbazine
- etoposide
- gemcitabine
- ifosfamide
- irinotecan
- taxol
- taxotene
- topotecan.

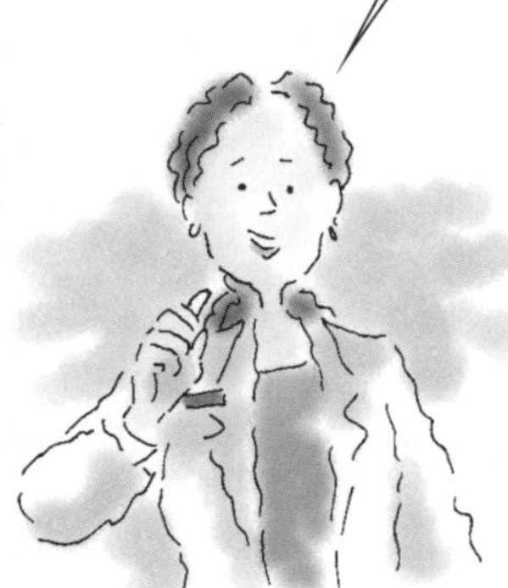

Obtaining I.V. access

Peripheral I.V. catheters are appropriate for most chemotherapeutic infusions. Peripheral I.V. catheters shouldn't be used for continuous vesicants because of the risk of infiltration and extravasation. Butterfly needles pose an extremely high risk for infiltration and shouldn't be used for chemotherapy infusion.

Gather 'round

Assemble the equipment you'll need for inserting of the peripheral I.V. catheter and preparing to administer the chemotherapeutic drug. If you're administering a vesicant, the extravasation kit should be immediately available. A chemotherapy spill kit should be readily available as well. Put on heavy chemotherapy gloves.

Preventing errors

Follow these precautions to prevent errors in chemotherapy administration:

- Only qualified personnel should write orders or administer chemotherapy. With rare exceptions, the administration of chemotherapy isn't an emergency procedure.
- All orders should be double-checked by the personnel preparing and administering the drugs.
- Repeatedly check the "five rights" of drug administration (right drug, right patient, right time, right dosage, right route).
- Any aspect of the order that's contrary to customary practice or to what has been done for the patient in the past should be questioned, especially when unusually high doses or unusual schedules are involved.
- The nurse shouldn't permit any distractions while checking an order or administering treatment.
- Orders for chemotherapy should be written only by the attending practitioner or oncology fellow who's responsible for the patient's care and most familiar with the drug regimen and dosing schedule.

(See *Equipment for administering chemotherapeutic drugs*, page 244.)

Who's there?

Check that you have the right patient. Call him by his first and last name, and ask for verification of his date of birth and address as a means of double-checking. Check the dose, and review potential adverse effects with the patient.

Choosing the right vein

Examine the possibilities for peripheral vein access by fully assessing the hand and forearm for an appropriate vein. Consider the following suggestions:

- Select a vein that's soft and pliable.
- Insert the I.V. catheter proximal to recent puncture sites, to prevent drug leakage through previously accessed sites.
- Avoid upper extremities that have impaired venous circulation.
- Avoid arms with functioning arteriovenous shunts, grafts, or fistulas for dialysis.
- Avoid using the arm on the same side as a mastectomy, if possible.
- To avoid damage to superficial tendons and nerves, use veins in the antecubital fossa and the back of the hand as a last resort.

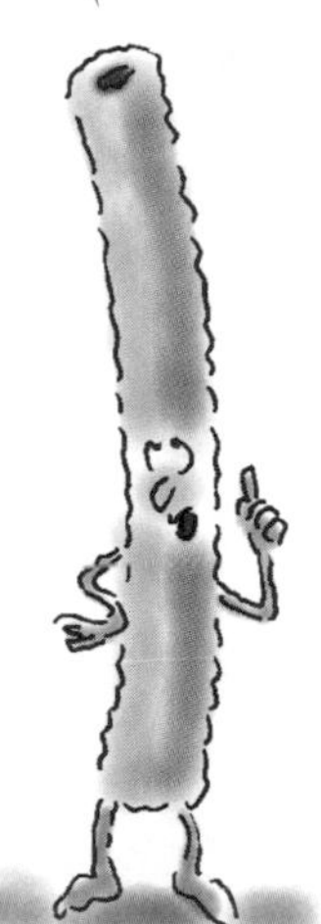

Gaining access

Select the venous access device with the smallest possible gauge (to accommodate the therapy and reduce the risk of infiltration), insert it into the vein, and then infuse 10 to 20 ml of free-flowing normal saline solution to confirm catheter placement within the vein.

Equipment for administering chemotherapeutic drugs

To administer chemotherapeutic drugs, gather the following equipment:

- prescribed drugs
- I.V. access supplies, if necessary
- sterile normal saline solution
- I.V. syringes and tubing with luer-lock connectors
- leakproof chemical waste container labeled CAUTION: BIOHAZARDOUS WASTE
- chemotherapy gloves
- chemotherapy spill kit
- extravasation kit.

Oh so many options

Patients receiving chemotherapeutic drugs have many vascular access device options. Patients receiving continuous vesicant infusions or multiple cycles of chemotherapeutic drugs or patients with poor peripheral vein access may require central venous access devices or implanted ports. Tunneled catheters and peripherally inserted central catheters are also options for chemotherapy administration.

Site-seeing encouraged

Apply a transparent dressing so that the site can be observed at all times for early signs of infiltration, extravasation, and vein irritation.

Giving drugs

Before administering a chemotherapeutic drug, connect an I.V. bag containing normal saline solution to the I.V. catheter.

A low-pressure situation

A low-pressure infusion pump should be used to administer vesicants through a peripheral vein to decrease the risk of extravasation. Central venous access devices are more appropriate for continuous vesicant infusions. (See *Preventing infiltration.*)

Administration variations

I.V. chemotherapeutic drugs can be administered in one of three ways:

 by direct I.V. push into an intermittent infusion device

Preventing infiltration

Follow these guidelines when giving vesicants:

- Use a distal vein that allows successive proximal venipunctures.
- Avoid using the hand, antecubital space, damaged areas, or areas with compromised circulation.
- Don't probe or "fish" for veins.
- Place a transparent dressing over the site.
- Start the push delivery or the infusion with free-flowing normal saline solution.
- Inspect the site for swelling and erythema.
- Tell the patient to report burning, stinging, pain, pruritus, or temperature changes near the site.
- After drug administration, flush the line with 20 ml of normal saline solution.

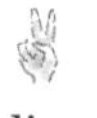

by indirect I.V. push through the side port of a running I.V. line

 as a continuous infusion.

No matter which method of administration is ordered, flush the vein with normal saline solution between the administration of each drug.

Investigating infiltration

Check for infiltration during administration as well as for signs of a hypersensitivity reaction. If swelling occurs at the I.V. site, the solution is infiltrating. Instruct the patient to report burning, stinging, or pain at or near the site. Observe around the site for streaky redness along the vein and other skin changes. Also, listen to what the patient has to say about his level of comfort; sudden discomfort during drug administration or flushing could indicate infiltration.

Keep in mind the expression, "When in doubt, take it out!"

Is your patient expressing discomfort?
When in doubt, take it out!

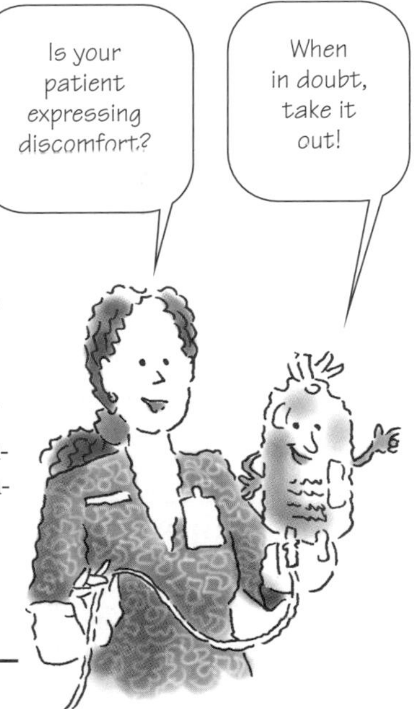

Finish with a flush

After drug administration is complete, infuse at least 20 ml of normal saline solution through the catheter before discontinuing the I.V. line. Doing so flushes the medication from the infusion delivery set, preventing drug leakage into the tissue as the catheter is removed (called "drug tracking") and helps minimize future vein damage.

Concluding treatment

After the I.V. line is removed, take the following steps:

- Dispose of all used needles and contaminated sharps in the red sharps container.
- Dispose of personal protective gear, glasses, and gloves in the yellow chemotherapy waste container.
- Dispose of unused medications, considered hazardous waste, according to your facility's policy.
- Wash your hands thoroughly with soap and water, even though you have worn gloves.
- Document the sequence in which the drugs were administered.
- Document the site accessed, the gauge and length of the catheter, and the number of attempts.
- Document the name, dose, and route of the administered drugs.
- Document the type and volume of the I.V. solutions and any adverse reactions and nursing interventions.

- According to facility policy and procedures, wear protective clothing when handling body fluids from the patient for 48 hours after the chemotherapy treatment.

Complications of chemotherapy

The properties that make chemotherapeutic drugs effective in killing cancer cells also make them toxic to normal cells. No organ system is untouched by chemotherapy. Therefore, all administration protocols strive to time the treatments and adjust the doses in a way that maximizes the effects against cancer cells while allowing time for normal cells to recover between courses of treatment.

Unfortunately, what makes chemotherapeutic drugs so effective in killing cancer cells also makes them toxic to normal cells like me.
RIP

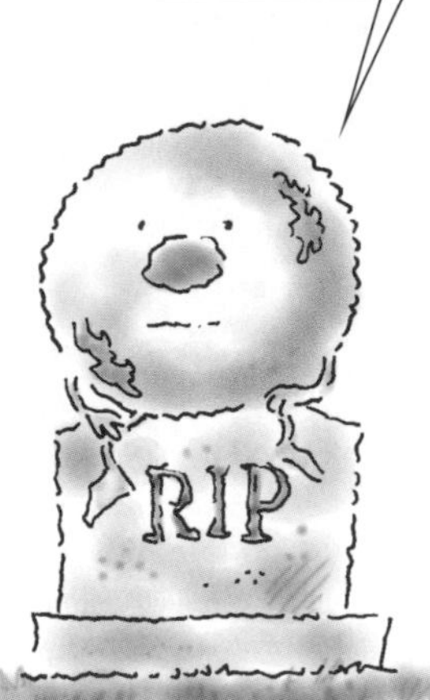

Categorizing complications

Complications resulting from chemotherapy can be categorized according to where or when exposure to the drug began. They're classified as:

- infusion-site related complications
- hypersensitivity or anaphylactic reactions
- short-term adverse effects
- long-term adverse effects.

Infusion-site-related complications

Infiltration, extravasation, and vein flare reactions are the most common infusion-site-related complications.

Infiltration

Infiltration is the inadvertent leakage of a nonvesicant solution or medication into the surrounding tissue. The main signs are swelling around the I.V. site, which will be cool to the touch, along with blanching and possibly a change in the I.V. flow rate.

Compression and compartment

Tightness in the patient's arm — he'll usually complain of numbness and tingling in the swollen area — due to large quantities of I.V. solutions entering the tissue indicates a nerve compression injury and can result in compartment syndrome. Notify the practitioner immediately.

Check, check, check

Check for infiltration before, during, and after the infusion by flushing the vein with normal saline solution. In the event of infiltration, remove the I.V. catheter and insert it in a new location.

Extravasation

Extravasation is the inadvertent leakage of a vesicant (a drug that can cause tissue necrosis and sloughing) solution into the surrounding tissue.

Stay hip to these tips

When assessing the patient for extravasation, keep these points in mind:

- Initial signs of extravasation may resemble those of infiltration—swelling, pain, and blanching.
- Blood return is an inconclusive test and shouldn't be used to determine if the I.V. catheter is correctly situated in the peripheral vein.
- To assess peripheral I.V. placement, flush the vein with normal saline solution and observe for site swelling.
- Symptoms can progress to blisters; skin, muscle, tissue, and fat necrosis; and tissue sloughing. The outer surface of veins, arteries, and nerves may also be damaged. Depending on the drug and the concentration of the drug in the solutions, blistering can be apparent within hours or days of the extravasation.
- Remember, "When in doubt, take it out!"

Emergency!

If a vesicant has extravasated, it's an emergency! Quickly take the following steps, designed to limit the damage:

- Stop the infusion. Check your facility's policy to determine if the I.V. catheter should be removed or left in place to infuse corticosteroids or a specific antidote. Treatment for extravasation should be in accordance with manufacturer's guidelines.
- Notify the practitioner.
- Instill the appropriate antidote according to facility policy. Usually, you'll give the antidote for extravasation either by instilling it through the existing I.V. catheter or by using a 1-ml syringe to inject small amounts subQ in a circle around the extravasated area. After the antidote has been injected, remove the I.V. catheter. (See *Antidotes to vesicant extravasation*, page 248.)

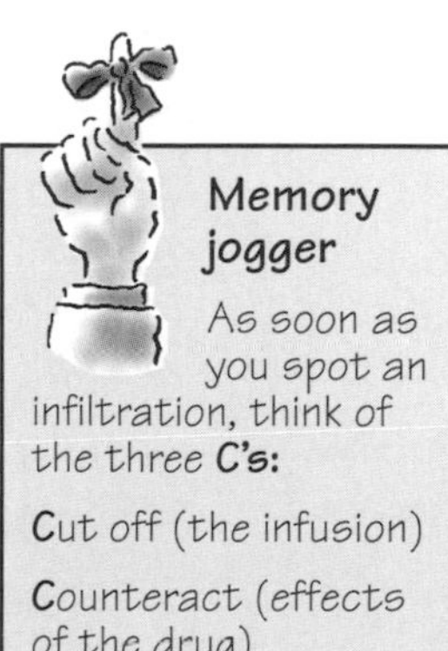

Memory jogger

As soon as you spot an infiltration, think of the three **C's:**

Cut off (the infusion)

Counteract (effects of the drug)

Contain (the affected area).

Don't forget the follow-up

Continue to visually monitor the site and document its appearance and the patient's response. Subsequent care of the extravasated area may include topical steroids or Silvadene cream. If

Antidotes to vesicant extravasation

Here are some examples of antidotes you may administer in the event of extravasation by a vesicant.

Infiltrating agent	Antidote	Nursing considerations
• daunorubicin • doxorubicin	dimethyl sulfoxide (DMSO)	• Apply a cold pack for at least 1 hour four times per day for 3 to 5 days. • DMSO 50% to 90% solution can be applied to the extravasation site every 6 hours for 14 days. Don't cover the application site; allow it to air-dry. • Injection of sodium bicarbonate is contraindicated.
• mechlorethamine (nitrogen mustard)	10% sodium thiosulfate	• Mix 4 ml of 10% sodium thiosulfate with 6 ml of sterile water for injection. • Inject 4 ml of the solution into the existing I.V. line that extravasated. • After the injection through the I.V. line, remove the catheter. • Inject 2 to 3 ml of the solution subcutaneously clockwise into the infiltrated area using a 25G needle. Change the needle with each new injection. • Apply ice for 6 to 12 hours.

the extravasation injury is severe, the patient may require skin debridement, skin grafts, or possibly amputation.

Vein flare

During infusion of an irritant into the vein, the patient may complain of burning pain or aching along the vein or up through the arm. A vein flare (marked by bright redness) may also appear in the vein along with blotches or hives on the affected arm. If the reaction is severe, injection of an I.V. steroid may be required. In some cases, the infusion of an irritant can result in damage to the lining of the vein wall, causing serious phlebitis or vein thrombosis.

Diluting the drug's effect

Irritants require large veins with good hemodilution to decrease the irritating properties of the drug. If the patient complains of pain or burning during the infusion, increase the dilution of the infused medication, decrease the infusion rate, or restart the I.V. catheter in a different vein.

Documentation

Be sure to document:

- location of the infiltration, extravasation, or vein flare
- size of the swollen area
- name of the drug and I.V. solution
- patient's complaints

- all nursing interventions
- time you notified the practitioner
- practitioner's response and orders.

Hypersensitivity or anaphylactic reactions

A hypersensitivity or anaphylactic reaction can occur at the initial dose of the drug or on subsequent infusions of the same drug. Some chemotherapeutic drugs put the patient at high risk for anaphylaxis. (See *Hypersensitivity risk of chemotherapeutic drugs*.)

Hypersensitivity reactions can occur at the beginning, middle, or end of the infusion. (See *Signs and symptoms of immediate hypersensitivity*, page 250.)

The specific treatment for a hypersensitivity reaction will depend on the severity of the reaction. Usually, you'll follow these five steps:

Stop the infusion.

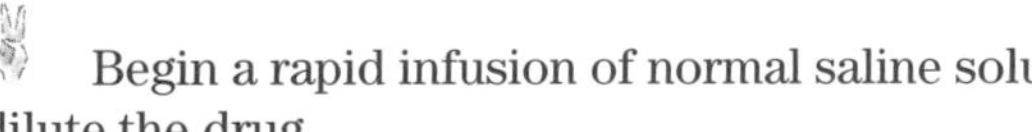
Begin a rapid infusion of normal saline solution to quickly dilute the drug.

Check the patient's vital signs.

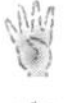
Notify the practitioner.

Administer emergency drugs as ordered by the practitioner.

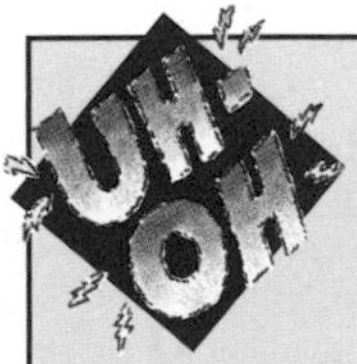

Warning!

Hypersensitivity risk of chemotherapeutic drugs

Note the risk levels associated with these chemotherapeutic drugs.

High risk
- asparaginase
- herceptin
- paclitaxel
- rituximab
- taxol
- taxotere

Moderate to low risk
- anthracyclines
- bleomycin
- carboplatin
- cisplatin
- cyclosporine
- etoposide
- melphalan
- methotrexate
- procarbazine
- teniposide

Low risk
- chlorambucil
- cyclophosphamide
- cytarabinc
- dacarbazine
- fluorouracil
- ifosfamide
- mitoxantrone

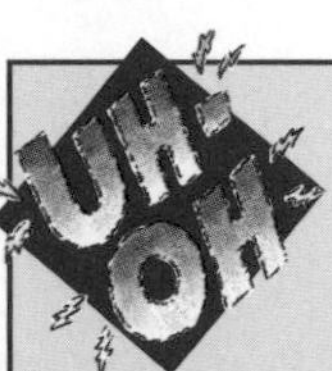

Warning!

Signs and symptoms of immediate hypersensitivity

An immediate hypersensitivity reaction to a chemotherapeutic drug will appear within 5 minutes after starting to administer the drug.

Organ system	Subjective complaints	Objective findings
Respiratory	Dyspnea, inability to speak, tightness in chest	Stridor, bronchospasm, decreased air movement
Skin	Pruritus	Cyanosis, urticaria, angioedema, cold and clammy skin
Cardiovascular	Chest pain, increased heart rate	Tachycardia, hypotension, arrhythmias
Central nervous system	Dizziness, agitation, anxiety	Decreased sensorium, loss of consciousness

What to give and when

Antihistamines are typically given first, followed by corticosteroids and bronchodilators. Epinephrine is given first in severe anaphylactic reactions. After you have administered the drug, monitor the patient's vital signs and pulse oximetry every 5 minutes until he's stable, and then every 15 minutes for 1 to 2 hours — or follow facility policy and procedures for acute treatment of allergic reactions.

Throughout the episode, maintain the patient's airway, oxygenation, and tissue perfusion. Life support equipment should be available in case the patient fails to respond. Document the drugs and dosage as well as the patient's response to the treatment.

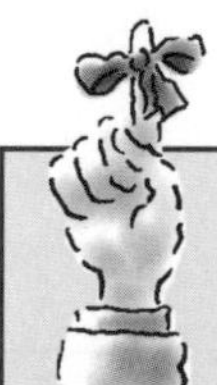

Memory jogger

When your patient has an immediate hypersensitivity reaction, guide your response with these three pairs of words:

- stop & stay (stop the infusion and stay with the patient)
- check & call (check vital signs and call the practitioner)
- open & ordered (open the I.V. line containing normal saline solution and administer ordered medications).

What the future holds in store...

The patient should discuss future drug infusions with the practitioner. The practitioner may reduce the dose of the drug or switch to a drug that targets the tumor type and is less toxic. If the practitioner continues the drug at a lower dose, premedication with an antihistamine and perhaps a corticosteroid will be required. Be sure to check with the practitioner for preinfusion treatments before subsequent therapy cycles.

Short-term adverse effects

The short-term adverse effects of chemotherapy include:
- nausea and vomiting
- hair loss (alopecia)
- diarrhea
- myelosuppression
- stomatitis.

These effects are produced by damage to tissues with a large proportion of frequently reproducing cells, including bone marrow, hair follicles, and GI mucosa.

All patients are different; not all experience these adverse effects, and some don't have any short-term adverse effects at all.

Nausea and vomiting

Nausea and vomiting can appear in three patterns:
- anticipatory
- acute
- delayed.

Each has its own cause. Because daily chemotherapy treatments may span several weeks, expect to see a mix of these three patterns. Managing them is a difficult balancing act but is crucial because of the effects that nausea and vomiting have on the patient's nutritional status, emotional well-being, and fluid and electrolyte balance.

Anticipatory nausea and vomiting may occur in a patient who had unpleasant symptoms after a previous dose of chemotherapy.

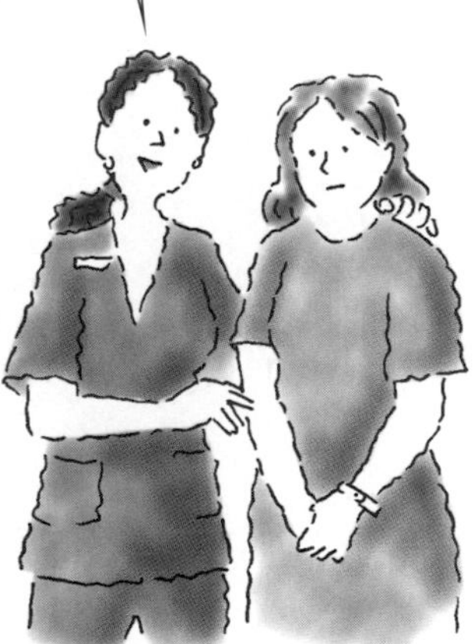

Anticipatory — it's enough to just think about it

The anticipatory pattern is a learned response from prior nausea and vomiting after a dose of chemotherapy. It's most likely to develop in people who experienced moderate to severe symptoms after previous doses of chemotherapy. These patients tend to have very high anxiety levels.

The key here is pretreatment. Aprepitant (Emend) is usually effective in preventing this type of nausea. The patient takes aprepitant before receiving chemotherapy, and continues it for two days after the chemotherapy. However, because some patients have overwhelming anxiety, I.V. lorazepam may be necessary before chemotherapy is administered.

Posttreatment control of nausea and vomiting can help prevent anticipatory nausea. The less nauseous a patient feels after treatment, the less anxiety he'll experience before the next treatment.

Acute — within the first 24 hours

Acute nausea and vomiting occur within the first 24 hours of treatment. A major factor is the emetogenic (vomit-inducing) potential of the drug or drugs administered. For example, cisplatin has a high potential; more than 90% of patients receiving it will experience nausea and vomiting. Bleomycin, however, has a low potential; only 10% to 30% of patients are affected.

Other factors that contribute to the occurrence and severity of nausea and vomiting include the combination of drugs, doses, rates of administration, and patient characteristics. There are many antiemetic drugs available. Ondansetron and granisetron are commonly used today. Other drugs, such as lorazepam or dexamethasone, may also be used.

Delayed but not out of the woods yet

Delayed nausea and vomiting is loosely designated as starting or continuing beyond 24 hours after chemotherapy has begun. Although its cause is less clearly understood than the anticipatory and acute patterns, the arsenal of drugs for treating it is larger. In addition to serotonin, antagonists, and corticosteroids, various antihistamines, benzodiazepines, and metoclopramide are usually effective.

Some patients are treated with antiemetic drugs for up to 3 days or longer after treatment.

Alopecia

Alopecia results from the destruction of rapidly dividing cells in the hair shaft or root. It may be minimal or severe depending on the type of chemotherapeutic drug and the patient's reaction.

Let them know it will regrow

Because so many patients find alopecia disturbing, reassurance about resumed hair growth is important. Inform the patient that his scalp will become sore at times due to the follicles swelling. Educate the patient on hair regrowth. Some patients will have hair growing back during the chemotherapy treatments whereas others will have no hair growth until 2 to 3 months after treatment is complete. Inform the patient that this new hair may be a different texture or color.

Give the patient sufficient time to decide whether to order a wig. This will also give him time to match the wig color up to his natural hair color before total hair loss occurs. The American Cancer Society has helped with the cost of wigs in the past and has even made donated wigs available.

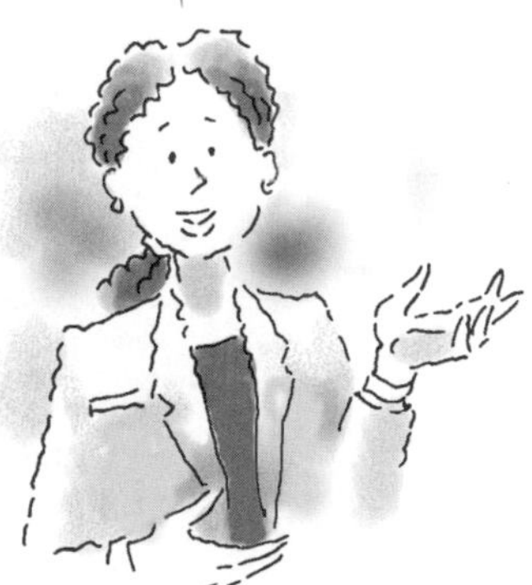

Diarrhea

Diarrhea — brought on because the rapidly dividing cells of the intestinal mucosa are killed — occurs in some patients receiving chemotherapy. Complications of persistent diarrhea include weight loss, fluid and electrolyte imbalance, and malnutrition. To minimize the effects of diarrhea, use dietary adjustments, anti-diarrheal medications, and ointments to the rectal area if irritated.

Myelosuppression

Myelosuppression is damage to the stem cells in the bone marrow. These cells are the precursors to cellular blood components — red and white blood cells and platelets — so their damage produces anemia, leukopenia, and thrombocytopenia. (See *Managing complications of chemotherapy*, page 254.)

Stomatitis

Stomatitis produces painful mouth ulcers 3 to 7 days after certain chemotherapeutic drugs are given, with symptoms ranging from mild to severe. Because of the accompanying pain, stomatitis can lead to fluid and electrolyte imbalance and malnutrition if the patient can't chew or swallow adequate food or fluid.

Oral hygiene is key

Treat stomatitis with scrupulous oral hygiene and topical anesthetic mixtures. Because pain may be severe, patients sometimes require opioid analgesics until ulcers heal. Allowing the patient to suck on ice chips while receiving certain drugs that cause stomatitis helps decrease the blood supply to the mouth, decreasing ulcer formation.

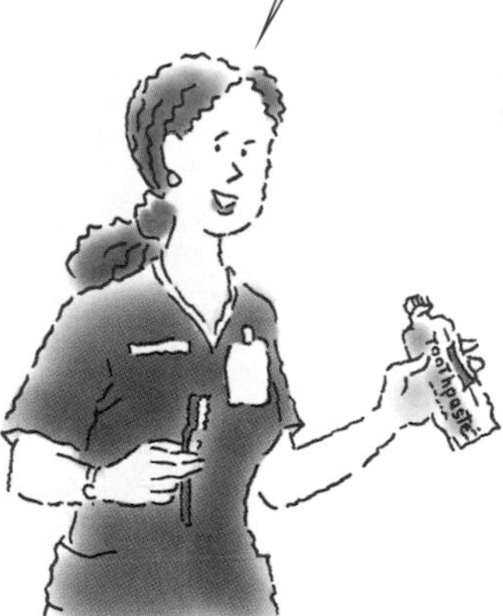

Long-term adverse effects

Organ system dysfunction, especially in the hematopoietic and GI systems, is common after chemotherapy. These effects are usually temporary, but some systems suffer permanent damage that manifests long after chemotherapy. The renal, pulmonary, cardiac, reproductive, and neurologic systems all show various temporary and permanent dysfunctions from exposure to chemotherapy.

Managing complications of chemotherapy

This chart identifies some common adverse effects of chemotherapy and offers ways to minimize them.

Adverse effect	Signs and symptoms	Interventions
Anemia	Dizziness, fatigue, pallor, and shortness of breath after minimal exertion; low hemoglobin and hematocrit; may develop slowly over several courses of treatment	• Monitor hemoglobin, hematocrit, and red blood cell count; report dropping values; remember that dehydration from nausea, vomiting, and anorexia will cause hemoconcentration, yielding falsely high hematocrit readings. • Be prepared to administer a blood transfusion or erythropoietin. • Instruct the patient to take frequent rests, increase intake of iron-rich foods, and take a multivitamin with iron as prescribed.
Leukopenia	Susceptibility to infections; neutropenia (an absolute neutrophil count less than 1,500 cells/µl)	• Watch for the nadir, the point of lowest blood cell count (usually 7 to 14 days after last treatment). • Be prepared to administer colony-stimulating factors. • Include the following information in patient and family teaching: good hygiene practices, signs and symptoms of infection, the importance of checking the patient's temperature regularly, how to prepare a low-microbe diet, and how to care for vascular access devices. • Instruct the patient to avoid crowds, people with colds or respiratory infections, and fresh fruit, fresh flowers, and plants.
Thrombocytopenia	Bleeding gums, increased bruising, petechiae, hypermenorrhea, tarry stools, hematuria, coffee-ground emesis	• Monitor platelet count: under 50,000 cells/µl means a moderate risk of excessive bleeding; under 20,000 cells/µl means a major risk and the patient may need a platelet transfusion. • Avoid unnecessary I.M. injections or venipunctures; if either is necessary, apply pressure for at least 5 minutes, and then apply a pressure dressing to the site. • Instruct the patient to avoid cuts and bruises, shave with an electric razor, avoid blowing his nose, stay away from irritants that would trigger sneezing, and not use rectal thermometers. • Instruct the patient to report sudden headaches (which could indicate potentially fatal intracranial bleeding).
Alopecia	Hair loss that may include eyebrows, lashes, and body hair	• Minimize shock and distress by warning the patient of the possibility of hair loss, discussing why hair loss occurs, and describing how much hair loss to expect. • Emphasize the need for appropriate head protection against sunburn and heat loss in the winter. • For patients with long hair, suggest cutting the hair shorter before treatment because washing and brushing cause more hair loss.

A devastating effect

One devastating long-term effect of chemotherapy is secondary malignancy. This can be caused by certain alkylating agents given to treat myeloma, Hodgkin's disease, and malignant lymphomas. A secondary malignancy can occur at any time. The prognosis is usually poor.

Teaching and documentation

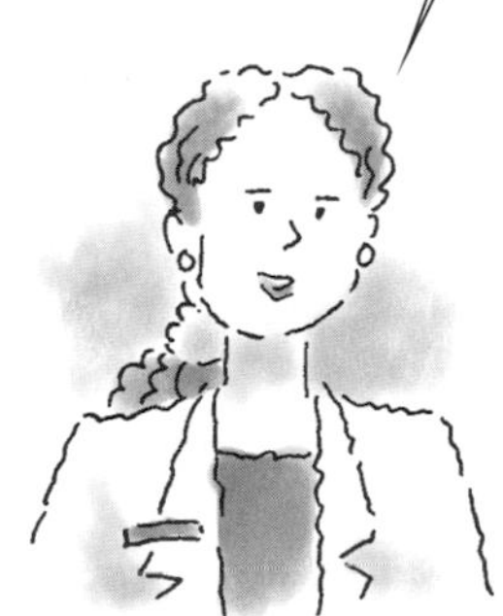

Not only is cancer a frightening and commonly lethal disease, but its treatment brings with it serious risks and fears as well. To give your patient some sense of control in the face of overwhelming odds, explain each procedure you do and teach him strategies for dealing with fear, pain, and the unwelcome adverse effects of chemotherapy.

Keep in mind that a positive attitude and a strong emotional support system will enable your patient to better endure — if not overcome — the disease and its treatments.

Building a strong chain of communication

Documentation is important for more than just legal reasons. Because the treatment for cancer can be prolonged, numerous health care providers and facilities may be involved over an extended period. Without clear and concise documentation of treatments given, actions taken, and patient responses, the chain of communication can break down. When communication is impaired, the patient will most certainly experience additional needless suffering.

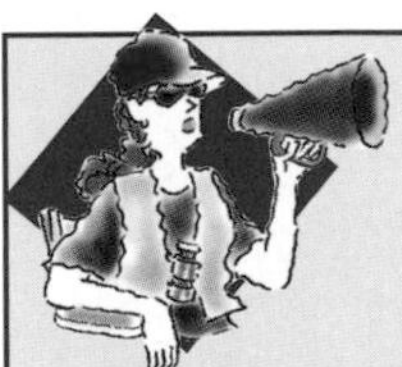

That's a wrap!

Chemotherapy infusions review

Chemotherapy infusion

- Usually calls for more than one drug to target different cancer cell phases
- Works best when the most effective drug is chosen as the first line
- Requires three treatment cycles for most patients

Chemotherapeutic drugs

- Categorized according to their action and how they interfere with cell production
- May be cycle-specific (act during specific phases of a cell cycle) or cycle-nonspecific (act on reproducing and resting cells)

(continued)

Chemotherapy infusions review *(continued)*

Immunotherapy
- Enhances the body's ability to destroy cancer cells
- Involves administration of monoclonal antibodies, which target tumor cells, or immunomodulatory cytokines, which affect immune response

Administering chemotherapy infusions
- Perform a preadministration check.
- Prepare chemotherapeutic drugs using appropriate protective measures.
- Establish I.V. access. (Peripheral catheters are appropriate; use smallest gauge possible.)
- Connect the I.V. bag containing normal saline solution to the I.V. catheter before giving the drug.
- Closely monitor the patient and I.V. site.
- Properly dispose of equipment.
- Document the procedure.

Chemotherapeutic drugs and tissue damage
- Vesicants—cause blisters and severe tissue damage
- Nonvesicants—don't cause irritation or tissue damage
- Irritants—cause a local venous response, with or without a skin reaction

Infusion-site complications

Infiltration
- Results from nonvesicant leaking into surrounding tissue
- Causes swelling, blanching, and possible flow-rate change

Extravasation
- Results from vesicant leaking into surrounding tissue
- Causes swelling, pain, and blanching

Vein flare
- Results from irritant drug
- Causes vein to become red and surrounded by hives

Adverse effects of chemotherapy
- Alopecia (hair loss)—may be minimal or severe
- Anaphylactic reaction—may occur any time during drug administration
- Diarrhea—may lead to weight loss, electrolyte imbalance, and malnutrition
- Myelosuppression—damage to precursors of WBCs, RBCs, and platelets
- Nausea and vomiting—may be anticipated, acute, or delayed
- Secondary malignancy—usually occurs after use of alkalating agents

Quick quiz

1. Which is *not* an advantage of administering chemotherapy by the I.V. route?

A. The drugs are completely absorbed.
B. The chances of acute nausea and vomiting are decreased.
C. The dose is highly accurate.
D. The drugs are systemically distributed.

Answer: B. Administering chemotherapeutic drugs I.V. doesn't decrease the chance of nausea and vomiting.

2. A drug that's cycle-specific will attack normal and malignant cells during specific phases of cell development, except for which phase?

A. Resting phase
B. Mitosis phase
C. Deoxyribonucleic acid synthesis phase
D. Ribonucleic acid synthesis phase

Answer: A. Cycle-specific drugs are effective only during specific phases of the cycle. When cell-cycle-specific chemotherapy is administered, cells in the resting phase survive.

3. OSHA requires that anyone administering chemotherapy must wear:

A. disposable gloves.
B. two pairs of latex surgical gloves.
C. any type of latex gloves.
D. chemotherapy gloves.

Answer: D. Chemotherapy gloves help prevent inadvertent exposure because they're thick and powderless and extend to the elbow.

4. Who's authorized to write chemotherapy orders?

A. The attending practitioner
B. The nurse
C. A fourth-year medical student
D. A pharmacist

Answer: A. Only a practitioner or an oncology fellow is allowed to write a chemotherapy order.

5. To treat extravasation, the first step is to:

A. give an antidote.
B. notify the practitioner.
C. stop the infusion.
D. notify the pharmacy.

Answer: C. The first step in treating extravasation is to stop the infusion. Check your facility's policy to determine whether the I.V. catheter should be removed. Notify the practitioner and pharmacy after stopping the infusion. Treatment for extravasation should always be in accordance with manufacturer's guidelines and should be appropriate according to facility policy.

Scoring

☆☆☆ If you answered all five questions correctly, congratulations! Now treat yourself to some extra time in your resting phase.

☆☆ If you answered three or four questions correctly, not bad! You are getting into the flow of things.

☆ If you answered fewer than three questions correctly, don't get discouraged! Sometimes it takes a few learning cycles before the information starts taking effect.

Parenteral nutrition

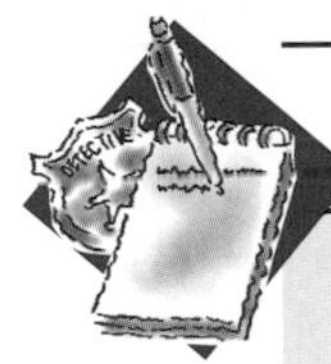

Just the facts

In this chapter, you'll learn:

- ♦ basic nutritional needs
- ♦ indications for parenteral nutrition
- ♦ nutritional solutions
- ♦ the proper way to perform a nutritional assessment
- ♦ the proper way to administer parenteral nutrition
- ♦ complications of parenteral nutrition.

Understanding parenteral nutrition

You may administer parenteral nutrition when illness or surgery prevents a patient from eating and metabolizing food. Common conditions that make parenteral nutrition necessary include:

- GI trauma
- pancreatitis
- ileus
- inflammatory bowel disease
- GI tract malignancy
- GI hemorrhage
- paralytic ileus
- GI obstruction
- short-bowel syndrome
- GI fistula
- severe malabsorption.

Critically ill patients may also receive parenteral nutrition if they're hemodynamically unstable or if GI tract blood flow is impaired.

Is your patient unable to eat and metabolize food?
Then serve me up!

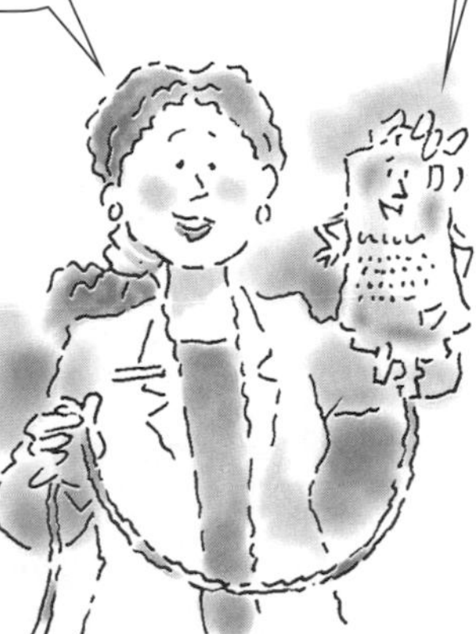

Nutritional needs

Essential nutrients found in food provide energy, maintain body tissues, and aid body processes, such as growth, cell activity, enzyme production, and temperature regulation.

Turning food into fuel

When carbohydrates, fats, and proteins are metabolized by the body, they produce energy, which is measured in calories (also called *kilocalories*). A normal healthy adult generally requires 2,000 to 3,000 calories per day. Specific requirements depend on an individual's size, sex, age, and level of physical activity.

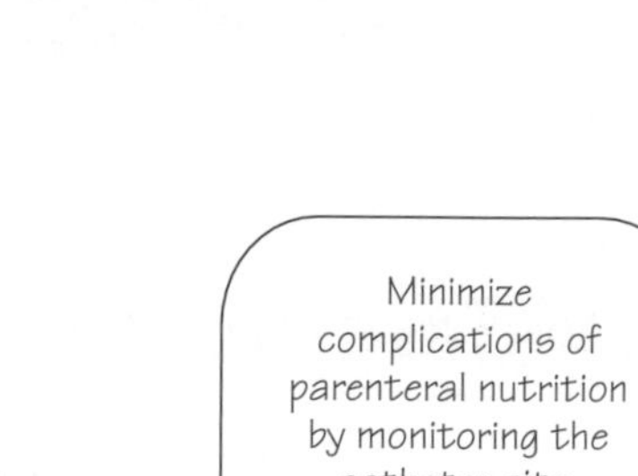

A nutritional solution — in more ways than one!

A parenteral nutrition solution — also known as *hyperalimentation* or *I.V. hyperalimentation* — may contain two or more of the following elements:

- dextrose
- proteins
- lipids
- electrolytes
- vitamins
- trace elements
- water.

It's a good thing...

Parenteral solutions can provide all necessary nutrients when a patient is unable to absorb nutrients through the GI tract. It enables cells to function despite the patient's inability to take in or metabolize food.

...but risky

Like all invasive procedures, parenteral nutrition incurs certain risks, including:

- catheter infection
- hyperglycemia (high blood glucose)
- hypokalemia (low blood potassium).

Complications of parenteral nutrition can be minimized with careful monitoring of the catheter site, infusion rate, and laboratory test results.

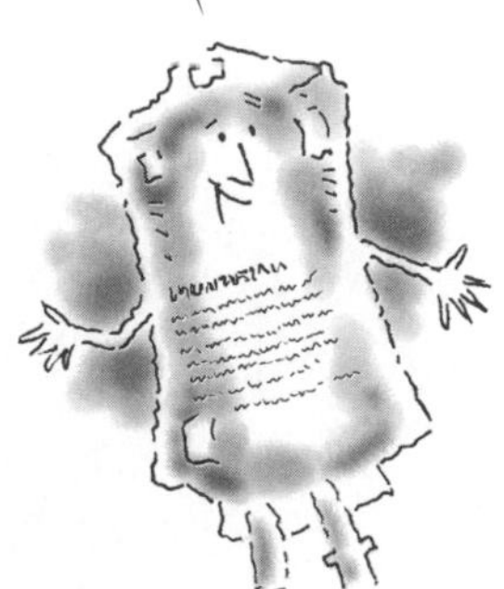

A matter of access

Another disadvantage of parenteral nutrition is the need for central venous (CV) access, which is used because the high dextrose concentration of parenteral nutrition solutions can cause vein sclerosis.

Price is a premium

Parenteral nutrition is expensive—about 10 times as expensive as enteral nutrition for the solutions alone. For this reason, it's used only when absolutely necessary.

Parenteral nutrition infusion methods

Depending on the type of therapy ordered, nutritional support solutions are administered through either a CV access device or peripheral infusion device.

CV infusion

If a patient needs long-term parenteral nutrition, he usually requires total parenteral nutrition (TPN). TPN with a final dextrose concentration of 10% or higher must be delivered through a CV access device, usually placed in the subclavian vein, with the tip of the catheter in the superior vena cava.

Peripheral infusion

Peripheral parenteral nutrition (PPN)—also called *partial parenteral nutrition*—is the delivery of nutrients through a short catheter inserted into a peripheral vein. Generally, PPN provides fewer nonprotein calories than TPN because lower dextrose concentrations are used. A much larger volume of fluid must be infused for PPN to deliver the same number of calories as TPN. Therefore, most patients who require parenteral nutrition therapy receive TPN, and PPN is reserved for short-term therapy (1 to 3 weeks).

Use TPN when lengthy or chronic illness leads to patient weight loss and decreased calorie and protein intake.

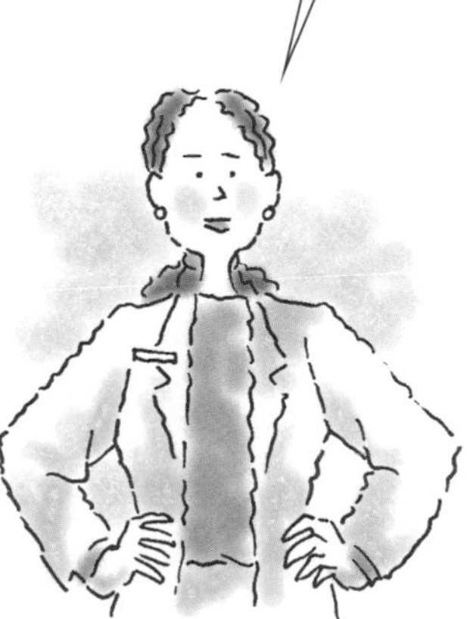

Indications for parenteral nutrition

The patient's condition determines whether TPN or PPN is used.

Indications for TPN

A patient may receive TPN for:

- debilitating illness lasting longer than 2 weeks.
- deficient or absent oral intake for longer than 7 days, as in cases of multiple trauma, severe burns, or anorexia nervosa.
- loss of at least 10% of pre-illness weight.
- serum albumin level below 3.5 g/dl.
- poor tolerance of long-term enteral feedings.
- chronic vomiting or diarrhea.
- inability to sustain adequate weight with oral or enteral feedings.

• GI disorders that prevent or severely reduce absorption, such as bowel obstruction, Crohn's disease, ulcerative colitis, short-bowel syndrome, cancer malabsorption syndrome, and bowel fistulas.
• inflammatory GI disorders, such as wound infection, fistulas, or abscesses.

Indications for PPN

Patients who don't need to gain weight, yet need nutritional support, may receive PPN for as long as 3 weeks. It's used to help a patient meet minimal calorie and protein requirements. PPN therapy may also be used with oral or enteral feedings for a patient who needs to supplement low-calorie intake or who can't absorb enteral therapy.

Use PPN to help the patient meet minimum calorie and protein requirements or to supplement oral or enteral feedings.

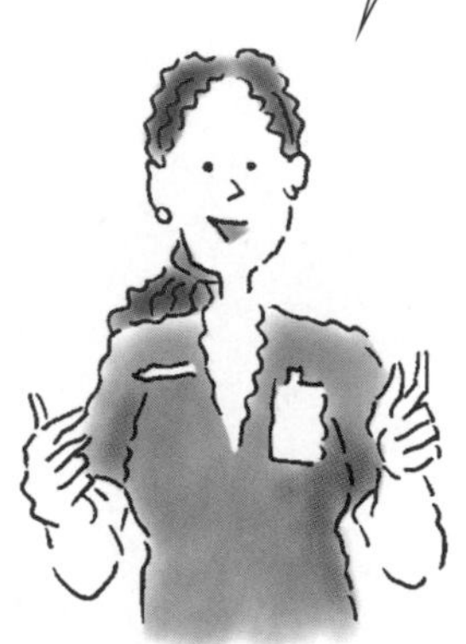

Putting PPN on hold

PPN shouldn't be used for patients with moderate to severe malnutrition or fat metabolism disorders, such as pathologic hyperlipidemia, lipid nephrosis, and acute pancreatitis caused by hyperlipidemia. In patients with severe liver damage, coagulation disorders, anemia, and pulmonary disease as well as those at increased risk for fat embolism, use parenteral nutrition cautiously.

Nutritional deficiencies

The most common nutritional deficiencies involve protein and calories. Nutritional deficiencies may result from a nonfunctional GI tract, decreased food intake, increased metabolic need, or a combination of these factors.

Hunger strike

Food intake may be decreased because of illness, decreased physical ability, or injury. Decreased food intake can occur with GI disorders, such as paralytic ileus, surgery, or sepsis.

Fever, burns, trauma, disease, and stress all increase metabolic activity, causing an increased need for caloric intake.

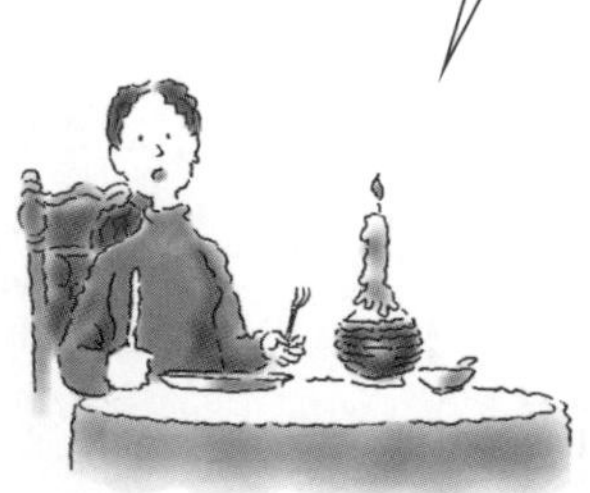

Metabolic activity up — need more calories!

An increase in metabolic activity requires an increase in calorie intake. Fever commonly increases metabolic activity. The metabolic rate may also increase in victims of burns, trauma, disease, or stress; patients may require up to twice the calories of their basal metabolic rate (the minimum energy needed to maintain respiration, circulation, and other basic body functions).

Effects of protein-calorie deficiencies

When the body detects protein-calorie deficiency, it turns to its reserve sources of energy. Reserve energy is drawn from three sources:

1. First, the body mobilizes and converts glycogen to glucose through a process called *glycogenolysis*.

2. Next, if necessary, the body draws energy from the fats stored in adipose tissue.

3. As a last resort, the body taps its store of essential visceral proteins (serum albumin and transferrin) and somatic body proteins (skeletal, smooth muscle, and tissue proteins). These proteins and their amino acids are converted to glucose for energy through a process called *gluconeogenesis*. When these essential body proteins break down, a negative nitrogen balance results (which means more protein is used by the body than is taken in). Starvation and disease-related stress contribute to this catabolic (destructive) state.

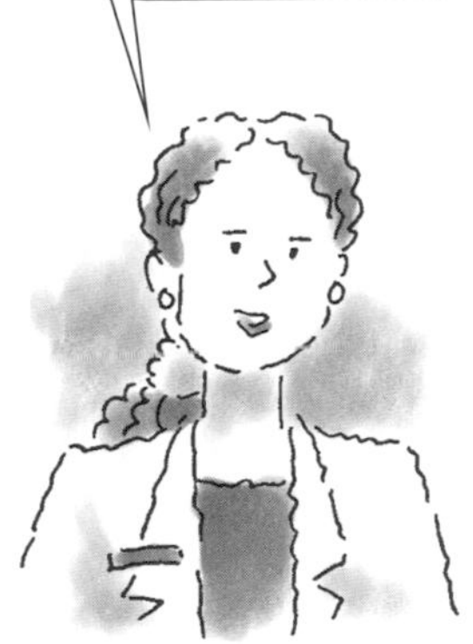

Protein-energy malnutrition

A deficiency of protein and energy (calories) results in protein-energy malnutrition (PEM), also called *protein-calorie malnutrition*. PEM refers to a spectrum of disorders that occur as a consequence of chronic inadequate protein or calorie intake or high metabolic protein and energy requirements.

PEM pals

Disorders that commonly lead to PEM include:

- cancer
- GI disorders
- chronic heart failure
- alcoholism
- conditions causing high metabolic needs such as burns.

The consequences of PEM may include:

- reduced enzyme and plasma protein production
- increased susceptibility to infection
- physical and mental growth deficiencies in children
- severe diarrhea and malabsorption
- numerous secondary nutritional deficiencies
- delayed wound healing
- mental fatigue.

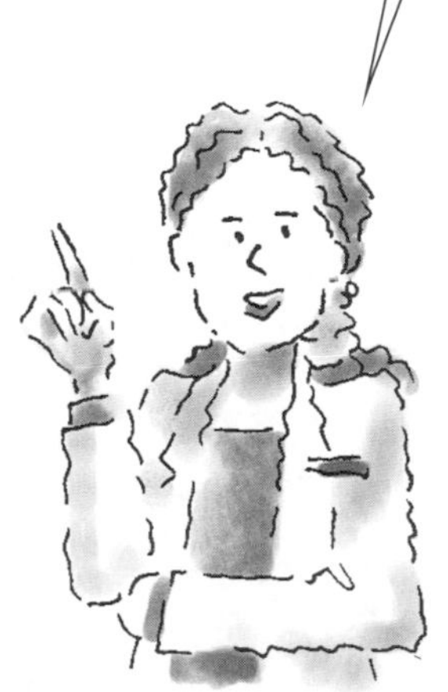

PEM forms

PEM takes three basic forms:

 iatrogenic PEM

 kwashiorkor

 marasmus.

Iatrogenic PEM

Commonly during hospitalization, a patient's nutritional status deteriorates because of inadequate protein or calorie intake, leading to iatrogenic PEM. Iatrogenic PEM affects more than 15% of patients in acute care centers. It's most common in patients hospitalized longer than 2 weeks.

Kwashiorkor

Kwashiorkor results from severe protein deficiency without a calorie deficit. It occurs most commonly in children ages 1 to 3. In the United States, it's usually secondary to:
- malabsorption disorders
- cancer and cancer therapies
- kidney disease
- hypermetabolic illness
- iatrogenic causes.

Marasmus

The third form of malnutrition, marasmus, is a prolonged and gradual wasting of muscle mass and subcutaneous fat. It's caused by inadequate intake of protein, calories, and other nutrients. Marasmus occurs most commonly in infants ages 6 to 18 months, after gastrectomy, and in patients with cancer of the mouth and esophagus.

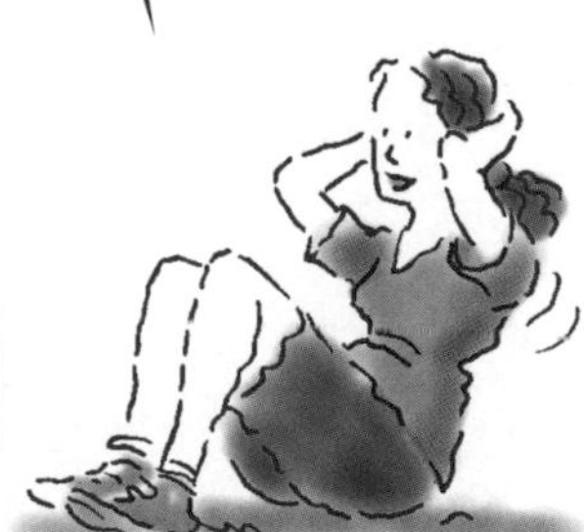

Nutritional assessment

When illness or surgery compromises a patient's intake or alters his metabolic requirements, you'll need to assess the relationship between nutrients consumed and energy expended. A nutritional assessment provides insight into how well the patient's physiologic need for nutrients is being met. Because poor nutritional status can affect most body systems, a thorough nutritional assessment helps you anticipate problems and intervene appropriately.

To assess nutritional status, follow these steps:

- Obtain a dietary history.
- Perform a physical assessment.
- Take anthropometric measurements.
- Review the results of pertinent diagnostic tests.

Dietary history

When obtaining a dietary history, check for signs of decreased food intake, increased metabolic requirements, or a combination of the two. Also check dietary recall, using a 24-hour recall or diet diary. Note any factors that affect food intake and changes in appetite. Obtain a weight history.

Physical assessment

When performing a physical assessment, be sure to include:

- chief complaint
- present illness
- medical history, including previous major illnesses, injuries, hospitalizations, or surgeries
- allergies and history of intolerance to food and medications
- family history, including familial, genetic, or environmental illnesses
- social history, including environmental, psychological, and sociologic factors that may influence nutritional status, such as alcoholism, living alone, or lack of transportation.

Are you missing anything?

Also, be sure to observe for subtle signs of malnutrition. (See *Signs of poor nutrition.*)

Measuring up

Anthropometry compares the patient's measurements with established standards. (See *Taking anthropometric measurements*, page 266.) It's an objective, noninvasive method for measuring overall body size, composition, and specific body parts. Commonly used anthropometric measurements include:

- height
- weight
- ideal body weight
- body frame size.

Triceps skinfold thickness, midarm circumference, and midarm muscle circumference are less commonly used anthropometric measurements because they tend to vary by age and race.

Signs of poor nutrition

When performing a physical assessment, note the patient's overall condition and inspect the skin, mouth, and teeth. Then look for these subtle signs of poor nutrition:

- poor skin turgor
- bruising
- abnormal pigmentation
- darkening of the mouth lining
- protruding eyes (exophthalmos)
- neck swelling
- adventitious breath sounds
- dental caries
- ill-fitting dentures
- signs of infection or irritation in and around the mouth
- muscle wasting
- abdominal wasting, masses, and tenderness and an enlarged liver.

Taking anthropometric measurements

Follow the steps below to measure midarm circumference, triceps skinfold thickness, and midarm muscle circumference.

Midarm circumference
Locate the midpoint on the patient's upper arm using a nonstretching tape measure, and mark the midpoint with a marking pen.

Triceps skinfold thickness
Determine the triceps skinfold thickness by grasping the patient's skin between the thumb and forefinger approximately 1 cm above the midpoint. Place the calipers at the midpoint and squeeze the calipers for about 3 seconds. Record the measurement registered on the handle gauge to the nearest 0.5 mm. Take two more readings, and then average all three to compensate for possible error.

Midarm muscle circumference
At the midpoint, measure the midarm circumference. Calculate midarm muscle circumference by multiplying the triceps skinfold thickness (in centimeters) by 3.143 and subtracting the result from the midarm circumference.

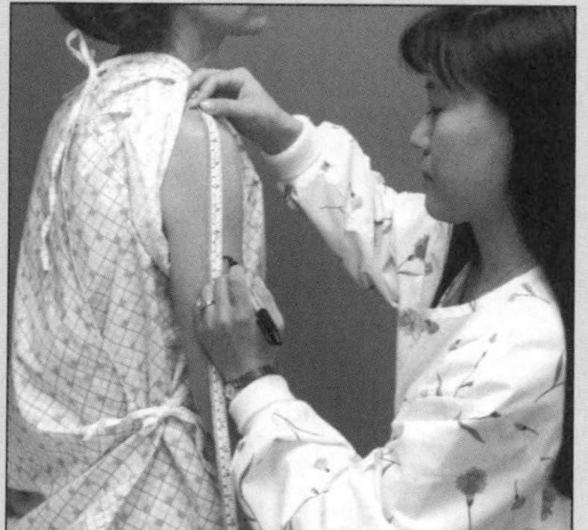

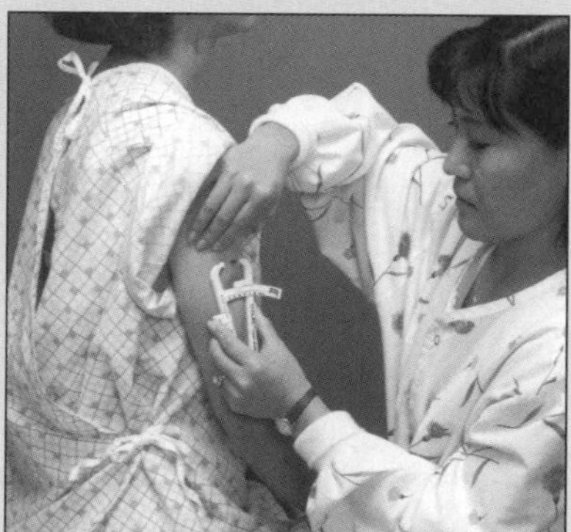

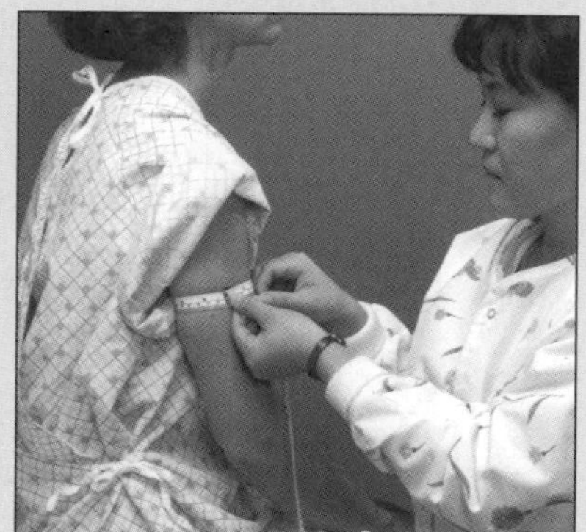

Interpreting your findings
Record all three measurements as percentages of the standard measurements using the following formula:

$$\frac{\text{Actual measurement}}{\text{Standard measurement}} \times 100$$

Compare the patient's percentage measurements with the standard. A measurement less than 90% of the standard indicates calorie deprivation; a measurement over 90% of the standard indicates adequate or more than adequate energy reserves.

Measurement	Standard	90%
Midarm circumference	Men: 29.3 cm Women: 26.5 cm	Men: 26.4 cm Women: 23.9 cm
Triceps skinfold thickness	Men: 12.5 mm Women: 16.5 mm	Men: 11.3 mm Women: 14.9 mm
Midarm muscle circumference	Men: 25.3 cm Women: 23.2 cm	Men: 22.8 cm Women: 20.9 cm

Not up to 90%?

A finding of less than 90% of the standard measurement may indicate a need for nutritional support.

Diagnostic studies

Evidence of a nutritional problem commonly appears in the results of a diagnostic test. Tests are used to evaluate:

- visceral protein status
- lean body mass
- vitamin and mineral balance.

Diagnostic studies are also used to evaluate the effectiveness of nutritional support. (See *Detecting deficiencies*.)

Detecting deficiencies

Laboratory studies help pinpoint nutritional deficiencies by aiding in the diagnosis of anemia, malnutrition, and other disorders. Check out this chart to learn about some commonly ordered diagnostic tests, their purposes, normal values, and implications. Albumin, prealbumin, transferrin, and triglyceride levels are the major indicators of nutritional deficiency.

Test and purpose	Normal values	Implications
Creatinine height index Uses a 24-hour urine sample to determine adequacy of muscle mass	• Determined from a reference table of values based on a patient's height or weight	• Less than 80% of reference value: moderate depletion of muscle mass (protein reserves) • Less than 60% of reference value: severe depletion, with increased risk of compromised immune function
Hematocrit Diagnoses anemia and dehydration	• Male: 42% to 50% • Female: 40% to 48% • Child: 29% to 41% • Neonate: 55% to 68%	• Increased values: severe dehydration, polycythemia • Decreased values: iron-deficiency anemia, excessive blood loss
Hemoglobin Assesses blood's oxygen-carrying capacity to aid in the diagnosis of anemia, protein deficiency, and hydration status	• Older adult: 10 to 17 g/dl • Adult male: 13 to 18 g/dl • Adult female: 12 to 16 g/dl • Child: 9 to 15.5 g/dl • Neonate: 14 to 20 g/dl	• Increased values: dehydration, polycythemia • Decreased values: protein deficiency, iron-deficiency anemia, excessive blood loss, overhydration
Serum albumin Helps assess visceral protein stores	• Adult: 3.5 to 5 g/dl • Child: same as adult • Neonate: 3.6 to 5.4 g/dl	• Decreased values: malnutrition, overhydration, liver or kidney disease, heart failure, excessive blood protein losses such as from severe burns
Serum transferrin (similar to serum total iron binding capacity [TIBC]) Helps assess visceral protein stores; has a shorter half-life than serum albumin and, thus, more accurately reflects current status	• Adult: 200 to 400 μg/dl • Child: 350 to 450 μg/dl • Neonate: 60 to 175 μg/dl	• Increased TIBC: iron deficiency, as in pregnancy or iron-deficiency anemia • Decreased TIBC: iron excess, as in chronic inflammatory states • Below 200 μg/dl: visceral protein depletion • Below 100 μg/dl: severe visceral protein depletion

(continued)

Detecting deficiencies *(continued)*

Test and purpose	Normal values	Implications
Serum triglycerides Screens for hyperlipidemia	• 40 to 200 mg/dl	• Increased values combined with increased cholesterol levels: increased risk of atherosclerotic disease • Decreased values: protein-energy malnutrition (PEM), steatorrhea
Total lymphocyte count Diagnoses PEM	• 1,500 to 3,000/µl	• Increased values: infection or inflammation, leukemia, tissue necrosis • Decreased values: moderate to severe malnutrition if no other cause, such as influenza or measles, is identified
Total protein screen Detects hyperproteinemia or hypoproteinemia	• 6 to 8 g/dl	• Increased values: dehydration • Decreased values: malnutrition, protein loss
Transthyretin (prealbumin) Offers information regarding visceral protein stores; should be used in conjunction with albumin level (Prealbumin has a shorter half-life [2 to 3 days] than albumin. This test is sensitive to nutritional repletion.)	• 16 to 40 mg/dl	• Increased values: renal insufficiency; patient on dialysis • Decreased values: PEM, acute catabolic states, postsurgery, hyperthyroidism
Urine ketone bodies (acetone) Screens for ketonuria and detects carbohydrate deprivation	• Negative for ketones in urine	• Ketoacidosis: starvation

Parenteral nutrition solutions

The solution you administer depends on the type of parenteral nutrition and the patient's status. (See *Parenteral solutions*.)

I'm not feeling very energetic today. Must be due to my solution's low dextrose content.

Element roll call

Parenteral nutrition solutions may contain the following elements, each offering a particular benefit:

- *Dextrose* provides most of the calories that can help maintain nitrogen balance. The number of nonprotein calories needed to maintain nitrogen balance depends on the severity of the patient's illness.

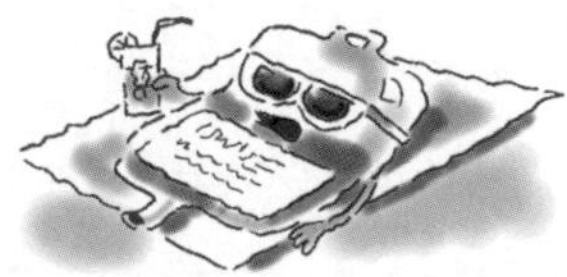

Parenteral solutions

Therapy and solution	Indications	Special considerations
Total parenteral nutrition • Dextrose, 20% to 70% (1 L dextrose 25% = 850 nonprotein calories) • Crystalline amino acids, 2.5% to 15% • Electrolytes, vitamins, micronutrients, insulin, and heparin as ordered • Fat emulsion, 10% or 20% (can be given peripherally or centrally) • Water	Long-term therapy (2 weeks or more) is used to: • supply large quantities of nutrients and calories (2,000 to 3,000 calories/day or more) • provide needed calories, restore nitrogen balance, replace essential vitamins, electrolytes, minerals, and trace elements • promote tissue synthesis, wound healing, and normal metabolic function • allow bowel rest and healing, reduce activity in the pancreas and small intestine • improve tolerance to surgery if severely malnourished.	• Is nutritionally complete • Requires surgical procedure for central venous (CV) access device insertion (can be done by a practitioner at the patient's bedside) • May result in metabolic complications (glucose intolerance or electrolyte imbalances) from hypertonic solution • May not be effective in severely stressed patients (such as those with sepsis or burns) • May interfere with immune mechanisms
Peripheral parenteral nutrition • Dextrose, 5% to 10% • Crystalline amino acids, 2.75% to 4.25% • Electrolytes, minerals, micronutrients, and vitamins as ordered • Fat emulsion, 10% or 20% • Heparin or hydrocortisone as ordered • Water	Short-term therapy (3 weeks or less) is used to: • maintain nutritional state in patients who can tolerate relatively high fluid volume, who usually resume bowel function and oral feedings in a few days, and who aren't candidates for CV access devices • provide approximately 1,300 to 1,800 calories/day.	• Is nutritionally complete for short-term therapy • Shouldn't be used in nutritionally depleted patients • Can't be used in volume-restricted patients because it requires high volumes of solution • Avoids insertion and maintenance of CV access device, but the patient must have good veins; I.V. site should be changed every 72 hours • Delivers less hypertonic solutions • May cause phlebitis • Offers lower risk of metabolic complications *I.V. lipid emulsion* • Has increased risk of hyperlipidemia • Irritates vein in long-term use

- *Amino acids* supply enough protein to replace essential amino acids, maintain protein stores, and prevent protein loss from muscle tissues.
- *Fats*, supplied as lipid emulsions, are a concentrated source of energy that prevent or correct fatty acid deficiencies. These are available in several concentrations and can provide 30% to 50% of a patient's daily calorie requirement.

- *Electrolytes and minerals* are added to the parenteral nutrition solution based on an evaluation of the patient's serum chemistry profile and metabolic needs.
- *Vitamins* ensure normal body functions and optimal nutrient use for the patient. A commercially available mixture of fat- and water-soluble vitamins, biotin, and folic acid may be added to the patient's parenteral nutrition solution.
- *Micronutrients*, also called *trace elements*, promote normal metabolism. Most commercial solutions contain zinc, copper, chromium, selenium, and manganese.
- *Water* is added to a parenteral nutrition solution based on the patient's fluid requirements and electrolyte balance.

Added features

Depending on the patient's condition, the practitioner may also order additives for the parenteral nutrition solution, such as insulin or heparin. (See *Understanding common additives.*)

Understanding common additives

Common parenteral nutrition solutions include dextrose 50% in water ($D_{50}W$), amino acids, and any of the additives listed here, which are used to treat a patient's specific metabolic deficiencies:

- Acetate prevents metabolic acidosis.
- Amino acids provide protein necessary for tissue repair.
- Calcium promotes development of bones and teeth and aids in blood clotting.
- Chloride regulates the acid-base equilibrium and maintains osmotic pressure.
- $D_{50}W$ provides calories for metabolism.
- Folic acid is needed for deoxyribonucleic acid formation and promotes growth and development.
- Magnesium aids carbohydrate and protein absorption.
- Micronutrients (such as zinc, manganese, and cobalt) help in wound healing and red blood cell synthesis.
- Phosphate minimizes the potential for developing peripheral paresthesia (numbness and tingling of the extremities).
- Potassium is needed for cellular activity and tissue synthesis.
- Sodium helps regulate water distribution and maintain normal fluid balance.
- Vitamin B complex aids the final absorption of carbohydrates and protein.
- Vitamin C helps in wound healing.
- Vitamin D is essential for bone metabolism and maintenance of serum calcium levels.
- Vitamin K helps prevent bleeding disorders.

Some of these additives may be ordered for your patient's parenteral nutrition solution.

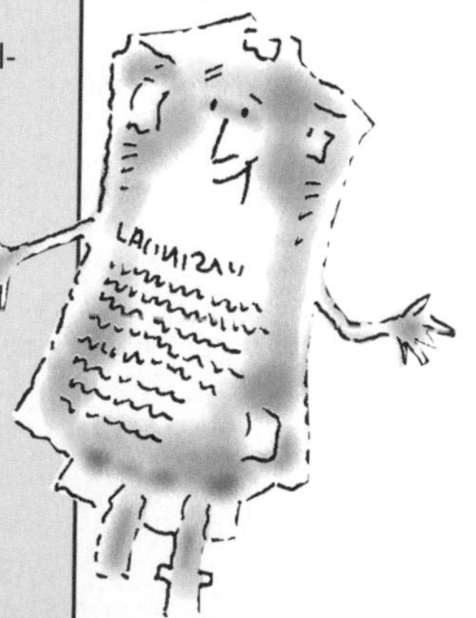

TPN solutions

Solutions for TPN are hypertonic, with an osmolarity of 1,800 to 2,600 mOsm/L. Electrolytes, minerals, vitamins, micronutrients, and water are added to the base solution to satisfy daily requirements. Lipids may be given as a separate solution or as an admixture with dextrose and amino acids.

When administering TPN, be sure to maintain the patient's glucose balance.

The 3:1 solution

Daily allotments of TPN solution, including lipids and other parenteral solution components, are commonly given in a single 3-L bag, called a *total nutrient admixture* or *3:1 solution.* (See *Understanding total nutrient admixture.*)

Maintaining glucose balance without adding insulin

Glucose balance is extremely important in a patient receiving TPN. Adults use 0.8 to 1 g of glucose per kilogram of body weight per hour. That means a patient can tolerate a constant I.V. infusion of hyperosmolar (highly concentrated) glucose without adding insulin to the solution. As the concentrated

Understanding total nutrient admixture

Total nutrient admixture is a white solution that delivers 1 day's worth of nutrients in a single 3-L bag. Also called *3:1 solution,* it combines lipids with other parenteral solution components.

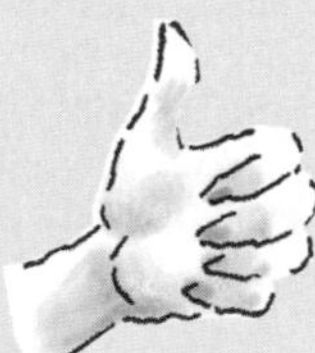

Advantages

The benefits of total nutrient admixture include:

- less need to handle the bag (lower risk of contamination)
- less time required
- less need for infusion sets and electronic infusion devices
- lower hospital costs
- increased patient mobility
- easier adjustment to home care.

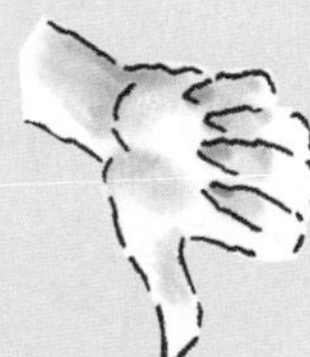

Disadvantages

The disadvantages of total nutrient admixture include:

- use of certain infusion devices precluded because of their inability to accurately deliver large volumes of solution
- 1.2-micron filter required (rather than a 0.22-micron filter) to allow lipid molecules through
- limited amount of calcium and phosphorus added because of the difficulty in detecting precipitate in the milky white solution.

glucose solution infuses, a pancreatic beta-cell response causes serum insulin levels to increase.

To allow the pancreas to establish and maintain the necessary increased insulin production, start with a slow infusion rate and increase it gradually as ordered. Abruptly stopping the infusion may cause rebound hypoglycemia, which calls for an infusion of dextrose.

Glucose balance may be further thrown off by:

- sepsis
- stress
- shock
- liver or kidney failure
- diabetes
- age
- pancreatic disease
- concurrent use of certain medications, including steroids.

PPN solutions

PPN solutions usually consist of dextrose 5% in water to 10% dextrose and 2.75% to 4.25% crystalline amino acids. Alternatively, PPN solutions may be slightly hypertonic, such as dextrose 10% in water ($D_{10}W$), with an osmolarity no greater than 600 mOsm/L. Lipid emulsions, electrolytes, trace elements, and vitamins may be given as part of PPN to add calories and other needed nutrients.

Lipid emulsions

In an oral diet, lipids or fats are the major source of calories, usually providing about 40% of the total calorie intake. In parenteral nutrition solutions, lipids provide 9 kcal/g. I.V. lipid emulsions are oxidized for energy as needed. As a nearly isotonic emulsion, concentrations of 10% or 20% can be safely infused through peripheral or central veins. Lipid emulsions prevent and treat essential fatty acid deficiency and provide a major source of energy.

In continuous delivery, I have to work day and night. In cyclic delivery, I get a few hours off. Gotta run now!

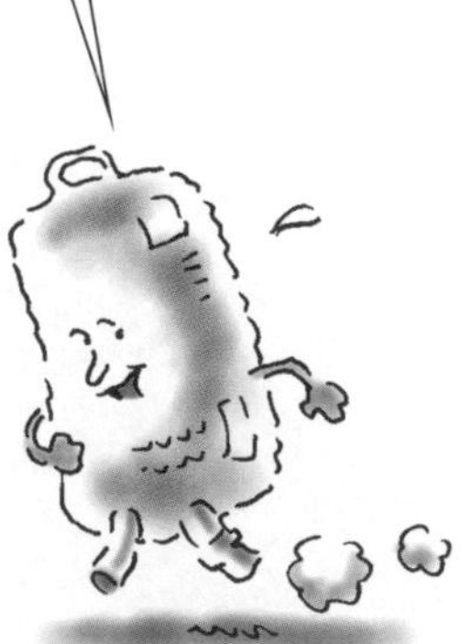

Administering parenteral nutrition

You may deliver parenteral nutrition in one of two ways:

 continuously

 cyclically.

Open for service 24 hours

With continuous delivery, the patient receives the infusion over a 24-hour period. The infusion begins at a slow rate and increases to the optimal rate as ordered. This type of delivery may prevent complications such as hyperglycemia caused by a high dextrose load.

Not-so-vicious cycle

A patient undergoing cyclic therapy receives the entire 24-hour volume of parenteral nutrition solution over a shorter period, perhaps 8, 10, 12, 14, or 16 hours. Home care parenteral nutrition programs have boosted the use of cyclic therapy. This type of therapy may be used to wean the patient from TPN. (See *Switching from continuous to cyclic TPN.*)

Switching from continuous to cyclic TPN

When switching from continuous to cyclic total parenteral nutrition (TPN), adjust the flow rate so the patient's blood glucose level can adapt to the decreased nutrient load. Do this by reducing the flow rate by one-half for 1 hour before stopping the infusion. Draw a blood glucose sample 1 hour after the infusion ends, and observe the patient for signs of hypoglycemia, such as sweating, shakiness, and irritability.

Administering TPN

TPN solutions must be infused in a central vein, using one of the following methods:

- peripherally inserted central catheter, with its tip lying in the superior vena cava
- CV access device
- implanted port.

In it for the long haul

Long-term therapy requires the use of one of the following devices:

- tunneled CV catheter, such as a Hickman, Broviac, or Groshong catheter
- implanted port, such as Infus-A-Port or Port-a-Cath.

The dilution solution

Because TPN fluid has about six times the solute concentration of blood, peripheral I.V. administration can cause sclerosis and thrombosis. To ensure adequate dilution, the CV access device is inserted into the superior vena cava, a wide-bore, high-flow vein.

Preparing the patient

To increase compliance, make sure that the patient understands the purpose of treatment and enlist his help throughout the course of therapy.

Taking TPN home

Understanding TPN and its goals helps a home care patient assume a greater role in administering, monitoring, and maintaining therapy. When instructing a home care patient, focus your teaching on signs and symptoms of:

- fluid, electrolyte, and glucose imbalances
- vitamin and trace element deficiencies and toxicities
- catheter infection, such as fever, chills, discomfort on infusion, and redness or drainage at the catheter insertion site.

To help prevent glucose imbalance, teach the home care patient receiving his first I.V. bag of TPN how to regulate the flow rate so he maintains the rate prescribed by the practitioner. Explain that a gradual increase in the flow rate allows the pancreas to establish and maintain the increased insulin production necessary to tolerate this treatment. When the goal rate of the TPN infusion is met, there should be no reason to adjust the rate.

Finally, review the details of the administration schedule, the equipment the patient will use and, to avoid incompatibilities, the prescribed and over-the-counter medications he takes.

To maintain glucose balance, teach your home care patient to increase the flow rate gradually.

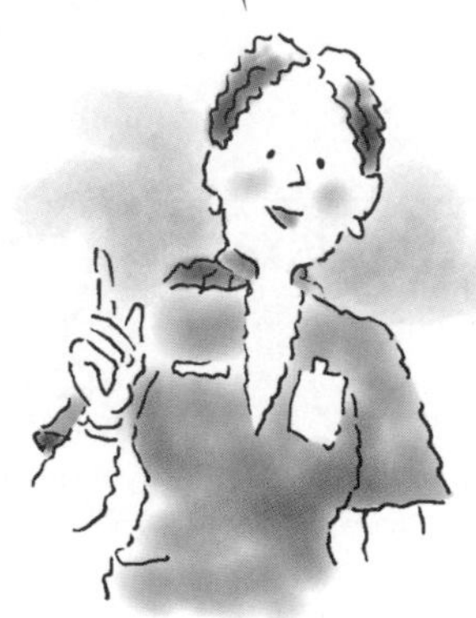

Be a compliance booster

To safely maintain this therapy, the prescribed regimen must be adhered to by the home care patient and his caregivers. Your teaching efforts and return demonstrations by the patient help boost compliance in all aspects of TPN therapy.

Preparing the equipment

Before TPN administration begins, the practitioner inserts a venous access device. The location of the catheter tip in the superior vena cava is confirmed by X-ray.

Gather the TPN solution, a pump, an administration set with a filter, alcohol swabs, gloves, and an I.V. pole. Be sure to wash your hands before preparing the TPN solution for administration, and prepare the administration set in a clean area.

Always use tubing with a filter when administering TPN. Filters are required by the Food and Drug Administration.

60-minute warm-up

The infusion of a chilled solution can cause discomfort, hypothermia, venous spasm, and venous constriction. Plan to remove the bag or bottle of TPN solution from the refrigerator about 60 minutes before hanging it to allow for warming.

Checking the order

Check the written order against the label on the bag or bottle. Make sure that the volumes, concentrations, and additives are included in the solution. Also check the infusion rate.

Infusate inspection is imperative

Careful inspection of the infusate should be a habit. Check for clouding, floating debris, or a change in color. Any of these phenomena could indicate contamination, problems with the integrity of the solution, or a pH change. If you see anything suspicious, notify the pharmacy. Inform the practitioner that there may be a delay in hanging the solution; he may want to order $D_{10}W$ until a new container of TPN solution is available. Also, be prepared to return the solution to the pharmacy.

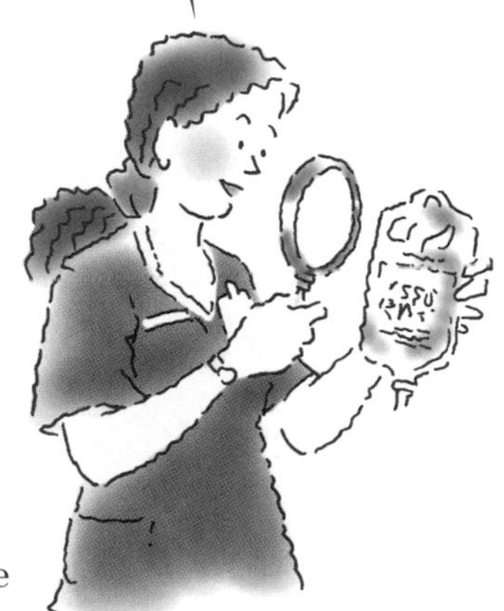

Handle with care

Most TPN solutions contain lipid emulsions, which call for special precautions. (See *Administering lipid emulsions.*)

Beginning the infusion

Before beginning the infusion, inspect the catheter insertion site for any signs or symptoms of infection. If none are seen, begin the infusion as ordered. Watch for swelling at the catheter insertion site. Swelling may indicate extravasation of the TPN solution, which can cause necrosis (tissue damage). If the patient reports discomfort at the start of the infusion, the catheter may be malpositioned or impaired, which requires a practitioner's follow-up. (See *Reducing the risk of infection,* page 276.)

Administering lipid emulsions

Most total parenteral nutrition solutions contain lipid emulsions. To safely administer them, follow these special precautions:

- Monitor the patient's vital signs and watch for adverse reactions, such as fever, a pressure sensation over the eyes, nausea, vomiting, headache, chest and back pain, tachycardia, dyspnea, cyanosis, and flushing, sweating, or chills. If the patient has no adverse reactions to the test dose, begin the infusion at the prescribed rate.
- Before the infusion, always check the parenteral nutrition containing lipids for separation or an oily appearance. If either condition exists, the lipid may have come out of emulsion and shouldn't be used.
- Because lipid emulsions are at high risk for bacterial growth, never rehang a partially empty bottle of emulsion.

Maintaining the infusion

If the patient tolerates the solution well the first day, the practitioner usually increases intake to the goal rate by the second day. To maintain a TPN infusion, follow these key steps:

- Check the order provided by the practitioner against the label on the TPN container.
- Label the container with the expiration date, time at which the solution was hung, glucose concentration, and total volume of solution. (If the bag or bottle is damaged and you don't have an immediate replacement, you can approximate the glucose concentration until a new container is ready by adding 50% glucose to $D_{10}W$.)
- Maintain flow rates as prescribed, even if the flow falls behind schedule.
- Don't allow TPN solutions to hang for more than 24 hours.
- Change the tubing and filter every 24 hours, using strict aseptic technique. Make sure that all tubing junctions are secure.
- Perform I.V. site care and dressing changes according to your facility's policy and protocol.
- Check the infusion pump's volume meter and time tape to monitor for irregular flow rate. Gravity should never be used to administer TPN.
- Record the patient's vital signs when you initiate therapy and every 4 to 8 hours thereafter (or more often, if necessary). Be alert for increased body temperature — one of the earliest signs of catheter-related sepsis.
- Monitor your patient's glucose levels as ordered using glucose fingersticks or serum tests.
- Accurately record the patient's daily fluid intake and output, specifying the volume and type of each fluid. This record is a diagnostic tool that you can use to assure prompt, precise replacement of fluid and electrolyte deficits.
- Assess the patient's physical status daily. Weigh him at the same time each morning (after voiding), in similar clothing, using the same scale. Suspect fluid imbalance if the patient gains more than 1 lb (0.45 kg) per day. If ordered, obtain anthropometric measurements.
- Monitor the results of routine laboratory tests, such as serum electrolyte, blood urea nitrogen, and glucose levels, and report abnormal findings to the doctor so appropriate changes in the TPN solution can be made.
- Check serum triglyceride levels, which should be in the normal range during continuous TPN infusion. Typically, alanine aminotransferase, aspartate aminotransferase, alkaline phosphatase, cholesterol, triglyceride, plasma-free fatty acid, and coagulation tests are performed weekly.

Need an emergency substitute for a damaged TPN bag? Try adding 50% glucose to $D_{10}W$.

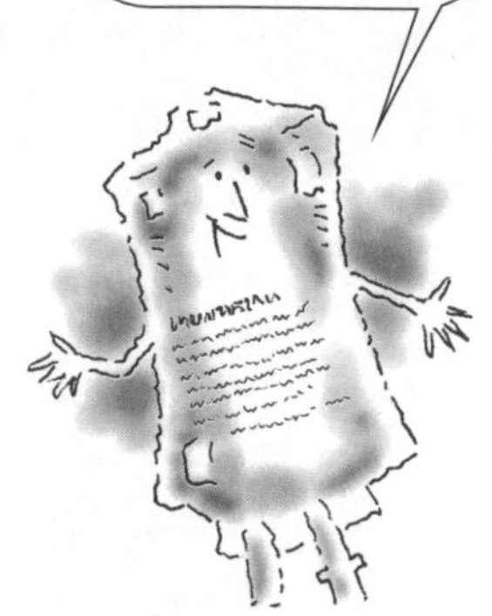

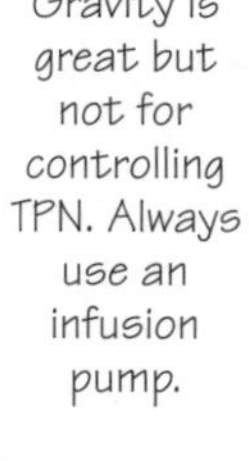

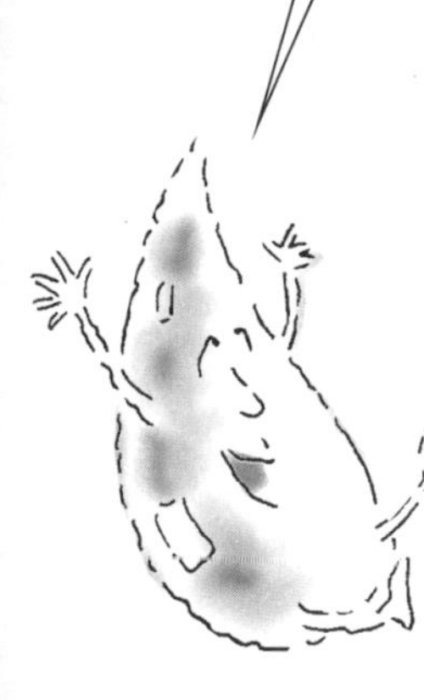

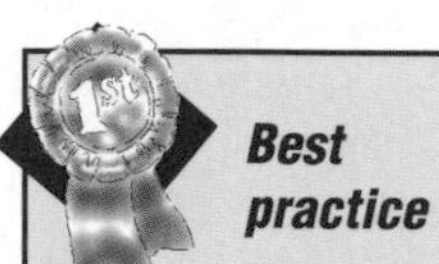

Best practice

Reducing the risk of infection

Because a total parenteral nutrition (TPN) solution serves as a medium for bacterial growth and a central venous line provides systemic access, the patient receiving TPN risks infection and sepsis. According to the Centers for Disease Control and Prevention, maintaining strict aseptic technique when handling the equipment used to administer therapy has been shown to reduce the number of TPN-related infections.

- Monitor the patient for signs and symptoms of nutritional aberrations, such as fluid and electrolyte imbalances and glucose metabolism disturbances. Some patients require supplementary insulin throughout TPN therapy; the pharmacy usually adds regular insulin directly to the TPN solution.
- Provide emotional support. Keep in mind that patients commonly associate eating with positive feelings and become disturbed when it's eliminated.
- Provide frequent mouth care for the patient.
- Document all assessment findings and nursing interventions.

Don't forget to record your assessment findings and nursing interventions throughout treatment.

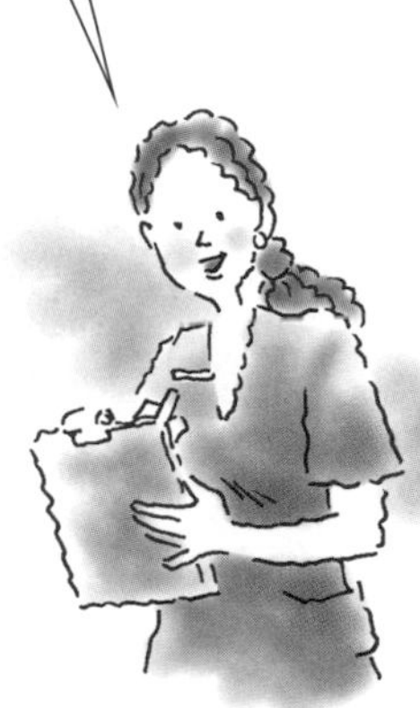

A port of last resort

Avoid using a TPN infusion port for another infusion. When using a single-lumen CV access device, don't use the line to piggyback or infuse blood or blood products, give a bolus injection, administer simultaneous I.V. solutions, measure CV pressure, or draw blood for laboratory tests. In unavoidable circumstances, the TPN port may be used for electrolyte replacement or insulin drips because these infusions are commonly additives to the solution. Remember, never add medication to a TPN solution container. Also, avoid using add-on devices, which increase the risk of infection.

Administering PPN

Using an amino acid, dextrose, and lipid emulsion solution, PPN fulfills a patient's basic calorie needs without the risks involved in CV access. Because PPN solutions have lower tonicity than TPN solutions, a patient receiving PPN must be able to tolerate infusion of large volumes of fluid. Administer PPN through a peripheral vein.

PPN solutions are less concentrated than TPN solutions...
...which means more fluid is needed to deliver nutrients.

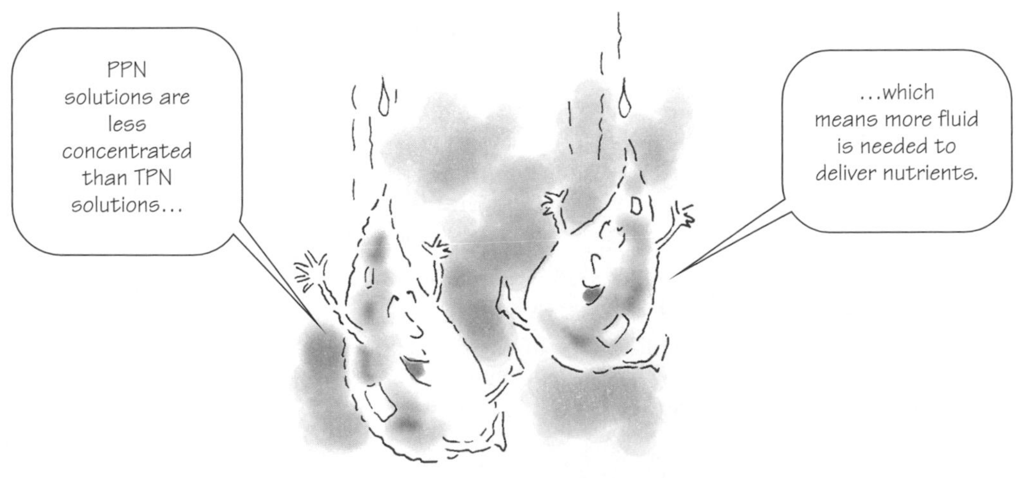

Preparing the patient

Make sure that the patient understands what to expect before, during, and after therapy.

Obtain the largest vein

Select the patient's largest available vein as the insertion site. Using a large vein enables the blood to adequately dilute the PPN solution, which can help avoid irritation. When using a short-term catheter, rotate the site every 48 to 72 hours, or according to your facility's policy and procedures.

Preparing the equipment

To administer PPN, gather the necessary equipment, including:

- ordered PPN solution (at room temperature)
- infusion pump
- administration set
- alcohol swabs
- I.V. pole
- venipuncture equipment, if needed.

Checking the order

Check the written order against the written label on the bag. Make sure that the solution is for peripheral infusion and that the volumes, concentrations, and additives are included in the solution. Also check the infusion rate.

A little lecture about lipids

In PPN therapy, lipid emulsions may be part of the solution. If given separately, piggyback the lipid emulsion below the in-line filter close to the insertion site to avoid having lipids clog the filtration system. When giving lipids, use controllers that can accommodate lipid emulsions.

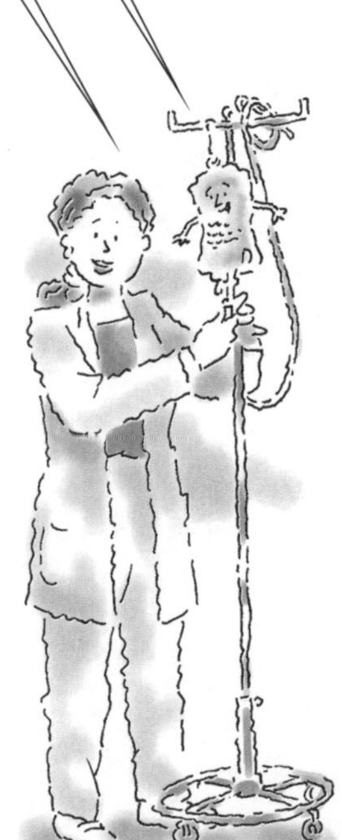

Beginning the infusion

Begin the PPN infusion as ordered. Watch for swelling at the peripheral insertion site. Swelling may indicate infiltration or extravasation of the PPN solution, which can cause tissue damage.

Maintaining the infusion

Caring for a patient receiving a PPN infusion involves the same steps required for any patient receiving a peripheral I.V. infusion. You need to maintain the infusion rate and care for the tubing, dressings, infusion site, and I.V. devices. In addition, monitor the patient for signs or symptoms of sepsis, including:

- glucose in the urine (glycosuria)
- chills
- malaise
- increased white blood cells (leukocytosis)
- altered level of consciousness
- elevated glucose levels, measured by fingerstick or serum chemistry
- elevated temperature (usually higher than 100.4° F [38° C], according to the Centers for Disease Control and Prevention).

Insulin insight

Because the synthesis of lipase (a fat-splitting enzyme) increases insulin requirements, the insulin dosage of a diabetic patient may need to be increased as ordered. Insulin is one of the additives that may be adjusted in the formulation of the PPN solution.

Hormone hint

For a patient with hypothyroidism who's receiving long-term TPN therapy, you may need to administer thyroid-stimulating hormone (TSH). TSH affects lipase activity and may prevent triglycerides from accumulating in the vascular system.

Patient reports

Patients receiving lipid emulsions commonly report a feeling of fullness or bloating; occasionally, they experience an unpleasant metallic or greasy taste. Some patients develop allergic reactions to the fat emulsion.

Lipid letdowns

Early adverse reactions to lipid emulsion therapy occur in fewer than 1% of patients. These reactions may include:

- fever
- difficulty breathing
- cyanosis
- nausea
- vomiting
- headache
- flushing
- sweating
- lethargy
- dizziness
- chest and back pain
- slight pressure over the eyes
- irritation at the infusion site.

Feeling full or bloated is a common response to lipid emulsions.

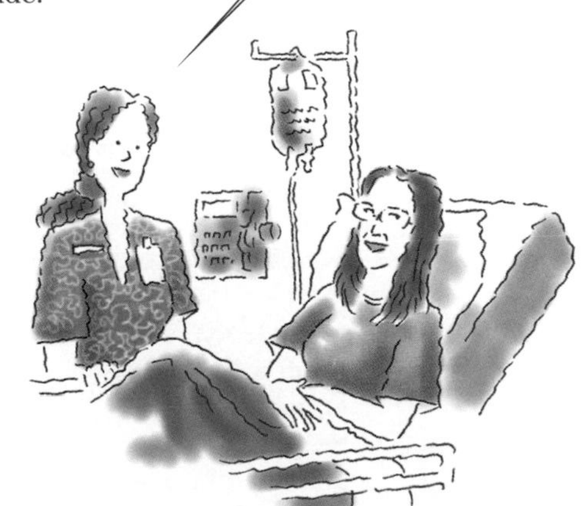

Changes in laboratory test results may also reveal problems when a patient receives lipid emulsions, including:
- hyperlipidemia
- hypercoagulability
- thrombocytopenia.

Considering clearance

The practitioner monitors the patient's lipid emulsion clearance rate. Lipid emulsion may clear from the blood at an accelerated rate in a patient with severe burns, multiple trauma, or a metabolic imbalance.

Precautions and complications

In this section, you'll find special considerations for administering parenteral nutrition to pediatric and elderly patients. You'll also find information about possible complications during therapy and pointers for discontinuing therapy safely.

Patients with special needs

Pediatric and elderly patients are particularly susceptible to fluid overload and heart failure. With these patients, be particularly careful to administer the correct volume of parenteral nutrition solution at the correct infusion rate.

Pediatric patients

Parenteral feeding therapy for children serves a dual purpose:

 It maintains a child's nutritional status.

 It fuels a child's growth.

An extra helping

Children have a greater need than adults for certain nutrients, including:
- protein
- carbohydrates
- fat
- electrolytes
- micronutrients
- vitamins
- fluids.

This greater need is an important consideration in accurately calculating solution components for pediatric patients.

Because they're growing, children need more of some nutrients than adults do.

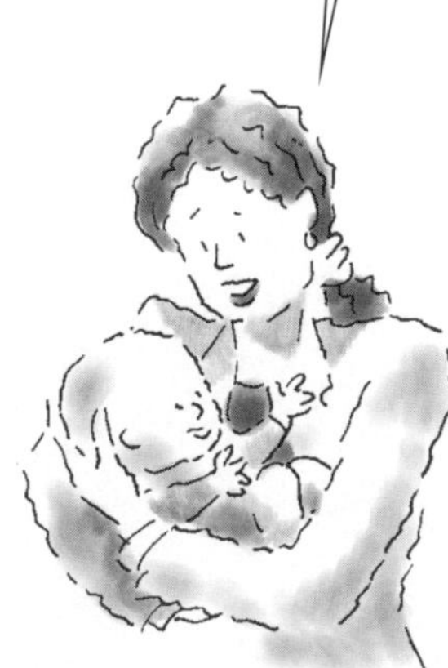

Factor these in

As with adults, children receiving TPN should be evaluated carefully by the nurse, practitioner, and nutritional support team. Keep in mind the following factors when planning to meet children's nutritional needs:

- age
- weight
- activity level
- size
- development
- calorie needs.

Lipid liabilities in little ones

Administering TPN with lipid emulsions in a premature or low-birth-weight neonate may lead to lipid accumulation in the lungs. Thrombocytopenia (platelet deficiency) has also been reported in infants receiving 20% lipid emulsions.

Elderly patients

Elderly patients are prone to fluid overload and drug interactions, so watch carefully when administering parenteral solutions.

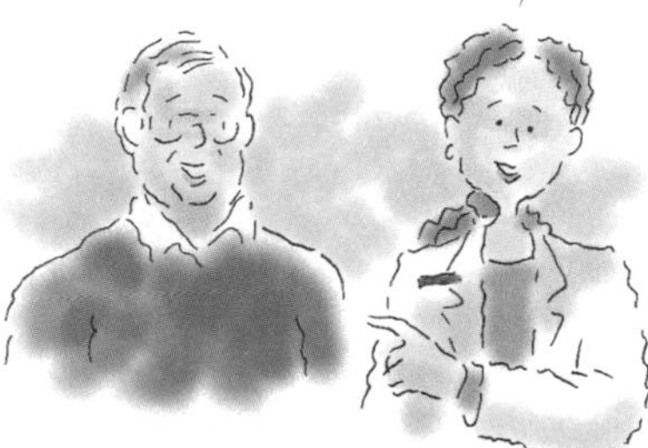

In elderly patients, overinfusion can produce serious adverse effects, so always monitor flow rates carefully. Elderly patients are also at risk for fluid overload when TPN or PPN is given.

What lies underneath

An elderly patient may have underlying clinical problems that affect the outcome of treatment. For example, he may be taking medications that can interact with the components in the parenteral nutrition solution. For this reason, ask the pharmacist about possible interactions with any drug the patient is taking.

Complications

Patients receiving parenteral nutrition therapy face many of the same complications as patients undergoing any type of peripheral I.V. or CV therapy. (See *Handling TPN hazards*, pages 282 and 283.)

Complications of any parenteral nutrition therapy may result from problems that are:

- catheter-related
- metabolic
- mechanical.

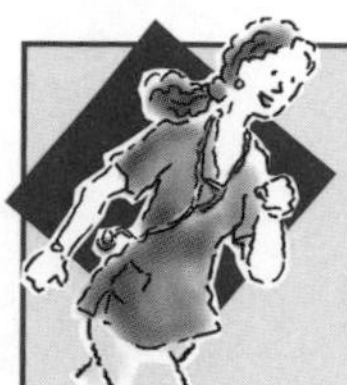

Running smoothly

Handling TPN hazards

Complications of total parenteral nutrition (TPN) therapy can result from catheter-related, metabolic, or mechanical problems. To help you treat these common complications, use this chart.

Complications	Interventions
Catheter-related complications	
Clotted catheter	• Reposition the catheter. • Instill alteplase (t-PA) to clear the catheter lumen as ordered.
Dislodged catheter	• Place a sterile gauze pad treated with antimicrobial ointment on the insertion site, and apply pressure.
Cracked or broken tubing	• Apply a padded hemostat above the break to prevent air from entering the line.
Pneumothorax	• Assist with chest tube insertion. • Maintain chest tube suctioning as ordered.
Sepsis	• Remove the catheter and culture the tip. • Give appropriate antibiotics as ordered.
Metabolic complications	
Hyperglycemia	• Start insulin therapy or adjust the TPN flow rate as ordered.
Hypoglycemia	• Infuse dextrose as ordered.
Hyperosmolar hyperglycemic nonketotic syndrome	• Stop dextrose. • Rehydrate with the ordered infusate.
Hypokalemia	• Increase potassium supplementation.
Hypomagnesemia	• Increase magnesium supplementation.
Hypophosphatemia	• Increase phosphate supplementation.
Hypocalcemia	• Increase calcium supplementation.
Metabolic acidosis	• Adjust the formula and assess for contributing factors.

Handling TPN hazards *(continued)*

Complications	Interventions
Metabolic complications	
Liver dysfunction	• Decrease carbohydrates and add I.V. lipids. • Consider cyclic infusions.
Hyperkalemia	• Decrease potassium supplementation.
Mechanical complications	
Air embolism	• Clamp the catheter. • Place the patient in Trendelenburg's position on the left side. • Give oxygen as ordered. • If cardiac arrest occurs, initiate cardiopulmonary resuscitation.
Venous thrombosis	• Notify the practitioner. • Administer heparin, if ordered. • Venous flow studies may be done.
Too rapid an infusion	• Check the infusion rate. • Check the infusion pump.
Extravasation	• Stop the I.V. infusion. • Assess the patient for cardiopulmonary abnormalities. Chest X-ray may be performed.
Phlebitis	• Apply gentle heat to the insertion site. • Elevate the insertion site, if possible.

Catheter-related complications

The most common catheter-related complications include:

- clotting
- dislodgment
- cracked or broken tubing
- pneumothorax
- sepsis.

Interrupted flow rate?

Suspect a clotted catheter if the infusion flow rate is interrupted. You may also notice that a greater pressure is needed to maintain the infusion at the desired infusion rate.

Discovering dislodgment

When the catheter comes out of the vein, catheter dislodgment may be obvious. You may note that the dressing is wet. The patient may report feeling cold or that his gown is wet. When the catheter is located peripherally, the area around the insertion site may be red or swollen from subcutaneous extravasation of the PPN solution. With a centrally inserted catheter, there may be swelling and redness around the insertion site. The most significant complications include bleeding from the insertion site or an air embolism.

Tubing trauma

If the catheter is damaged, infusate may leak from a cracked area or the insertion site. If the infusion tubing is damaged, the I.V. insertion site remains dry. Both situations require immediate attention because of the risk of bleeding, contamination, or air emboli.

Gasp! Air in the pleural cavity

Air in the pleural cavity (pneumothorax) usually results from trauma to the pleura during insertion of a CV access device. The patient may have dyspnea and chest pain; he may also develop a cough. Auscultation reveals diminished breath sounds, and the patient may be sweating and appear cyanotic. Assessment may also reveal unilateral chest movement. Pneumothorax should be confirmed by X-ray for the best treatment results.

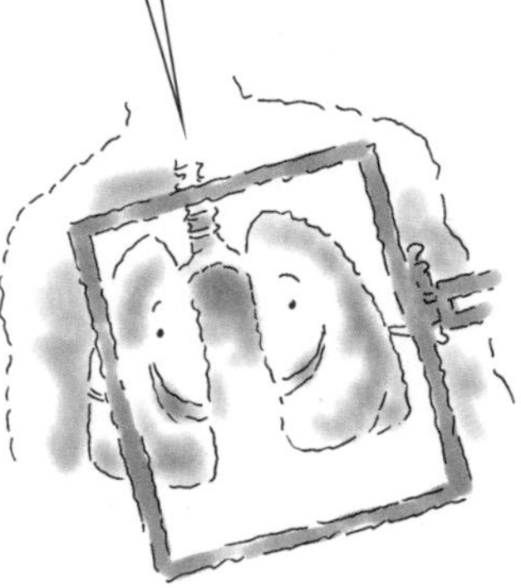

Sepsis alert

Sepsis, the most serious catheter-related complication, can be fatal. You can prevent it by providing meticulous, consistent catheter care.

If the patient is developing catheter-related sepsis, he'll develop an unexplained fever, chills, and a red, indurated area around the catheter site. The patient may also have unexplained hyperglycemia, commonly an early warning sign of sepsis.

Metabolic complications

Metabolic complications include:

- hyperglycemia or hypoglycemia (high or low blood glucose level)
- hyperosmolar hyperglycemic nonketotic syndrome (HHNS)
- hyperkalemia or hypokalemia (high or low blood potassium level)
- hypomagnesemia (low blood magnesium level)

- hypophosphatemia (low blood phosphate level)
- hypocalcemia (low blood calcium level)
- metabolic acidosis
- liver dysfunction.

Glucose — feast or famine

The patient may develop hyperglycemia if the formula's glucose concentration is excessive, the infusion rate is too rapid, or his glucose tolerance is compromised by diabetes, stress, or sepsis. Signs and symptoms of hyperglycemia include fatigue, restlessness, and weakness. The patient may become anxious, confused and, in some cases, delirious or even comatose. He'll be dehydrated and have polyuria and elevated blood and urine glucose levels.

Conversely, the patient may develop hypoglycemia if parenteral nutrition is interrupted suddenly or if he receives excessive insulin. Signs and symptoms may include sweating, shaking, confusion, and irritability.

S.O.S.! It's HHNS!

An acute complication of hyperglycemic crisis, HHNS is caused by hyperosmolar diuresis resulting from untreated hyperglycemia. A patient with HHNS has a high serum osmolarity, is dehydrated, and has extremely high glucose levels — as high as 4,800 mg/dl. If untreated, he can develop glycosuria and electrolyte disturbances and even become comatose. Suspect HHNS if your patient becomes confused or lethargic or experiences seizures.

Glucose levels ranging from 600 to 4,800 mg/dl indicate HHNS.

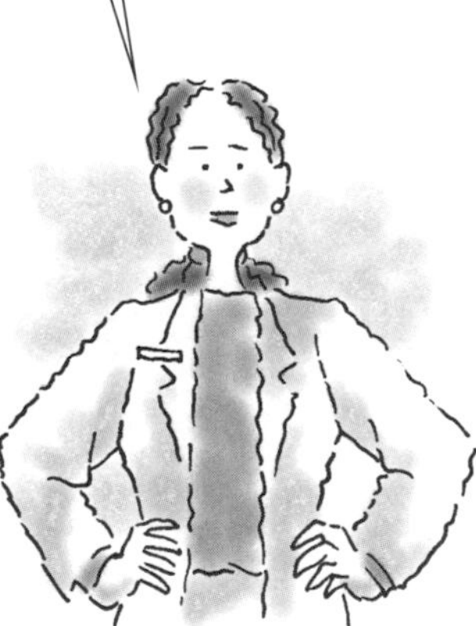

Potassium — a plethora or pittance

Patients develop hyperkalemia because of too much potassium in the TPN formula, renal disease, or hyponatremia. Look for skeletal muscle weakness, decreased heart rate, irregular pulse, and tall T waves.

Patients develop hypokalemia because of too little potassium in the solution, excessive loss of potassium brought on by GI tract disturbances or diuretic use, or large doses of insulin. Look for muscle weakness, paralysis, paresthesia, and cardiac arrhythmias.

Magnesium mayhem

Hypomagnesemia results from insufficient magnesium in the solution. Suspect hypomagnesemia if your patient complains of tingling around the mouth or paresthesia in his fingers. He may also show signs of mental changes, hyperreflexia, tetany, and arrhythmias.

Phosphate funk

Hypophosphatemia results from insulin therapy, alcoholism, and the use of phosphate-binding antacids. Suspect hypophosphatemia if the patient shows irritability, weakness, and paresthesia. In extreme cases, coma and cardiac arrest can occur. Very rarely, a patient develops hyperphosphatemia. Patients with renal insufficiency are prone to hyperphosphatemia.

Calcium calamity

Hypocalcemia, a rare complication, results from too little calcium in the solution, vitamin D deficiency, or pancreatitis. The patient may develop numbing or tingling sensations, tetany, polyuria, dehydration, and arrhythmias.

Acid-base balance blues

Metabolic acidosis can occur if the patient develops an increased serum chloride level and a decreased serum bicarbonate level.

Last but not least, liver dysfunction

Increased serum alkaline phosphatase, lactate dehydrogenase, and bilirubin levels can indicate liver dysfunction.

Mechanical complications

Mechanical complications that can plague parenteral nutrition therapy include:

- air embolism
- venous thrombosis
- extravasation
- phlebitis.

Sounds like an air embolism

Suspect an air embolism if the patient develops apprehension, chest pain, tachycardia, hypotension, cyanosis, seizures, loss of consciousness, or cardiac arrest. Auscultation may also reveal the classic sign of an air embolism: a churning heart murmur.

A churning heart murmur is a classic sign of air embolism.

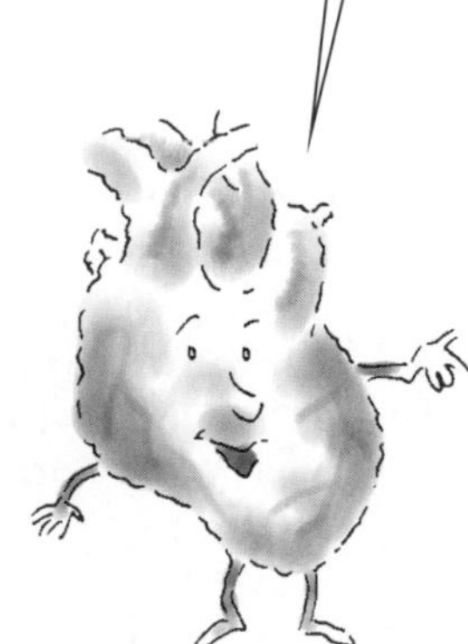

Looks like thrombosis

Suspect thrombosis when you see swelling at the catheter insertion site or swelling of the hand, arm, neck, or face on the same side as the catheter. Other signs and symptoms include pain at the insertion site and along the vein, malaise, fever, and tachycardia.

The risk of rushing

If TPN is infused too rapidly, the patient may feel nauseated, have a headache, and become lethargic. Heart failure is also a risk because of fluid overload.

An intimation of extravasation

If you observe swelling of the tissue around the insertion site, it may indicate extravasation. The patient may also complain of pain at the insertion site.

Feels like phlebitis

Pain, tenderness, redness, and warmth at the insertion site and along the vein path may indicate phlebitis.

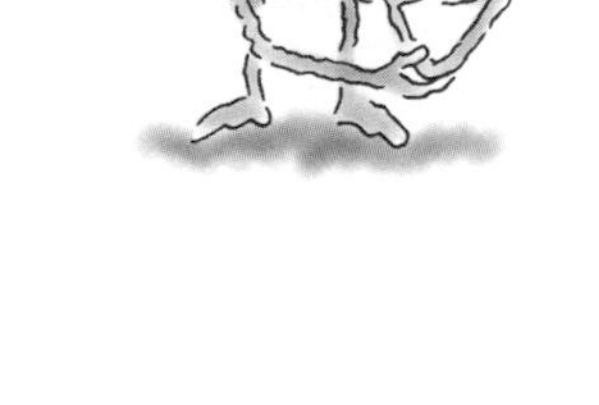

Other complications

PPN and lipid emulsion administration pose distinct risks.

Particular PPN problems

Significant complications of PPN therapy include phlebitis, infiltration, and extravasation.

Lipid low points

Prolonged administration of lipid emulsions can produce delayed complications, including an enlarged liver or spleen, blood dyscrasia (thrombocytopenia and leukopenia), and transient increases in results of liver function studies. A small number of patients receiving 20% I.V. lipid emulsion develop brown pigmentation due to fat pigmentation.

Discontinuing therapy

One major difference exists between the procedures for discontinuing TPN and PPN therapy. A patient receiving TPN should be weaned from therapy and should receive some other form of nutritional therapy such as enteral feedings.

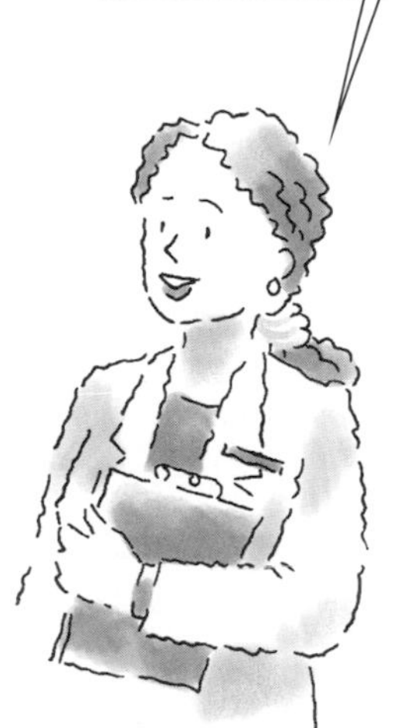

When to wean and when not to wean

When the patient is receiving PPN, therapy can be discontinued without weaning because the dextrose concentration is lower than in TPN. When discontinuing TPN therapy, however, you should wean the patient over 24 hours to prevent rebound hypoglycemia.

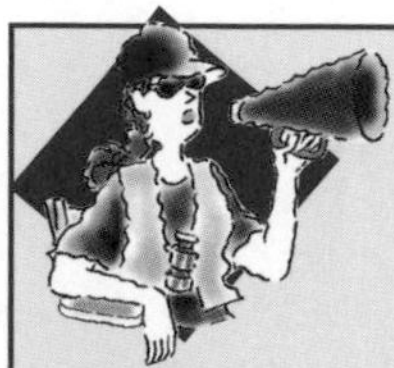

That's a wrap!

Parenteral nutrition review

Benefits
- Provides nutrition for patients who can't take nutrients through the GI tract because of illness or surgery
- Can be used when the patient is hemodynamically unstable or has impaired blood flow to the GI tract

Drawbacks
- Carries certain risks (catheter infection, hyperglycemia, hypokalemia)
- Requires vascular access
- Costs about 10 times more than enteral nutrition

Protein-energy malnutrition
Iatrogenic
- Inadequate protein and calorie intake during hospitalization

Kwashiorkor
- Severe protein deficiency without a calorie deficiency
- Typically occurs in children ages 1 to 3

Marasmus
- Inadequate intake of protein, calories, and other nutrients
- Typically occurs in infants ages 6 to 18 months, in patients with mouth and esophageal cancer, and after gastrectomy

Assessing nutritional status
Dietary history
- Check for decreased intake.
- Check for increased metabolic requirements.

Physical assessment
- Check for subtle signs of malnutrition.
- Obtain anthropometric measurements.

Diagnostic tests
- Major indicators of malnutrition are changes in the albumin, prealbumin, transferrin, and triglyceride levels.

TPN vs. PPN
TPN
- Dextrose 20% to 70%
- Administered through a central venous access device
- May be given in a 3-L bag with lipids daily
- Requires starting slow infusion with gradual increase

PPN
- Dextrose 5% to 10%
- Administered through a peripheral catheter
- Requires larger volume of fluid to meet nutritional needs
- Doesn't require starting with slow infusion rate

Potential complications
- Problems related to catheter (clotting, dislodgment, infection, pneumothorax, damaged tubing)
- Metabolic problems
- Mechanical complications (air embolism, venous thrombosis, extravasation, phlebitis)

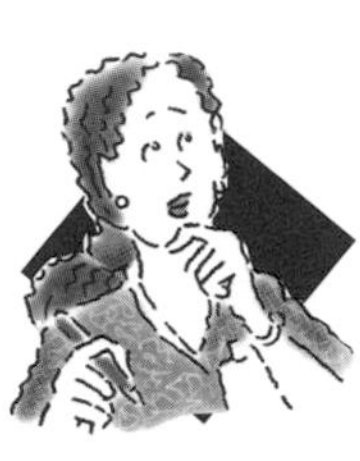

Quick quiz

1. What's the maximal amount of time that TPN solutions are permitted to infuse before the bag must be replaced?

A. 24 hours
B. 48 hours
C. 12 hours
D. 72 hours

Answer: A. Don't allow TPN solutions to hang for more than 24 hours.

2. When administering TPN, which of the following conditions is one of the first signs of catheter-related sepsis?

A. Hypothermia
B. Pruritus
C. Increased temperature
D. Hypoglycemia

Answer: C. When administering TPN, be alert for increased temperature, one of the earliest signs of catheter-related sepsis.

3. The first step in troubleshooting a clotted catheter is to:

A. perform a dye study.
B. remove the catheter.
C. stop the I.V. infusion.
D. reposition the catheter.

Answer: D. Reposition the catheter and attempt to aspirate the clot. If that doesn't work, instill alteplase (t-PA) to clear the catheter lumen.

4. A commonly used anthropometric measurement that helps determine nutritional status is:

A. biceps skinfold.
B. lean body mass.
C. midarm muscle circumference.
D. head circumference.

Answer: C. Weight, midarm muscle circumference, and triceps skinfold measurement are all anthropometric measurements that help to determine nutritional status.

5. Most of the calories in TPN are contributed by which element?
   A. Fats
   B. Dextrose
   C. Amino acids
   D. Electrolytes

Answer: B. Most calories in TPN solutions come from dextrose.

6. Which type of solution is usually used for TPN?
   A. Isotonic
   B. Hypotonic
   C. Hypertonic
   D. Emulsion

Answer: C. Solutions for TPN are hypertonic with an osmolarity of 1,800 to 2,600 mOsm/L.

7. A common laboratory test that indicates protein status is:
   A. hemoglobin.
   B. albumin.
   C. total protein.
   D. triglycerides.

Answer: B. Albumin, with a half-life of 21 days, is a good marker of nutritional status over time.

Scoring

☆☆☆ If you answered all seven questions correctly, feel fulfilled! You've metabolized the chapter components and converted them to cerebral energy.

☆☆ If you answered five or six questions correctly, sit back and digest! Your mind has been well nourished.

☆ If you answered fewer than five questions correctly, have a snack and review this book! There's nothing wrong with enhancing your diet of knowledge with a fact-filled supplement.

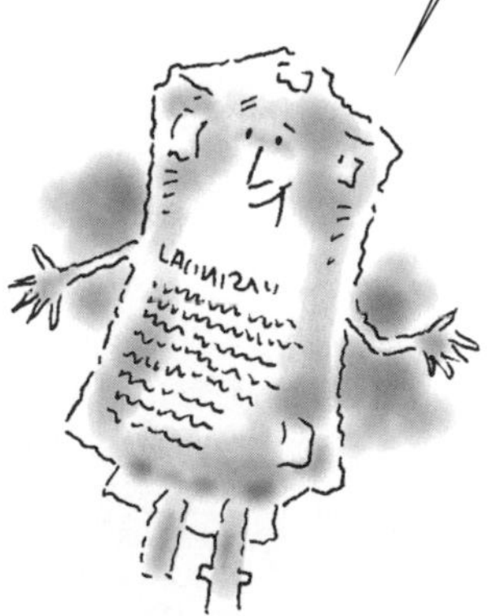

Pediatric I.V. therapy

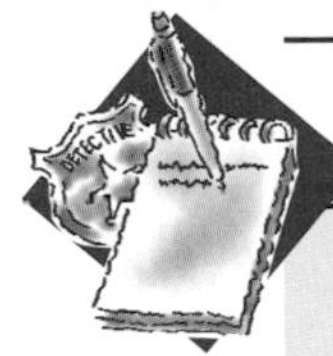

Just the facts

In this chapter, you'll learn:

- ♦ common uses of I.V. therapy in pediatric patients
- ♦ how to calculate children's fluid needs
- ♦ how to select an appropriate I.V. site in infants and older children
- ♦ appropriate I.V. insertion techniques to use with pediatric patients
- ♦ monitoring techniques and complications to watch for
- ♦ alternative fluid delivery systems used with children.

Delivering I.V. therapy to children

One of your most challenging experiences related to I.V. therapy will occur when caring for a child. It may also be a memorable event for the child because your I.V. therapy skills and knowledge can have a lasting effect on his future hospitalizations and experiences with I.V. therapy.

Chill! It's simply a child challenge . . .

In children, I.V. therapy is typically prescribed to administer medications or to correct a fluid deficit, improve serum electrolyte balance, or provide nourishment. Your first nursing concern related to pediatric I.V. therapy includes correlating the I.V. site and equipment with the reason for therapy and the patient's age, size, and activity level. For example, a scalp vein is a typical I.V. site for an infant, whereas a peripheral hand, wrist, or foot vein may suit older children.

. . . or is it?

You'll find that choosing an appropriate site can be more difficult than in an adult because the child's veins are smaller and have more subcutaneous tissue covering them. When you know a child's vein anatomy, it will make palpating for veins and documenting the location of an I.V. site easier.

Finding an appropriate site for I.V. therapy in a child can be more difficult than in an adult . . . a child's veins are smaller and there's usually more subcutaneous tissue surrounding the vein so it's harder to pin down the site.

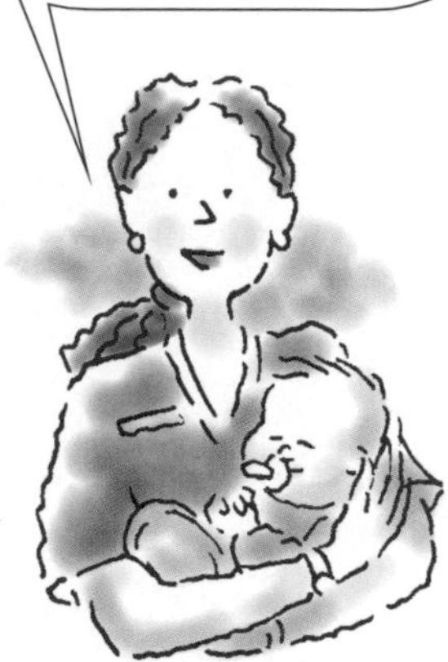

Why I.V. therapy is needed

The most common reasons for providing I.V. therapy to a child include:

- replacement of body fluids and prevention or correction of electrolyte imbalances
- blood and blood product administration
- nutrition maintenance
- medication administration.

Replacing body fluids and preventing or correcting electrolyte imbalances

Children can quickly become dehydrated and develop electrolyte imbalances — for example, when they have vomiting, diarrhea, fever, or other disorders that affect body fluid or electrolyte levels. (See *Common fluid and electrolyte imbalances in pediatric patients*, page 293.)

Read the signs

Clinical symptoms of dehydration (such as decreased skin turgor, sunken eyes or fontanels, and dry mucous membranes) and symptoms of electrolyte imbalance (such as arrhythmias, altered respiratory effort, and muscle spasms) can give an estimation of the severity of the child's condition. To maintain fluid and electrolyte balance, remember that you'll need to adjust the maintenance fluid volume based on the child's condition, treatments, and ongoing losses (such as from vomiting, diarrhea, and insensible losses through respiration and sweating).

Pay attention to signs of dehydration and electrolyte imbalances, and adjust the fluid volume accordingly.

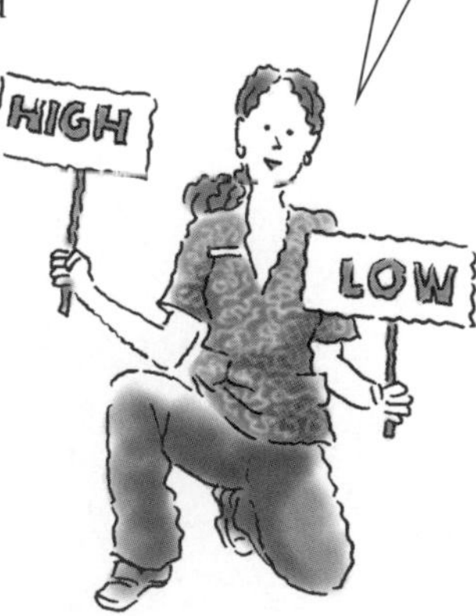

Administering blood or blood products

Expect to administer blood or blood products to a child who has:

- bone marrow failure
- severe anemia
- a sudden loss of blood
- a low hemoglobin level before, during, or after surgery.

Common fluid and electrolyte imbalances in pediatric patients

Imbalance	Causes	Signs and symptoms	Treatment
Hypovolemia (fluid volume deficit)	Dehydration, vomiting, diarrhea, decreased oral intake, and excessive fluid loss	Thirst, oliguria or anuria, dry mucous membranes, weight loss, sunken eyes, decreased tears, depressed fontanelles (in infants), tachycardia, and altered level of consciousness	Oral rehydration (in mild to moderate dehydration), I.V. fluid administration (in severe dehydration), or electrolyte replacement
Hypernatremia (serum sodium >145 mEq/L [>145 mmol/L])	Water loss in excess of sodium loss, diabetes insipidus (insufficient antidiuretic hormone [ADH] production or reduced response to ADH), insufficient water intake, diarrhea, vomiting, fever, renal disease, and hyperglycemia	Decreased skin turgor; tachycardia; flushed skin; intense thirst; dry, sticky mucous membranes; hoarseness; nausea; vomiting; decreased blood pressure; confusion; and seizures	Gradual replacement of water (in excess of sodium) or ADH replacement or vasopressin administration (for patients with diabetes insipidus)
Hyponatremia (serum sodium <138 mEq/L [<138 mmol/L])	Syndrome of inappropriate antidiuretic hormone (SIADH), edema (from cardiac failure), hypotonic fluid replacement (for diarrhea), cystic fibrosis, malnutrition, fever, and excess sweating	Dehydration, dizziness, nausea, abdominal cramps, and apprehension	Sodium replacement, water restriction, diuretic administration, or fluid replacement (with ongoing fluid loss, such as with diarrhea)
Hyperkalemia (serum potassium >5 mEq/L [>5 mmol/L])	Acute acidosis, hemolysis or rhabdomyolysis, renal failure, excessive administration of I.V. potassium supplement, and Addison's disease	Arrhythmias, weakness, paresthesia, electrocardiogram (ECG) changes (tall, tented T waves; ST segment depression; prolonged PR interval and QRS complex; and absent P waves), nausea, vomiting, hoarseness, flushed skin, intense thirst, and dry, sticky mucous membranes	Dialysis (for renal failure), sodium polystyrene (Kayexalate) (to remove potassium via the GI tract), I.V. calcium gluconate (antagonizes cardiac abnormalities), I.V. insulin or hypertonic dextrose solution (shifts potassium into the cells), bicarbonate (for acidosis), or restricted potassium intake
Hypokalemia (serum potassium <3.5 mEq/L [<3.5 mmol/L])	Vomiting, diarrhea, nasogastric suctioning, diuretic use, acute alkalosis, kidney disease, starvation, and malabsorption	Fatigue, muscle weakness, muscle cramping, paralysis, hyporeflexia, hypotension, tachycardia or bradycardia, apathy, drowsiness, irritability, decreased bowel motility, and ECG changes (flattened or inverted T waves, presence of U waves, and ST segment depression)	Oral or I.V. potassium administration (I.V. infusions must be diluted and given slowly)

A whole lot o' blood . . . and O_2

Whole blood transfusion replenishes both the volume and the oxygen-carrying capacity of the circulatory system by increasing the mass of circulating red cells. Transfusion of packed red blood cells, from which 80% of the plasma has been removed, restores only the oxygen-carrying capacity. Both types of transfusion treat decreased hemoglobin levels and hematocrit.

Portioned-out products

Other blood transfusion products that you may give to a child include albumin, fresh frozen plasma, platelets, and Factor VIII concentrate. (See *Blood administration guidelines*.)

Maintaining nutrition

When a child is unable to obtain adequate nutritional requirements orally or through a gastrostomy tube, you'll need to administer parenteral nutrition. Conditions that can make this necessary include cancer, burns, GI disorders or surgery, and malnutrition.

A formula for success

Nutritional formulas are typically delivered by an I.V. infusion pump and contain water, glucose, amino acids, lipids, electrolytes, vitamins, and minerals.

Administering medications

An I.V. medication may be prescribed for a child when:

- the child can't take medications orally
- the oral route changes the drug or interferes with its ability to be absorbed by the GI tract
- the drug isn't available in another form or is too irritating for I.M. administration
- rapid therapeutic action is needed, such as during an emergency.

Quick and highly efficient

Compared with other routes of administration, the I.V. route is the fastest, most efficient way to deliver medications throughout the body. When you administer an I.V. medication, it will typically be either a bolus injection (a concentrated dose of medication given all at once) or an I.V. drip or piggyback infusion (a drug that's diluted with I.V. solution and given over a predetermined time). Most chemotherapeutic drugs that you'll administer will be given by I.V. infusion.

Blood administration guidelines

This chart lists some of the common blood products you may give to a child.

Component	Indications	Rate	Administration guidelines
Whole blood Single-donor anticoagulated blood	• Massive blood loss • Exchange transfusion • Special procedures (extracorporeal membrane oxygenation [ECMO] to prime the circuit, apheresis)	• As rapidly as necessary to reestablish blood volume • 45 to 60 minutes (longer if hemodynamically unstable)	• Always administer ABO group and Rh type specific.
Packed red blood cells (RBCs) Concentrated RBCs with most of the plasma, leukocytes, and platelets removed	• Severe anemia • Surgical blood loss • Suppression of erythropoiesis (such as thalassemia or sickle cell anemia) • ECMO — blood loss from bleeding or multiple sampling for laboratory analysis	• 5 ml/kg/hour	• Administer ABO group and Rh type specific if possible. If not, compatible group and type can be transfused safely. • O-negative uncrossmatched blood may be used for infants up to age 4 months.
Albumin Plasma protein available in 5% and 25% solutions	• 5% solution: hypoproteinemia, volume deficits • 25% solution: severe burns, cerebral edema	• 5%: 1 to 2 ml/minute (60 to 120 ml/hour); can be administered as fast as possible to correct shock • 25%: 0.2 to 0.4 ml/minute (12 to 24 ml/hour)	• No blood filter is needed. • Only one person must identify the product and the patient. • 25% albumin rapidly mobilizes large volumes of fluid into circulation. Watch for pulmonary edema or other symptoms of fluid overload. • Product is stored at room temperature and has a very long shelf life. • Administer within 6 hours of thawing to preserve clotting factor activity.
Fresh frozen plasma Contains all the clotting factors and some fibrinogen	• Massive hemorrhage • Hypovolemic shock • Multiple clotting deficiencies	• Hemorrhage: as indicated by patient's condition • Clotting deficiency: over 2 to 3 hours	• Donor's plasma should be ABO compatible with recipient's RBCs. • Rh compatibility isn't required because product doesn't contain RBCs.

(continued)

Blood administration guidelines *(continued)*

Component	Indications	Rate	Administration guidelines
Platelets Platelets suspended in a small amount of plasma	• Severe thrombocytopenia (platelet count less than 20,000) • Platelet count less than 50,000 in a child who requires surgery or in a child with hemorrhage or imminent bleeding • Cardiac surgery with massive blood replacement • Platelet count less than 80,000 to 100,000 in a child undergoing ECMO	• May be given by I.V. push (5 to 10 minutes/unit); if volume overload is a concern, transfuse the total dose over 2 to 3 hours using an infusion pump	• Rh compatibility is required; ABO plasma compatibility is preferred. • Platelets may be irradiated to inactivate donor lymphocytes that cause graft-versus-host disease in immunocompromised patients. • If single-donor or HLA platelets are ordered, obtain 1-hour and 24-hour platelet counts after the transfusion to determine adequate platelet response. • Gently agitate every hour because platelets tend to clump.
Factor VIII concentrate Sterile lyophilized powder containing blood coagulation factor VIII, which is prepared from pooled human plasma	• Hemophilia A	• I.V. push over about 5 minutes (2 ml/minute maximum) • If patient complains of headache: slow the rate because product is high in protein	• Dose is ordered in units. • No compatibility testing is required. • Administer within 1 hour of reconstitution.

Calculating fluid needs

Calculating the fluid replacement needs for a child is complex and requires the practitioner to perform a thorough assessment and consider many factors when ordering the type and amount of fluid to be infused. As the nurse administering the fluids, you're responsible for double-checking the order for accuracy and ensuring that it meets the child's needs but doesn't put him at risk for fluid overload.

Double-checking the order for accuracy and determining whether it meets the child's fluid needs . . . Now that's one tall order!

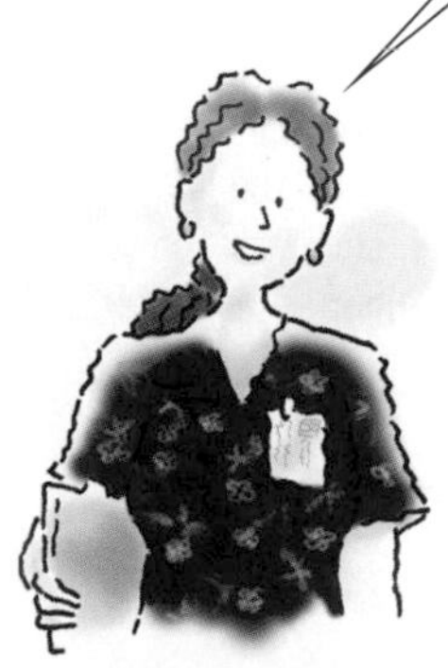

Replacement therapy

Generally, replacement therapy will be based on the child's stage of dehydration, which is measured as mild, moderate, or severe. The most accurate way to determine this is by obtaining the child's current and immediate pre-illness weights in kilograms, if known. (See *Formula for calculating percentage of fluid loss.*)

Dehydration double-check

Make sure you correlate your findings with the child's clinical symptoms. If you can't accurately determine the child's weights, estimate his dehydration severity by clinical signs alone. (See *Clinical signs and dehydration severity*, page 298.)

Daily fluid fill-up

After you've determined the percentage of fluid the child has lost, and before you calculate the amount of fluid replacement required, you first need to determine the child's daily maintenance fluid requirements. Check your facility's protocol because many

Formula for calculating percentage of fluid loss

To determine the child's percentage of fluid loss, or dehydration, first calculate his weight change, which will provide his fluid deficit in kilograms:

Deficit = Pre-illness weight (kg) – current weight (kg)

Then, use the fluid deficit to determine the percent of dehydration:

Dehydration percent = (deficit ÷ pre-illness weight [kg]) × 100

The percent of dehydration will then tell you if a child has mild, moderate, or severe dehydration:

- Mild dehydration — 3% to 5%
- Moderate dehydration — 6% to 9%
- Severe dehydration — greater than 10%

Example

A child is admitted to your facility with signs of dehydration. His current weight is 30 lb (13.6 kg) and his mother tells you that his weight before he became ill (obtained 1 week earlier at the doctor's office) was 32 lb (14.5 kg).

First, determine the amount of the child's fluid deficit:
Deficit = 14.5 kg – 13.6 kg
Deficit = 0.9 kg

Then, determine the percentage of dehydration:
Dehydration percentage = (0.9 kg ÷ 14.5 kg) × 100
Dehydration percentage = (0.06) × 100
Dehydration percentage = 6

This child's dehydration percentage, 6%, places him within the range of moderate dehydration. *Remember:* Always correlate this finding with the child's clinical status.

Clinical signs and dehydration severity

Use the information below to help correlate the child's dehydration severity with his clinical status. This chart can also be used alone to help determine the severity of dehydration.

	Severity		
Sign	**Mild (3% to 5%)**	**Moderate (6% to 9%)**	**Severe (greater than 10%)**
Level of consciousness	Alert	Lethargic, confused	Unconscious
Heart rate	Normal	Slightly increased	Rapid, weak
Blood pressure	Normal	Normal; possibly orthostatic hypotension	Hypotension
Pulse	Normal	Thready	Faint
Respirations	Normal	Slightly increased	Increased
Skin	Normal turgor	Decreased turgor	Tenting
Extremities	Normal temperature and color; possible muscle fatigue and weakness	Cool temperature; normal color or mottling; extreme fatigue and muscle cramping	Cool to cold temperature; mottling or gray color; muscle spasms
Capillary refill	Normal (less than 2 seconds)	Slow (2 to 4 seconds)	Greater than 4 seconds
Mucous membranes	Slightly dry	Very dry	Parched or cracked
Eyes and tears	Normal eyes; presence of tears	Sunken eyes; decreased tears	Sunken eyes; absence of tears
Anterior fontanelle	Normal	Slightly depressed	Sunken
Urine	Slightly decreased output; dark yellow color	Moderately decreased output; very dark yellow color	Oliguria or anuria

facilities use charts listing the amount of maintenance fluid therapy required based on the child's weight. (To figure this amount yourself, see *Calculating maintenance and replacement fluid requirements*.) Once you've determined the maintenance fluid therapy the child requires, you can calculate the amount of replacement fluid needed.

Calculating maintenance and replacement fluid requirements

To calculate a pediatric patient's maintenance fluid requirements, use the appropriate formula based on the child's current status from the chart below.

Child's status	Formula
Neonate (0 to 72 hours)	60 to 100 ml/kg/24 hours
0 to10 kg	100 ml/kg/24 hours
11 to 20 kg	1,000 ml for first 10 kg + 50 ml/kg/24 hours for each kilogram over 10 kg
21 to 30 kg	1,500 ml for first 20 kg + 20 ml/kg/24 hours for each kilogram over 20 kg

Example

A child is admitted to your facility after several days of vomiting and diarrhea. He has no signs of dehydration, is afebrile and, according to his mother, hasn't lost any weight. The vomiting and diarrhea have resolved, but his practitioner has ordered that he receive maintenance I.V. fluids. His current weight is 22 kg.

The formula to calculate the 24-hour maintenance fluid requirements for this child is:

$$(1{,}500 \text{ ml for each of the first 20 kg}) + (20 \text{ ml for each kg over 20})$$

$$1{,}500 \text{ ml} + (2 \times 20)$$

$$(1{,}500 \text{ ml}) + (40 \text{ ml}) =$$

$$1{,}540 \text{ ml/24 hours}$$

Once you've determined the amount of replacement fluid needed and you know the child's severity of dehydration, you can calculate his replacement fluid requirements using the chart below.

Fluid deficit (dehydration severity)	Formula for calculating amount of replacement fluid/24 hours
Mild	Maintenance + (maintenance × 0.5)/24 hours
Moderate	Maintenance + (maintenance × 1.0)/24 hours
Severe	Maintenance + (maintenance × 1.5)/24 hours

(continued)

Calculating maintenance and replacement fluid requirements *(continued)*

To continue the example from above, the child's clinical assessment indicates that he has mild dehydration. Therefore, his maintenance fluid need is 1,540 ml / 24.

$$1{,}540 \text{ ml} + (1{,}540 \text{ ml} \times 0.5) / 24 \text{ hours}$$

$$1{,}540 \text{ ml} + 770 \text{ ml} / 24 \text{ hours}$$

$$2{,}310 \text{ ml} / 24 \text{ hours}$$

The child's total replacement fluid requirement is 2,310 ml/24 hours.

Tally those losses, too

When calculating replacement fluid needs, it's important to consider ongoing losses, such as those occurring from vomiting, diarrhea, diaphoresis, hyperthermia, and fluids collected from nasogastric tubes and drains. Ongoing fluid losses should be measured, if possible, and replaced with physiologic equivalents of the fluids.

Don't forget to account for us ongoing losses when calculating a child's replacement fluid needs.

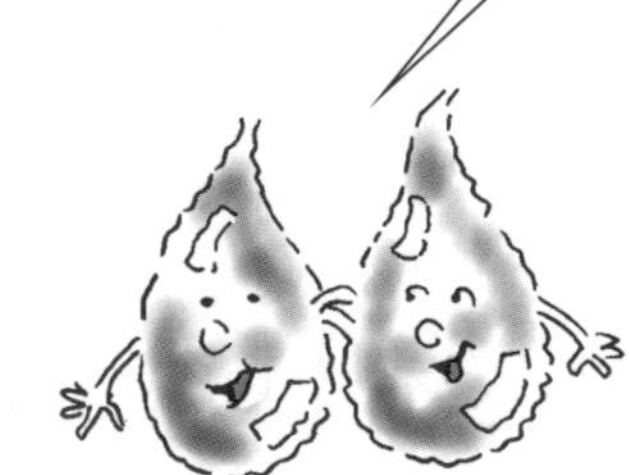

A stickler for scheduling

Replacement fluids are given based on the child's condition. The practitioner may order you to administer one or more bolus fluid injections, followed by the remainder at a specified drip rate, or he may order all of the fluids to be administered over a specified time period.

Following a typical replacement schedule, you'll administer one-half of the deficit plus the maintenance amount over the first 8 hours of therapy and the remaining one-half of the deficit plus the maintenance amount over the next 16 hours. The child should be monitored at least every 2 hours for ongoing losses and fluid excess, which will necessitate adjustment of the replacement amounts.

Administering I.V. therapy

A child requires special care during I.V. catheter insertion and throughout therapy. Although your venipuncture technique will be basically the same for most pediatric patients, your approach, restraint method, and manner of securing the I.V. catheter will depend on the child's age and medical condition. You'll need to monitor the child closely during therapy to determine whether the fluid is infusing correctly to prevent fluid overload, infiltration, and other complications.

Selecting an I.V. catheter site

Perhaps your greatest challenge in providing I.V. therapy to a child will be choosing an appropriate vein. The veins of infants and toddlers are usually difficult to visualize or palpate, especially when the child is dehydrated or hypovolemic from another medical condition. Also, toddlers and prepubescent children have more subcutaneous tissue covering their veins than adults, which makes finding a suitable vein more difficult.

Only the best will do

When you're choosing the best I.V. site for a child, first consider his age, activity level, and the reason for the I.V. therapy. An ideal vein for a 10-year-old child may not be the best choice for an 8-month-old child. Other factors to consider include how difficult the venipuncture will be for you and the patient and which site carries the lowest risk of device-related systemic infection. You should always avoid previously used or sclerotic veins.

Infants

Until a child is about 12 months old, the scalp veins are readily accessible for a short peripheral catheter because they have no valves and are easy to stabilize for catheter insertion. However, they're best reserved for infants younger than 6 months old because they can easily be dislodged by the child's hands. To locate an appropriate scalp vein, carefully palpate the site for arterial pulsations. If you feel these pulsations, select another site. (See *Identifying scalp veins.*) However, in hypotensive or premature infants, the pulse may be more difficult to detect.

Other veins can be gold mines, too

The dorsal surface of the foot and the lower leg are also good I.V. sites for children prior to walking age. Femoral veins can be used for children of all ages, but when used in a child with a diaper, remember to keep the site as clean as possible to decrease the risk of infection.

Children over age 1

Palpate for a suitable vein in the hands, forearms, or upper arms when selecting an I.V. site in a child or adolescent, and always try

Identifying scalp veins

This illustration shows the scalp veins most commonly used for venipuncture in infants.

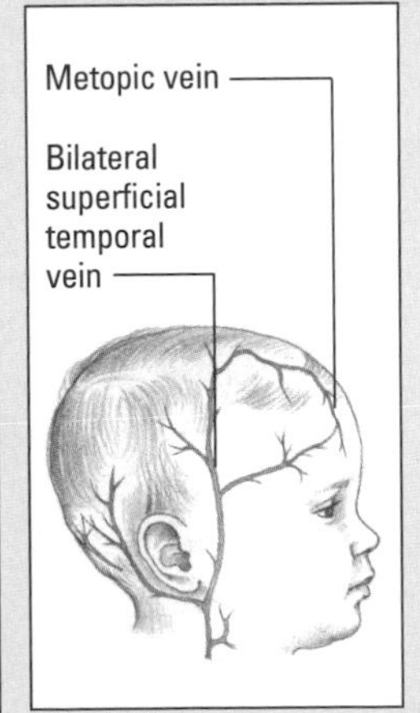

to select the most distal site available. Start with the child's non-dominant side to avoid interference with self-care or other activities, and move to the dominant side if necessary. Also keep in mind whether the child is young and sucks his thumb; if so, make sure to use the opposite side.

Always consider the child's age and activity level when choosing an I.V. site, especially if he's young and still sucks his thumb.

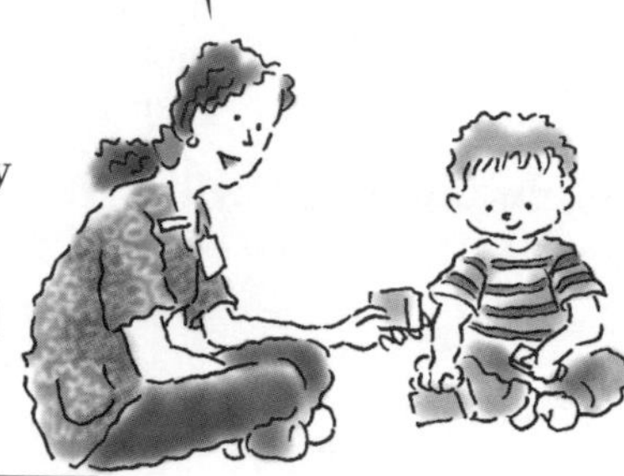

Anti-antecubital

Although antecubital veins are appropriate for children of all ages and are usually easy to view and palpate, you should try to avoid their use for peripheral I.V. therapy. Antecubital sites can be uncomfortable for the child, and they must be securely supported at all times.

For the mobile guitar hero

For a mobile patient, select an I.V. site on the upper extremity so that he can still get out of bed. Also avoid starting the I.V. in the same arm as the patient's identification band. Remove the band and replace it on the other arm, to prevent potential circulatory impairment.

Preparing for insertion

The preferred venous access device for infants and young children, no matter which vein you are using, is a small-diameter, winged catheter. This device is less likely to cause traumatic injury to the vein.

Tailored to size and need

Choose the needle and catheter that you'll use to obtain I.V. access based on the size of the child's veins and the type of fluid he'll be receiving. Use the smallest-gauge catheter in the shortest length possible to allow blood to flow around the catheter while I.V. fluids are infusing. When you're administering blood products, you'll typically use a larger catheter to prevent hemolysis.

Forewarned and forearmed

Explain to the child's parents what you'll be doing when inserting the I.V. catheter and why it's necessary. Forewarn them if you'll be using a scalp vein, and tell them that you may have to clip the hair from a small section of the infant's head. Give an age-appropriate explanation to the child when the time is right. If the child is at least 1 month old, you can lessen his anxiety, reduce his pain, and improve compliance during I.V. catheter insertion by applying a transdermal anesthesia cream before the venipuncture. (See *Easing the pain of venipuncture.*) You may also consider placing warm packs on the site for 10 minutes prior to insertion to enhance vein dilation.

1st

Best practice

Easing the pain of venipuncture

For some children, receiving a needle stick— especially during venipuncture—can be a traumatic experience. You can lessen your pediatric patient's anxiety, reduce his pain, and improve compliance during the procedure by applying a transdermal anesthesia cream before the venipuncture. The Infusion Nurses Society recommends using a transdermal anesthetic for all pediatric patients when possible. Here are a few guidelines for the use of this cream:

- Transdermal anesthesia cream (commonly known by the brand name EMLA cream) is supplied in a eutectic mixture of lidocaine 2.5% and prilocaine 2.5%. A eutectic mixture has a melting point below room temperature, allowing it to penetrate intact skin as far as the fat layer. The onset, depth, and duration of the anesthesia depend on how long the cream is allowed to stay on the skin. The minimum duration of application is 60 minutes; the maximum is 180 minutes.
- Apply the cream in a thick layer to clean, dry, intact skin at the intended venipuncture site. Then cover it with a transparent occlusive dressing, being careful not to spread the cream.
- Note the time of application on the dressing with a marking pen. When you're ready to perform the venipuncture, carefully remove the dressing. Wipe off the cream, clean the site with an antiseptic solution, and perform the venipuncture as usual.
- EMLA cream is also indicated for pain relief for various other procedures, including lumbar puncture, port access, bone marrow aspiration, insertion of a peripherally inserted central venous access device, withdrawal of blood samples for arterial blood gas analysis and other laboratory tests, I.M. injection, and superficial skin surgery. It can be used on adults and on children who are at least 1 month old. Local reactions may include erythema and edema. Avoid administering EMLA cream to individuals with a known sensitivity to lidocaine or prilocaine.

Restrain for safety's sake

At times, you may have to restrain the child to ensure that you obtain I.V. access and for the child's safety. If possible, enlist the aid of a coworker, and try to avoid having the parents assist with restraint. Encourage them to talk to the child and comfort him by holding his hand or stroking his arm instead of involving them directly in what may be a frightening experience. Provide the child with a favorite toy or blanket for comfort.

If the child is an infant, wrap him in a blanket with the site exposed. If he's a toddler or school-age child, seat him across from you or in your assistant's lap. You can also have him lie down on the bed or a treatment table. Ask your assistant to hold the extremity chosen for the I.V. in one hand while restraining the other extremities. The assistant's hand can be also be used as a tourniquet while restraining the child.

Provide an age-appropriate explanation about the venipuncture when the time is right. Oops . . . I think I might have jumped the gun a bit with this one.

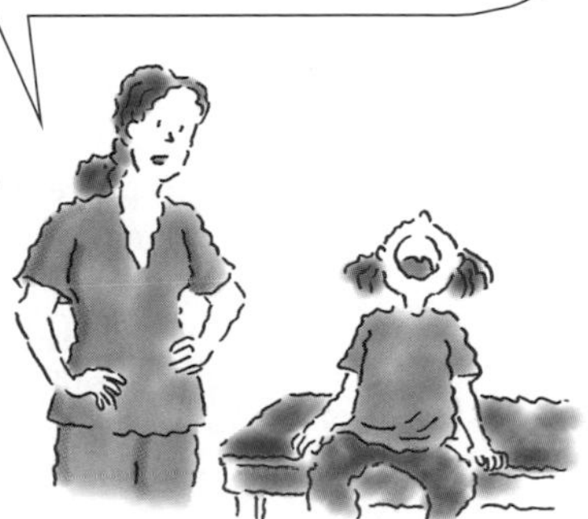

Inserting the catheter

If you need to use a tourniquet to dilate a vein, make sure it's appropriately sized for that particular child. When accessing a scalp vein, use a special rubber band with a tape tab and place it above the child's eyes and ears. Check for the child's pulse to make sure that you haven't overtightened the tourniquet.

Having a flashback to childhood

Insert the I.V. needle and catheter into the vein, and watch for blood to flow backward through the catheter or butterfly tubing, which confirms that the needle is in the vein. In children, blood return in the flashback chamber may be minimal. When you see a blood return, advance the needle about 1/8″ (0.3 cm) and slowly thread the catheter into the vein. If you feel resistance, allow the child to relax for a few seconds and try again. Loosen the tourniquet, and attach the I.V. tubing to the hub of the catheter to begin the infusion.

Keeping it just right

Make sure that the I.V. tubing is connected to a small volume reservoir, volume-control set with microdrip tubing, or an electronic infusion pump with an anti-free-flow feature to reduce the risk of fluid overload.

Securing the site

Stabilizing the I.V. site can be a little tricky with pediatric patients. Always begin by applying a catheter securement device and then taping the site as you would for an adult so the skin over the access site is easily visible.

Finger-proof and protect

In addition to securing the I.V. catheter with a catheter securement device and tape, you must take care to make sure the I.V. insertion site is inaccessible to the child's prying fingers and that the tubing is safely secured. Several types of protective devices to place over the I.V. site are available commercially, including plastic covers, fabric wraps, and elastic netting. (See *Protecting an I.V. site.*)

To safeguard the catheter, loop the tubing and tape it so that if it's pulled, the strain will be exerted on the tubing and not the catheter. If possible, thread the tubing through the child's shirt to exit out the back, where it can't be reached, and to help prevent an accidental strangulation with the tubing.

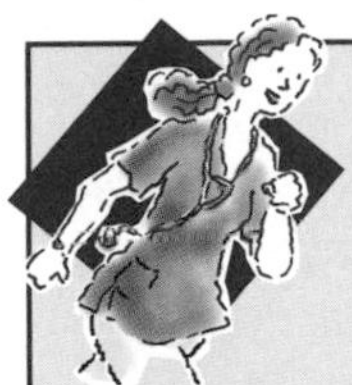

Running smoothly

Protecting an I.V. site

Protecting a child's I.V. site can be a challenge. An active child can easily dislodge an I.V. catheter, which will necessitate your reinserting it — thus causing him further discomfort. A child may also injure himself by dislodging the I.V. catheter.

To prevent a child from dislodging an I.V. catheter, first secure the catheter carefully. Tape the I.V. site as you would for an adult, so that the skin over the tip of the venipuncture device is easily visible. However, avoid overtaping the site because doing so makes it harder to inspect the site and the surrounding tissue.

If the child is old enough to understand, warn him not to play with or jostle the equipment, and teach him how to walk with an I.V. pole to minimize tension on the line. If necessary, you can restrain the extremity.

You should also create a protective barrier between the I.V. site and the environment using one of the following methods.

Paper cup

Consider using a small paper cup to protect a scalp site. First, cut off the cup's bottom. (Make sure there are no sharp edges that could damage the child's skin.)

Next, cut a small slot through the top rim to accommodate the I.V. tubing. Place the cup upside down over the insertion site, so the I.V. tubing extends through the slot. Then, secure the cup with strips of tape (as shown at right). The opening you cut in the cup allows you to examine the site.

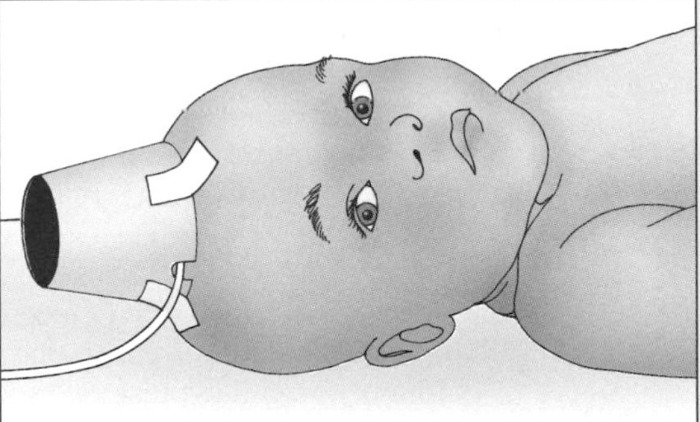

Stockinette

Cut a piece of 4″ (10.2-cm) stockinette the same length as the patient's arm. Slip the stockinette over the patient's arm, and lay the arm on an arm board. Then grasp the stockinette at both sides of the arm, and stretch it under the arm board. Securely tape the stockinette beneath the arm board (as shown at right).

Note: You may also protect a scalp site by placing a stockinette on the patient's head, leaving a hole to allow access to the site.

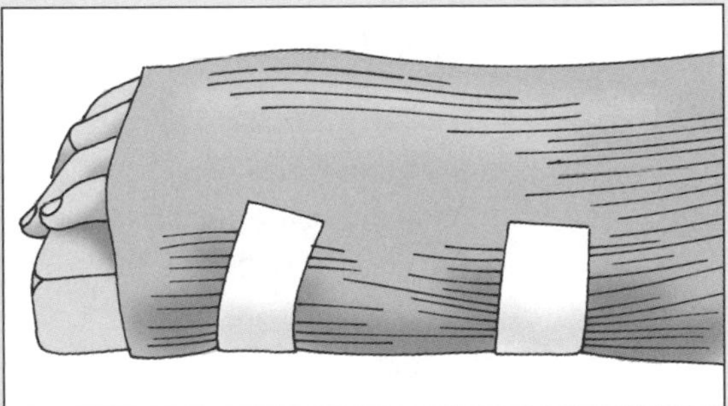

I.V. shield

Peel off the strips covering the adhesive backing on the bottom of the shield. Position the shield over the site so that the I.V. tubing runs through one of the shield's two slots. Then firmly press the shield's adhesive backing against the patient's skin (as shown at right). The shield's clear plastic composition allows you to see the I.V. site clearly.

If the shield is too large to fit securely over the site, just cut off the shield's narrow end below the two air holes. Now you can easily shape the device to the patient's arm.

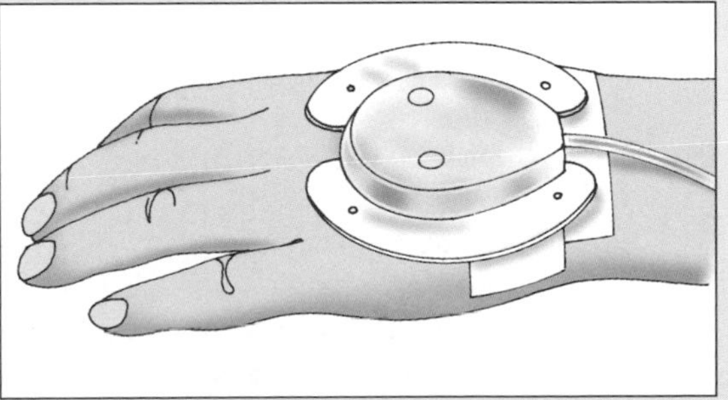

Still stuck on stickers

After inserting the I.V. catheter, remember to reward your preschool or school-age patient. Colorful stickers to wear on clothes or on the I.V. dressing are always popular with this age-group.

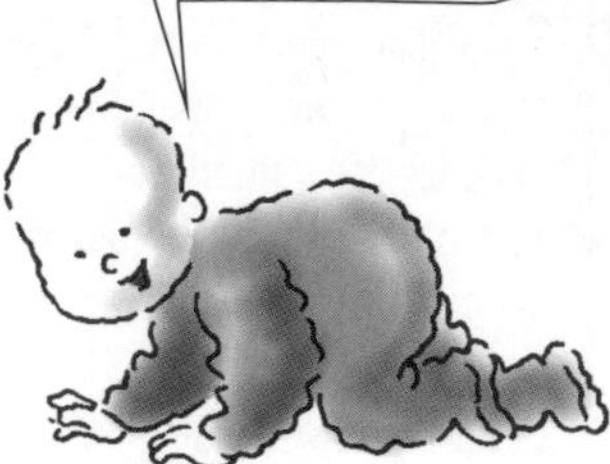

Assessment and management

The frequency of monitoring will depend on the child's condition, age, and the reason for I.V. therapy. For instance, a child who's receiving replacement fluids for dehydration will require continuous monitoring, whereas a child with an I.V. access site for medication administration will require less frequent monitoring. You'll need to assess the I.V. site of an infant or toddler frequently because he's more likely to dislodge the catheter than the adolescent who understands the necessity of the I.V. and the discomfort associated with having it reinserted.

Dehydration demands diligence

When you assess the child receiving I.V. therapy for dehydration, be sure to compare your results with the child's baseline findings. Monitor the child's pulse rate and volume, blood pressure, temperature, capillary refill, urine output, and laboratory test results. Also assess the child's peripheral pulses, skin color, and the temperature of his extremities.

Timely weights and measures

All children receiving I.V. therapy should be weighed before the fluid administration is started and once per shift throughout the course of treatment. Blood tests should include serum electrolytes and glucose levels, depending on the type of fluid being infused.

Count on calculating

When you're monitoring a child receiving I.V. therapy, calculate the amount of fluid that has been infused to ensure that the child is receiving the ordered amount. Also verify that the flow rate corresponds with the most recent practitioner's orders.

Around-the-clock assessments

Assess the child's I.V. site at least hourly, observing for redness, streaking, edema, and soiled dressings. Palpate for hardening of the accessed blood vessel and note the temperature of the surrounding skin. Make sure that you also assess the areas above and below the insertion site. Check that the dressing and I.V. tubing are secure to prevent the child from dislodging the device or becoming tangled in the tubing. Don't reinforce wet or soiled dressings, tapes, or protective devices. Change them if they become loose or dislodged or if there's blood or fluid leakage.

Check that pain!

Use a standardized assessment tool or a face rating scale, where the child points to the face that describes how he feels, to determine whether the child is experiencing pain at the I.V. site. Observe closely for facial or body language reactions when you assess the site. Ask the child if the access site hurts and give him permission to tell you that it does. Some children may be reluctant to admit that they're having pain. You should constantly be aware of the amount of discomfort that I.V. therapy can cause and work to minimize the pain as quickly as possible.

Use a standardized pain assessment tool to rate your patient's pain, and do whatever it takes to ease his discomfort. Even if it means drawing faces or wearing a corny cape, it's worth it, right?

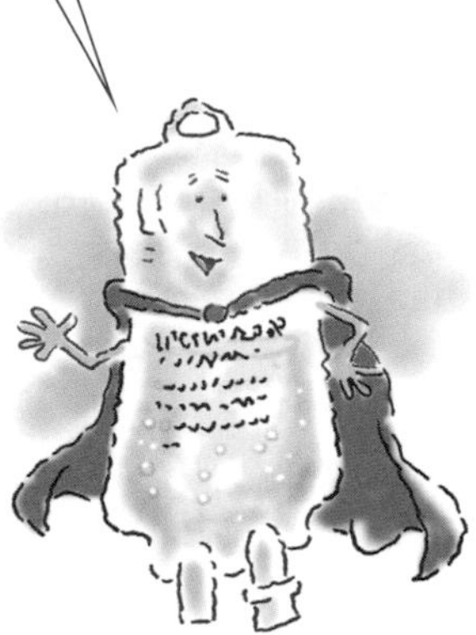

Flushed and duly noted

Flush the I.V. line after each medication delivery or at least every 8 hours when it isn't in use to maintain patency and prevent complications. Make sure that if saline flushes are ordered, you use preservative-free normal saline solution.

Be sure to document all of your findings and interventions, according to facility policy, on flow sheets and in the nurses' notes.

Dealing with complications

The potential complications associated with I.V. therapy are similar in children and adults. However, some aren't as common in children as they are in adults and others occur more frequently. The most common complications associated with I.V. therapy in children include infection, infiltration or extravasation, fluid overload, and allergic reactions. Although phlebitis and emboli can also occur, they're not as common as in adults.

Infection

Infection can occur at the I.V. insertion site for several reasons, including:

- improper cleansing before the venipuncture
- contaminated equipment
- disruption of the occlusive dressing, which allows bacteria to enter the area
- moist or wet dressings that encourage bacteria colonization.

That moist dressing . . . over there . . . looks like a good place to start the colony.

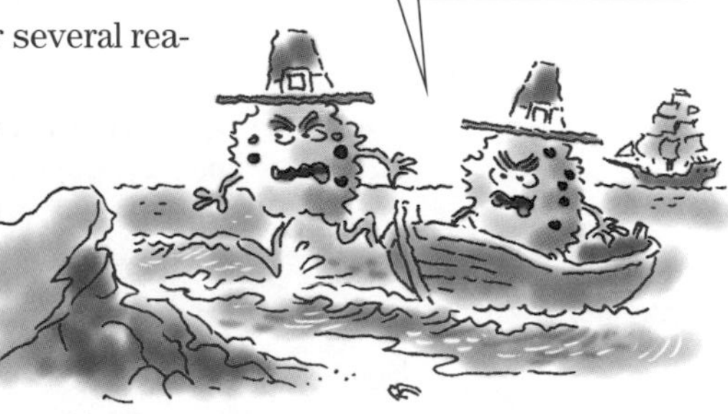

Taking the local or septic route

Infection of I.V. sites is usually local, resulting in redness, warmth, and swelling of the area. The child may also develop a fever. Septicemia, though rare, can also occur if bacteria enter the bloodstream, especially in children who have compromised immune systems.

Strictly aseptic

You can usually prevent I.V. site infection if you use strict aseptic technique during I.V. insertion, provide safeguards to prevent the child from playing with or removing the dressing, and frequently monitor the integrity of the dressings and change them as soon as they become moist.

Infiltration and extravasation

Infiltration and extravasation occur when the I.V. fluid or medication infuses into the tissue surrounding the vein, instead of entering the venous circulation. It typically occurs as a result of an accidental vein puncture from the needle, dislodgment of the catheter from the vein, or leakage between the catheter and the wall of the vein. Infiltration involves a substance that's a nonvesicant, whereas extravasation involves a vesicant substance.

Give it a grade

Signs of infiltration include localized swelling, pain, and coolness to the touch. It's usually graded on a scale ranging from 0, in which there are no symptoms, to 4, which presents with translucent or blanched, tight skin; leaking around the insertion site, usually identified by wet dressings; edema measuring greater than 6″ (15 cm); and moderate to severe pain.

Cease and desist

When you identify an infiltrated I.V., you should immediately stop the infusion and remove the catheter. Removal of an extravasated I.V. varies, depending on the substance being infused. Treatment depends on the severity of the infiltration and whether the substance is a vesicant or nonvesicant.

Fluid overload is probably the most severe complication of administering I.V. therapy to children. It can happen very suddenly and have fatal consequences.

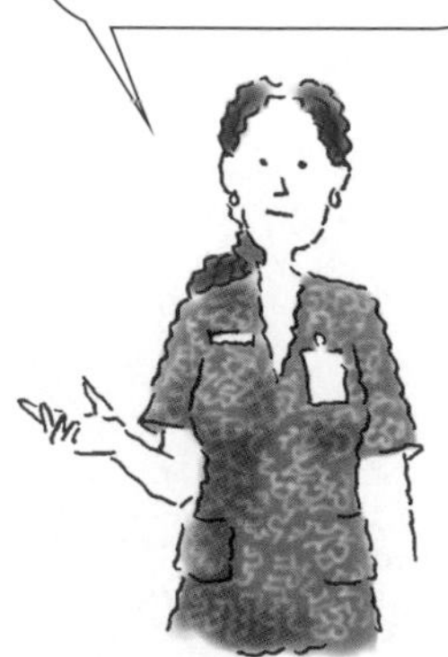

Fluid overload

Fluid overload occurs when fluids are given at a higher rate or in a larger volume than the child's system can absorb or excrete. It's potentially the most severe complication of pediatric I.V. therapy because it can occur in a very short time and can be life-threatening.

Beware the ominous signs!

Signs of fluid overload include edema, dyspnea, hypertension, weight increase, a third heart sound, and crackles. Careful monitoring of the child and rapid notification of the practitioner when the child's status changes can help prevent the infusion of too much fluid in too short of a time. Consequently, you should check the I.V. flow rate frequently, even when you're using a volume-control set or infusion pump.

Allergic reactions

Allergic reactions are typically caused by the antiseptics used to cleanse the site, dressings applied to cover the site, or tape used to secure the site. Some children are also allergic to the materials used in the manufacturing or packaging of the catheters.

Most reactions present as local inflammation, redness and, possibly, a rash. If the child has been previously exposed to the allergen, anaphylactic shock is possible, though rare.

Preventing and predicting occurrences

You can't always prevent an allergic reaction or accurately predict which child will experience one. Make sure that you ask the parents whether the child has any known allergies or has ever had a previous reaction. Whenever possible, make sure that you're using latex-free gloves and equipment, including the I.V. catheter.

Severe I.V. therapy complications can be prevented through diligent monitoring and thorough assessments. Early identification of problems and prompt interventions to correct them can prevent minor complications from becoming serious ones.

Other fluid delivery systems

In some instances, it may not be possible or in the child's best interest to insert a peripheral I.V. catheter. In these situations, other types of fluid delivery systems, such as an intraosseous infusion, a peripherally inserted central catheter (PICC), or an umbilical vessel catheter, may be used.

Intraosseous infusion

Usually performed in an emergency, an intraosseous infusion may be necessary to provide resuscitative fluids, medication, and blood until a vein can be accessed by I.V. administration. An intraosseous needle, or if one isn't available, a 16G or 19G straight needle, is placed in the medullary cavity of a bone, usually in the distal end of the femur or the proximal or distal ends of the tibia. The I.V. solution is then infused directly into the cavity, which is rich in blood. (See *Understanding intraosseous infusion*, page 310.)

Understanding intraosseous infusion

During intraosseous infusion, the bone marrow serves as a noncollapsible vein; thus, fluid infused into the marrow cavity rapidly enters the circulation by way of an extensive network of venous sinusoids. Here, the needle is shown positioned in the patient's tibia.

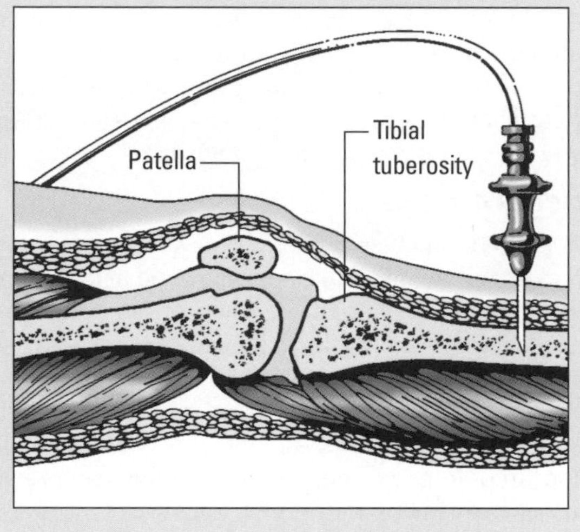

Peripherally inserted central catheter

A PICC is a catheter that's inserted percutaneously into a peripheral vein. The catheter tip resides in the lower one-third of the superior vena cava, at the junction of the superior vena cava and right atrium.

PICC a peck of reasons

PICC placement is indicated for intermediate to long-term I.V. access for the administration of antibiotics, pain medications, chemotherapy or other vesicants, parenteral nutrition or other hyperosmolar solutions, or blood products. The early use of PICCs may also spare peripheral veins and limit the pain of repeated needle sticks, which can be traumatic to children. Another reason to use a PICC is that PICCs are also associated with fewer complications in infants and children.

Generally, good to go

In general, to maintain good blood flow around the catheter, children are encouraged to use the arm with the PICC as usual, rather than guard it. However, very active children are at a greater risk for breaking or dislodging a PICC; immobilization of the extremity may be necessary in these children.

Hmm . . . may not be an ideal candidate for a PICC. Let me think about it another minute.

Umbilical vessel catheter

An umbilical catheter may be inserted into the neonate's umbilical artery or vein for I.V. therapy, when necessary.

Arterial access

An umbilical artery catheter is commonly inserted for:

- taking frequent blood samples
- providing direct arterial blood pressure measurement
- administering fluids and medications.

This type of catheter is contraindicated in neonates older than 7 days and in those who have abdominal wall defects, necrotizing enterocolitis, peritonitis, or vascular compromise in the buttocks or lower limbs.

Vote for venous

An umbilical venous catheter may be inserted to administer fluids and medications and to provide venous access for exchange transfusions. It's also typically the first choice of intravascular access in neonatal resuscitation.

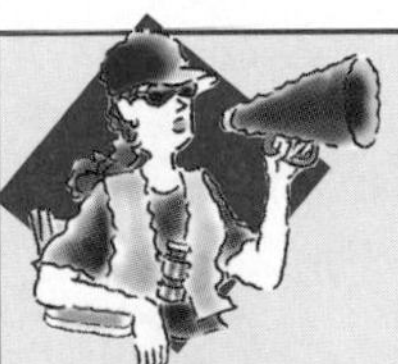

That's a wrap!

Pediatric I.V. therapy review

Reasons for I.V. therapy in children

- Replacement of body fluids
- Prevention or correction of electrolyte imbalances
- Blood and blood product administration
- Nutrition maintenance
- Medication administration

Calculating fluid needs

- Amount of fluid replacement is based on child's stage of dehydration.
- If available, obtain the child's current and immediate pre-illness weights in kilograms.
- Determine the child's dehydration percentage.
- Correlate the results with the child's clinical symptoms.
  –If precise weights aren't available, estimate the dehydration severity by clinical signs alone and adjust percentage based on whether the child weighs more or less than 10 kg.
  –Determine the child's daily maintenance fluid requirements.
  –Adjust the maintenance fluid amounts based on the child's condition, activity level, treatments, and insensible fluid losses.

(continued)

Pediatric I.V. therapy review *(continued)*

- Add the child's replacement amounts to his maintenance amounts to determine daily fluid needs.
- Consider ongoing losses, such as those occurring from vomiting, diarrhea, diaphoresis, and hyperthermia and fluids collected from nasogastric tubes and drains, when determining fluid replacement needs.
- Typical replacement schedule is to administer one-half of the deficit plus the maintenance amount over the first 8 hours of therapy and the remaining one-half of the deficit plus maintenance over the next 16 hours.
- Monitor the child at least every 2 hours for ongoing losses and fluid excess, to determine if adjustment of the replacement amounts is necessary.

Site selection

- Consider the child's age, activity level, and the reason for the I.V. therapy when choosing the best I.V. site.
- Avoid previously used or sclerotic veins.

Scalp veins

- Reserve use for infants younger than 6 months old.
- Be aware that they have no valves and are easy to stabilize for catheter insertion.
- Palpate the site for arterial pulsations; if you feel these pulsations, select another site.

Hand, forearm, and upper arm veins

- Choose the most distal site available.
- Start with the child's nondominant side and move to the dominant side if necessary.
- Make sure that you use the opposite hand if the patient is a young child who sucks his thumb.
- Avoid starting the I.V. in the same arm as the patient's identification band.
- Keep in mind that hand veins are ideal sites for long-term therapy.
- Immobilize the arm with an arm board if you insert the catheter near the wrist or elbow.
- Avoid using antecubital, wrist, knee, and axillary veins.

Foot and leg veins

- Use the dorsal surface of the foot and the lower leg for children prior to walking age.
- Immobilize an I.V. site on the foot with a padded board and place padding under the foot.
- Remember that femoral veins can be used for children of all ages.

I.V. catheter insertion

- Choose the needle and catheter based on the size of the child's veins and the type of fluid he'll be receiving.
- Use the smallest-gauge catheter in the shortest length that will allow blood to flow around the catheter while the I.V. fluid is infusing.
- Make sure that the I.V. tubing is connected to a small volume reservoir, volume-control set with micro-drip tubing, or an electronic infusion pump with an anti-free-flow feature.
- Give an age-appropriate explanation to the child when the time is right.
- Apply a transdermal anesthesia cream before the venipuncture to lessen the child's anxiety, reduce his pain, and improve compliance, if he's older than 1 month.
- Place warm packs on the site for 10 minutes to enhance vein dilation.
- Restrain the child, as necessary.
- In children, the blood return in the flashback chamber may be minimal after inserting the I.V. needle and catheter into the vein.
- Using sterile tape, secure the device.
- Cover the insertion site and device with a transparent semipermeable dressing.
- Place a protective device over the I.V. site to prevent dislodgment by the child.
- Loop the tubing and tape it so that, if it's pulled, the strain will be exerted on the tubing and not the catheter.

Assessment and management

- Frequency of monitoring depends on the child's condition, age, and the reason for I.V. therapy.
- Monitor the child's pulse rate and volume, blood pressure, temperature, capillary refill, urine output, peripheral pulses, skin color, extremities temperature, and laboratory test results.
- Compare your results with the child's baseline findings. Weigh the child before fluid administration is started and once per shift throughout the course of treatment.
- Monitor the amount of fluid infused and confirm flow rates.
- Assess the child's I.V. site at least hourly for signs of complications.

Pediatric I.V. therapy review *(continued)*

- Determine if the child is having pain.
- Document all findings and interventions according to facility policy, on flow sheets and in the nurses' notes.

Complications

- Infection
- Infiltration or extravasation
- Fluid overload
- Allergic reactions
- Phlebitis and emboli (uncommon)

Other fluid delivery systems

- Intraosseous infusion
- Peripherally inserted central catheters
- Umbilical vessel catheters

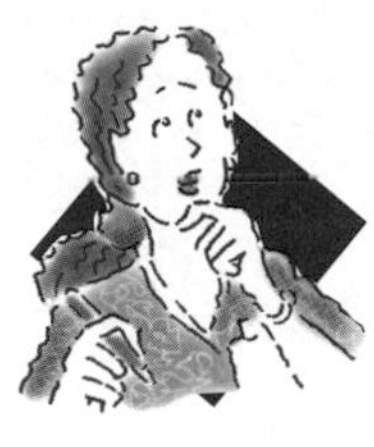

Quick Quiz

1. A child with moderate dehydration will have:
A. normal skin turgor.
B. a rapid, weak pulse.
C. extreme fatigue and muscle cramping.
D. normal capillary refill.

Answer: C. A child with moderate dehydration has cool extremities and experiences extreme fatigue and muscle cramping.

2. A child's pre-illness weight was 12 kg and his current weight is 11 kg. What is his percent of dehydration?
A. 1%
B. 8%
C. 20%
D. 25%

Answer: B. To determine the child's percent of dehydration, subtract his current weight (11 kg) from his pre-illness weight (12); divide your answer (1 kg) by the child's pre-illness weight (12 kg), and then multiply that number (0.08) by 100 to arrive at 8%.

3. When you're providing maintenance I.V. fluids to a child, it's important to:
A. use the child's current weight as the basis for determining the child's fluid needs.
B. determine the child's percent of dehydration.
C. administer bolus injections, followed by the remaining amount of fluid.
D. adjust the amounts based on the child's activity level, treatments, and insensible fluid losses.

Answer: D. The child's activity level, treatments, and insensible fluid losses affect the amount of maintenance fluids required.

4. A scalp vein is usually an ideal I.V. site for the:
- A. neonate.
- B. 10-month-old child.
- C. 2-year-old child.
- D. adolescent.

Answer: A. Scalp veins are best reserved for infants younger than 6 months old because they can easily be dislodged by the child's hands.

5. How long should EMLA cream remain on the skin to provide anesthesia for venipuncture?
- A. 15 minutes
- B. 30 minutes
- C. 45 minutes
- D. 60 minutes

Answer: D. The onset, depth, and duration of the anesthesia of EMLA cream depend on how long the cream is allowed to stay on the skin. For venipuncture, the recommended duration of application is 60 minutes.

6. The most common complications associated with I.V. therapy in children include:
- A. infection, infiltration or extravasation, fluid overload, and allergic reactions.
- B. infection, infiltration or extravasation, phlebitis, and allergic reactions.
- C. infection, emboli, fluid overload, and allergic reactions.
- D. infection, infiltration or extravasation, fluid overload, and deep vein thrombosis.

Answer: A. Infection, infiltration or extravasation, fluid overload, and allergic reactions are the complications of I.V. therapy that are most often seen in children.

Scoring

☆☆☆ If you answered all six answers correctly, two toddler thumbs up! You're practically a pediatric parenteral pro!

☆☆ If you answered four or five questions right, great goin'. You earned yourself an I.V. bagful of M & Ms!

☆ If you answered fewer than four questions correctly, no worries. Have a little snack, then begin your chapter infusion over again. You'll do better next time!

Geriatric I.V. therapy

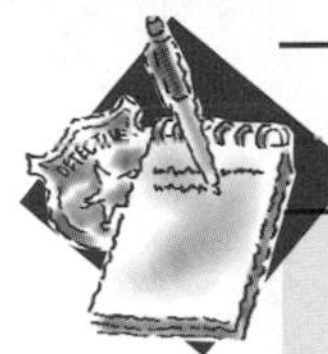

Just the facts

In this chapter, you'll learn:

- physiologic changes associated with aging
- considerations for administering I.V. therapy to older adults
- potential complications to watch for
- patient teaching considerations and techniques to use with elderly patients
- what to document when providing I.V. therapy.

The older adult

Chances are that many of the patients you will be required to perform I.V. therapy on will be older adults. People age 65 and older require health care services more frequently than any other age group; they account for over one-third of all hospital stays. Because so much of the health care population is elderly, it's important to recognize how to tailor your I.V. therapy to this population.

Modify your technique

When caring for older patients, you must make certain modifications to the techniques you normally use for other adults. You need to take into account the physiologic changes that normally occur during aging, and you need to understand how these changes affect I.V. therapy.

Physiologic changes of aging

With aging come the loss of some body cells and the reduced metabolism of others. These changes lead to altered body composition and reductions in certain body functions. Consequently, the older patient is more susceptible to complications with I.V. therapy.

Skin, hair, and nails

Perhaps some of the most obvious signs of aging occur with changes to the integumentary system.

The skinny on skin changes

Age-related subcutaneous fat loss, dermal thinning, and decreasing collagen lead to the development of facial lines around the eyes, mouth, and nose. Cell replacement decreases by 50%. Mucous membranes become drier, and sweat gland output reduces as the number of active sweat glands decrease.

Skin also loses elasticity with age, to the point were it may seem almost transparent. As the thickness and amount of connective tissue in the dermal layer (where veins reside) decreases, veins become more fragile. Typically, veins will appear tortuous because of the increased transparency and decreased elasticity of the skin. (See *Aging and its effect on skin.*)

Aging alters the body composition and reduces certain bodily functions, so it makes sense that you'll need to modify your nursing technique.

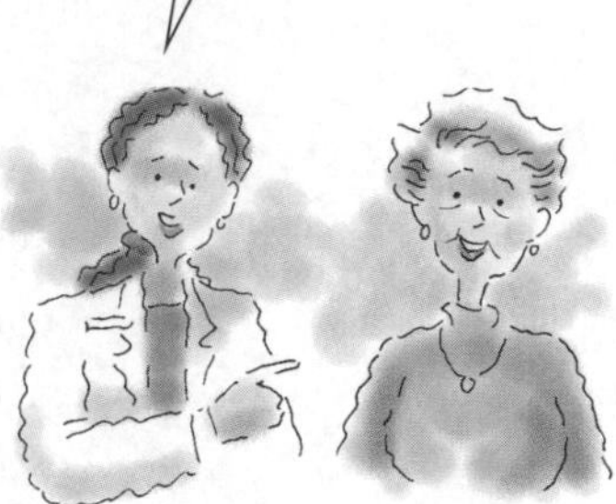

Aging and its effect on skin

Although the effects of aging vary with the specific tissue or organ, all older adults eventually become more susceptible to fatigue and disease. Some of the physiologic changes that occur in skin with aging include:

- gradual loss of subcutaneous fat and elastin, which causes the skin to wrinkle and sag.
- decreased dermal thickness.

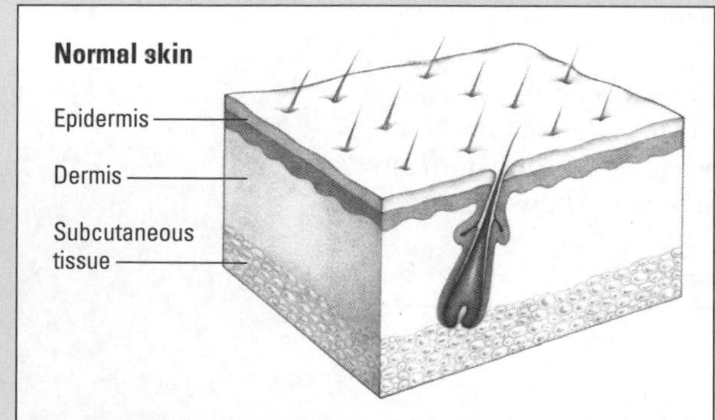

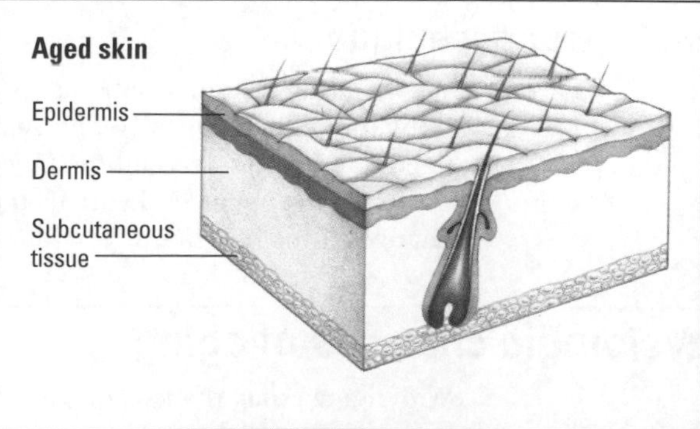

Hair . . . it's neither here nor there

Hair pigment decreases with age as the number of melanocytes decreases, so the hair may turn gray or white. Hair also thins as the patient ages.

Tough toenails

With age, nail growth slows and longitudinal ridges, thickening, brittleness, and malformations may increase.

Slow to heal

Besides wounds taking longer to heal, other common skin conditions in elderly people include:
- senile keratosis — overgrowth and thickening of the horny epithelium
- acrochordon — benign skin tags
- senile angiomas — benign tumors made up of blood vessels or lymph vessels.

Eyes and vision

Aging causes changes to the both the eye structure and visual acuity. The eyes sit deeper in the orbital socket and the eyelids lose their elasticity, becoming baggy and wrinkled. As the lacrimal apparatus loses fatty tissue, tears diminish in quantity.

The incredible shrinking pupil

The pupil shrinks, decreasing the amount of light that reaches the retina. To see objects, older adults need about three times as much light as younger people.

Who dimmed the lights?

Aging also diminishes night vision and depth perception. Many older adults develop presbyopia, a vision defect in which objects very close to the eye can't be seen clearly without corrective lenses.

Now here's an enlightening statistic: Older people require about three times as much light to see as younger people.

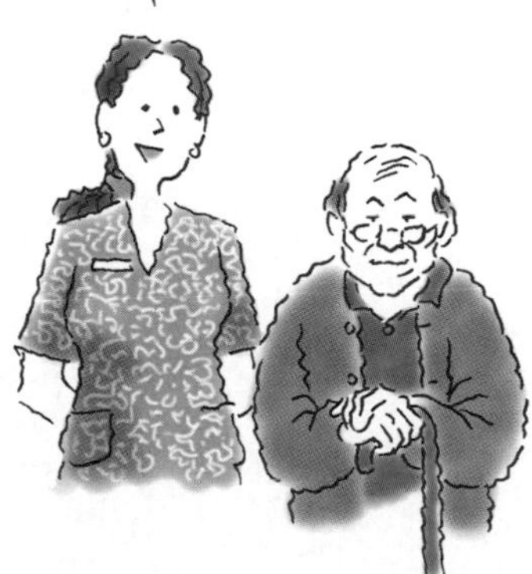

Ears and hearing

Many elderly persons lose some degree of hearing. By age 60, most adults have difficulty hearing about 4,000 Hz. (The normal range for speech recognition is 500 to 2,000 Hz.) Many older adults have trouble distinguishing higher-pitched consonants, such as *s*, *sh*, *f*, *ph*, *ch*, *z*, *t*, and *g*.

Some people may not be immediately aware of the onset or progression of a hearing defect. Others may recognize it but view it as a natural part of aging. Both vision changes and hearing changes need to be taken into account when preparing and teaching an elderly patient about I.V. therapy.

Impaired ventilation of the lungs' basal areas causes an elderly patient to have less tolerance for excess fluid. This puts her at increased risk for fluid-load complications with I.V. therapy.

Respiratory system

Age-related changes occur in all areas of the respiratory system. In the upper airway, the nose enlarges from continued cartilage growth and the tonsils atrophy. Many patients also experience some degree of tracheal deviation. In the thorax, the anteroposterior chest diameter increases, which may result in decreased chest wall mobility. Respiratory muscle degeneration or atrophy may also occur, reducing pulmonary function.

Airway closed

Aging also results in the closing of some airways, which impairs ventilation of the basal areas of the lungs and reduces the maximum breathing capacity, forced vital capacity, and inspiratory reserve. This decreases the elderly patient's tolerance of excess fluid, and increases the risk for complications due to fluid overload.

Cardiovascular system

The heart usually decreases slightly with age. The heart muscle becomes less efficient and loses contractile strength, and fibrotic and sclerotic changes thicken the heart valves and reduce their flexibility. The aorta grows more rigid, causing systolic blood pressure to rise proportionately more than diastolic blood pressure.

Fluid shifting sensitivity

By age 70, many people experience a 35% decrease in cardiac output at rest. This decrease in cardiac output makes the older patient more sensitive to fluid shifts that may occur with I.V. therapy.

GI system

Normal age-related changes in the GI system include diminished mucosal elasticity and reduced GI secretions, which in turn may alter digestion and absorption. GI tract motility, esophageal sphincter tone, and abdominal muscle strength may also decrease with age. These changes may result in appetite loss, esophageal reflux, constipation, and an increased risk of dehydration. (See *Preventing dehydration in elderly patients.*)

Preventing dehydration in elderly patients

To maintain adequate hydration, an elderly patient needs 1,000 to 3,000 ml of fluid daily. Less than 1,000 ml daily may lead to constipation, which can contribute to urinary incontinence. It may also result in more concentrated urine, which predisposes the patient to urinary tract infections. Follow these guidelines to make sure the patient is adequately hydrated.

Monitoring

- Monitor intake and output. Ensure an intake of at least 1,500 ml of oral fluids and urine output of 1,000 to 1,500 ml per 24 hours.
- Check skin turgor and mucous membranes.
- Monitor vital signs, especially pulse rate, respiratory rate, and blood pressure. An increase in pulse and respiratory rates with decreased blood pressure may indicate dehydration.
- Monitor laboratory test results, such as serum electrolyte, blood urea nitrogen, and creatinine levels; hematocrit; and urine and serum osmolarity. Check for signs of acidosis.
- Weigh the patient at the same time daily, using the same scale and with the patient wearing the same type of clothes.
- Auscultate bowel sounds for any increase in activity. Monitor stools for character: Hard stools may indicate dehydration; loose, watery stools indicate loss of water.
- Be aware of diagnostic tests that affect intake and output (for example, laxative or enema use, which cause fluid loss), and replace any lost fluids.

Providing fluids

- Provide fluids often throughout the day, for example, every hour and with a bedtime snack.
- Provide modified cups that the patient can handle; help those who have difficulty.
- Offer fluids other than water; find out the types of beverages the patient likes and the preferred temperatures (for example, ice cold or room-temperature drinks).
- Monitor coffee intake; coffee acts as a diuretic and may cause excessive fluid loss.
- If the patient is unable to take oral fluids, request an order for I.V. hydration.

Hematologic and immune systems

The older person's immune system is less responsive to foreign bodies and antigens, including vascular access devices. Because the body reacts more slowly under such adverse conditions, the patient is at increased risk for health-care acquired infections and generally requires more time to heal.

Fluid balance and aging

As the body ages, its fluid reserves become limited and the total amount of body water is decreased by 6%. This places the patient at higher risk for developing a fluid volume deficit.

Further fluid factors

Other contributing factors for fluid volume deficit in an elderly patient include:

- decreased saliva
- decreased thirst mechanism
- electrolyte imbalances (See *Common fluid and electrolyte imbalances in elderly patients.*)
- increased urination.

Common fluid and electrolyte imbalances in elderly patients

The following chart lists some of the common fluid and electrolyte imbalances you may encounter while caring for elderly patients.

Imbalance	Causes	Signs and symptoms	Treatment
Hypervolemia (fluid volume excess)	Renal failure, heart failure, cirrhosis, increased oral or I.V. sodium intake, mental confusion, seizures, and coma	Edema, weight gain, jugular vein distention, crackles, shortness of breath, bounding pulse, elevated blood pressure, and increased central venous pressure	Diuretics, fluid restriction (less than 1 qt [1 L]/day), sodium restriction, or hemodialysis (for patients with renal failure)
Hypovolemia (fluid volume deficit)	Dehydration, vomiting, diarrhea, fever, polyuria, chronic kidney disease, diabetes mellitus, diuretic use, hot weather, decreased oral intake secondary to anorexia, nausea, diminished thirst mechanism, and inadequate water intake (common in nursing home patients)	Dry mucous membranes, oliguria or concentrated urine, anuria, orthostatic hypotension, dizziness, weakness, confusion or altered mental status, and possible severe hypotension, increased hemoglobin, hematocrit, blood urea nitrogen, and serum creatinine levels	Fluid administration (may be oral or I.V., depending on degree of deficit and patient's response; a urine output of 30 to 50 ml/hour usually signals adequate renal perfusion)
Hypernatremia (serum sodium greater than 145 mEq/L [greater than 145 mmol/L])	Water deprivation, hypertonic tube feedings without adequate water replacement, diarrhea, and low body weight	Dry mucous membranes, restlessness, irritability, weakness, lethargy, hyperreflexia, seizures, hallucinations, and coma	Gradual infusion of hypotonic electrolyte solution or isotonic saline solution
Hyponatremia (serum sodium less than 138 mEq/L [less than 138 mmol/L])	Diuretics, loss of GI fluids, kidney disease, excessive water intake, and excessive I.V. fluids or parenteral feedings	Nausea and vomiting, lethargy, confusion, muscle cramps, diarrhea, delirium, weakness, seizures, coma	Gradual sodium replacement, water restriction (1 to 1.5 L/day), or discontinuation of diuretic therapy (if ordered)

Common fluid and electrolyte imbalances in elderly patients *(continued)*

Imbalance	Causes	Signs and symptoms	Treatment
Hyperkalemia (serum potassium greater than 5 mEq/L [greater than 5 mmol/L])	Renal failure, impaired tubular function, potassium-conserving diuretic use (in patients with renal insufficiency), rapid I.V. potassium administration, metabolic acidosis, and diabetic ketoacidosis	Arrhythmias, weakness, paresthesia, electrocardiogram (ECG) changes (tall, tented T waves; ST segment depression; prolonged PR interval and QRS complex; shortened QT interval, absent P waves)	Dialysis (for renal failure); sodium polystyrene (Kayexalate) (to remove potassium), I.V. calcium gluconate (antagonizes cardiac abnormalities), I.V. insulin or hypertonic dextrose solution (shifts potassium into the cells), bicarbonate (for patients with acidosis); or potassium intake restriction
Hypokalemia (serum potassium less than 3.5 mEq/L [less than 3.5 mmol/L])	Vomiting, diarrhea, nasogastric suction, diuretic use, digoxin toxicity, and decreased potassium intake	Fatigue, weakness, confusion, muscle cramps, ECG changes (flattened T waves, presence of U waves, ST segment depression, prolonged PR interval), ventricular tachycardia or fibrillation	Oral or I.V. potassium administration (I.V. infusions must be diluted and given slowly)

Mind your elders!

When caring for an elderly patient, especially one who is receiving I.V. therapy, remain mindful of his fluid volume status. (See *Assessing fluid volume status.*)

Assessing fluid volume status

Your usual assessments of fluid volume status need to be adjusted when caring for an older patient because of the normal changes associated with aging. For example, instead of testing skin turgor on the forearm, you should test skin turgor on the patient's forehead or sternum. The normal decrease in skin elasticity is diminished in these areas compared to the forearm. Other assessments used to assess fluid volume status include:

- Temperature — a decrease in temperature may indicate a decrease in fluid volume
- Decreased filling of veins in hands
- Intake and output
- Weight (daily)
- Tongue — should be moist, midline, and pink
- Blood pressure — normal for patient without orthostatic hypotension
- Mental assessment — fluid volume deficit may result in confusion

Administering I.V. therapy

Because of the age-related skin changes and often fragile condition of older adults, administering I.V. therapy to geriatric patients can be particularly challenging. The nurse must pay close attention to not only to the mechanical aspects of accessing a vein and administering I.V. fluids but also to the patient's tolerance of the fluids and the therapy's overall ensuing physiologic effects.

Make sure to monitor the patient often during therapy for subtle changes that can signal intolerance or impending complications.

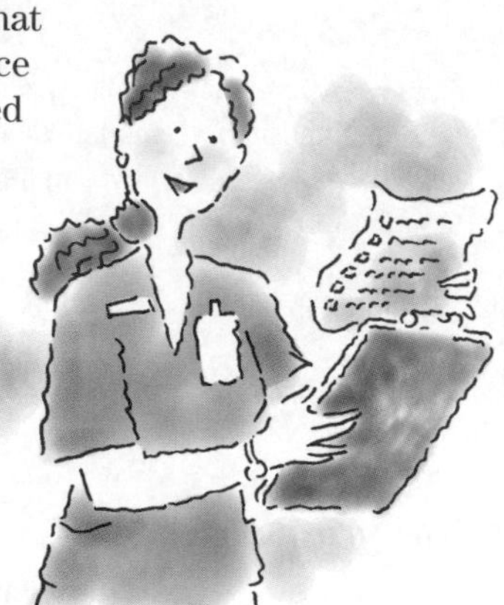

Keen on assessment

Ongoing assessment plays a crucial role when administering I.V. therapy to elderly patients. After you complete your initial assessment, you'll need to check the practitioner's orders to ensure that they don't conflict with your assessment findings or any advance directives the patient may have. Throughout therapy, you'll need to assess the patient frequently for signs of intolerance or complications.

Subtle signals

Remember that older adults have a decreased tolerance for too much or too little fluid, but their bodies tend to manifest symptoms slowly in response to such extremes. Therefore, you're responsible for monitoring for subtle changes that could signal a potential problem and alerting the practitioner before they escalate to a more serious condition.

Selecting an I.V. site

Many of the same principles used in selecting a site for younger patients also apply for older patients. However, avoid sites that are already bruised. Also avoid areas of flexion — especially the hands, if possible — to reduce the risk of dislodgment, which can lead to infiltration and phlebitis.

Integral site integrity

Vein preservation in the elderly patient is difficult, but it's almost always necessary to accomplish successful treatment. Review the length and type of treatment the patient needs and assess the need for alternative access, such as a peripherally inserted central catheter (PICC) or central venous access device.

Inserting the I.V. catheter

Inserting an I.V. catheter into an elderly patient follows the same steps as with a younger patient.

Avoid thick, ropelike veins. They're too thick-walled and occluded, making it hard for me to thread my way through them. Hey . . . thanks for listening!

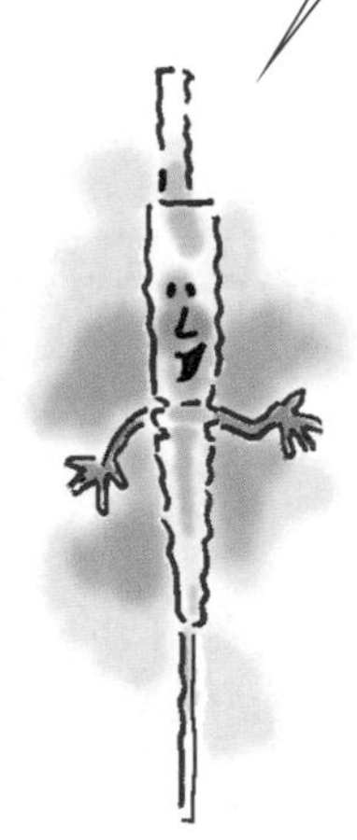

Palpating the vein

After choosing an appropriate site, carefully palpate the patient's veins. Although a tourniquet may be necessary for some patients, you may find that many elderly patients have easily visible veins. If the patient is taking an anticoagulant, avoid using a tourniquet as it may cause bleeding or hematoma formation. If possible, avoid veins that are thick and ropelike; this indicates thick, occluded vein walls and inserting and threading a catheter into them may be difficult.

Preparing the site

Site preparation is an important aspect with older adults. Their skin is typically dry and loose and can't tolerate many of the antiseptics needed for cleansing. Recommended skin disinfectants appropriate for elderly patients include chlorhexidine, povidone-iodine, alcohol, and 2% tincture of iodine. Apply the antiseptic with a careful friction motion, and allow the area to dry completely before inserting the catheter.

Inserting the device

Because the older patient has looser tissue, you may find stabilizing the vein difficult. To help stabilize a vein for insertion, stretch the skin proximal to the insertion site and anchor it firmly with your nondominant hand.

Veni, Vedi, Vici!

Also, because the patient's veins are more fragile, you'll need to perform venipuncture quickly and efficiently to avoid excessive bruising. A smaller gauge needle, such as 24G ¾″ needle, may be more appropriate and easier to insert.

Tank the tourniquet

If you use a tourniquet, remove it promptly to prevent bleeding through the vein wall around the infusion device, which may result from increased vascular pressure.

Securing the catheter

When securing the catheter, pay special attention to the patient's skin. Because elderly skin is thinner and more fragile, don't use more adhesive than is necessary. Secure the catheter using a catheter securement device and a transparent semipermeable dressing. If appropriate, use a skin barrier and allow it to dry before securing the catheter.

Seeing is believing

The insertion site must remain visible at all times, but padding under the catheter with gauze can help protect the skin. It's also more comfortable for the patient.

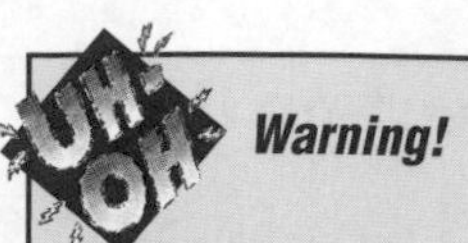

Don't go too fast with fluids

Elderly patients can develop heart failure if I.V. fluids are infused too rapidly. Therefore, use caution when administering I.V. fluids to replace fluid losses in these patients.

Controlling the flow

When administering I.V. therapy to an elderly patient, be sensitive to rapid variations of fluid volume and their effect on the patient. Keep in mind that the infusion of too much fluid at a too-rapid rate can trigger severe and often irreversible complications. (See *Don't go too fast with fluids.*)

Better safe than sorry

To control the flow of I.V. solution, you'll need to ensure that the administration tubing has additional safety features, in the form of either electronic or mechanical flow devices, in place. Make sure the tubing is long enough to provide adequate range of movement for the patient, but not so long that it drags on the floor and creates a fall hazard.

Use an electronic or mechanical flow device to control the flow rate of I.V. solution, and keep the tubing at a reasonable length to allow movement but prevent falls. Safety first!

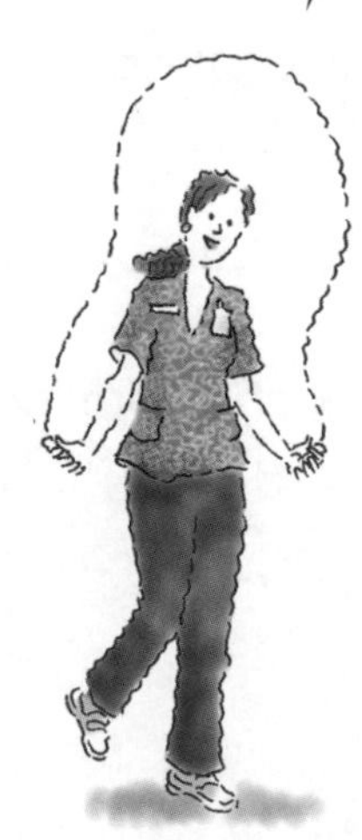

Removing the catheter

Although it's recommended to remove I.V. catheters and insert a new catheter every 72 hours, in older patients it may acceptable to continue using the same catheter as long as no signs or symptoms of infection are present.

It ain't *over* till it's *over*

Remove the catheter as soon as I.V. therapy is complete and the patient no longer needs I.V. access. This helps decrease the risk of infection, a prime consideration for older patients, who are more prone to it.

A little TLC won't hurt

Catheter removal can be difficult, especially when the skin is very thin. Take extra care when removing the catheter and use an adhesive remover; this will help alleviate pain and prevent any skin tearing that can occur.

Checking for complications

Older adults are extremely sensitive to the complications of I.V. therapy. Changes in metabolic systems, fluid and electrolyte imbalances, chronic disease, malnutrition, and changes to the integumentary system all contribute to this sensitivity.

The usual suspects

Some of the complications that are more likely to occur in an elderly patient include phlebitis, infiltration, extravasation, occlusion, pulmonary edema, air embolism, and speed shock.

Elderly patients are more prone to phlebitis, but they can develop any of the usual complications of I.V. therapy, so assess for signs and symptoms often.

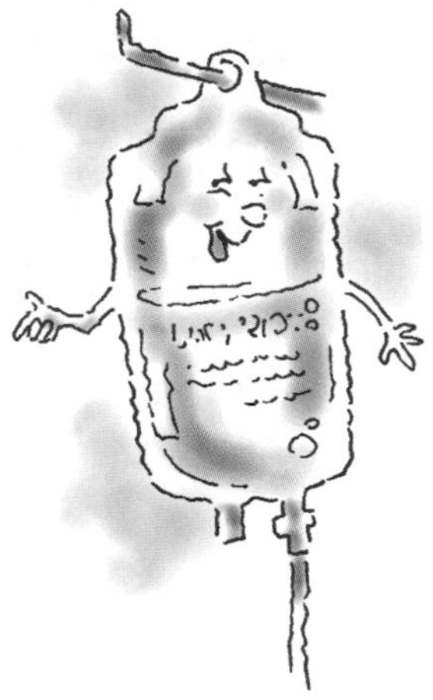

Can't feel the pain

Be aware that older patients may have a diminished pain sensation, especially in their hands and extremities. As a result, they may be unable to feel the pain caused by phlebitis and infiltration of I.V. fluid. Carefully assess the I.V. insertion site every 2 hours. Also remember to assess for signs and symptoms of fluid overload, hypersensitivities, and other complications on a frequent basis.

Patient teaching

When teaching elderly patients about I.V. therapy, you need to tailor your approach to account for their different learning styles, abilities, and needs. To help ensure successful sessions, keep in mind how the aging process may affect their mental capacity, sensory perception, and psychomotor function.

Mental capacity changes

A person's intellectual ability changes with age. Some factors of intelligence, such as those associated with experience and learning over time, increase with age. However, as degenerative processes occur, other mental processes decline, causing such changes as slowed processing time and slowed response time.

Have a chat

Talk to the patient and determine his previous experiences with I.V. therapy. Use this existing knowledge as a beginning for your teaching.

Divvy times repeat equals . . .

Older people generally need more time to process and react to information, especially when learning something new and complex. Modify your teaching sessions accordingly by:

- avoiding long explanations
- dividing your teaching into short segments of information
- providing plenty of time for the patient to comprehend what you have said (allow extra time to answer your questions)
- repeating information if the patient seems confused or hesitant to answer questions.

Sensory losses

The ability to discriminate high-frequency sounds begins to diminish around age 60. Severe impairment can make the patient feel isolated, suspicious, or even paranoid. The older person may nod his head and agree with everything you say when you look like you're expecting a response.

I said, "I think we'd better postpone the patient-teaching session until I can assess what's up with your hearing aid."

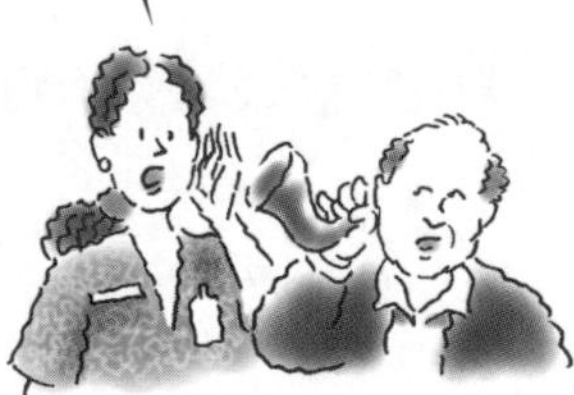

Can you hear me now?

If the patient speaks loudly or tilts his head when listening, assess for deafness. If he has a hearing aid, make sure he's wearing it and that it's turned on and functioning. Speak slowly, clearly, and in a normal tone; don't raise your voice. Also, use a quiet room for teaching sessions.

A bright idea

Impaired vision may prevent the patient from being able to read any patient-teaching handouts you give him, so take time to read the information with him if necessary. If possible, provide large-print handouts. Make sure that reading lights are properly placed and that they supply bright but diffused light.

More info, please!

Whenever possible, use the opportunity to teach the patient about his I.V. therapy and to answer any questions he may have. Being informed and receiving regular updates about his treatment will help foster his sense of control over his environment and situation.

Documentation

Documentation of I.V. therapy for elderly patients is the same as for younger ones. In your nurse's notes or on the appropriate I.V. sheets, record the date and time of the venipuncture; the type, gauge, and length of the cannula; the anatomic location of the insertion site; the length of the catheter; and, if applicable, the reason the I.V. site was changed. Also document the number of attempts at venipuncture (if you made more than one), the type and flow rate of the I.V. solution, the name and amount of medication in the solution (if any), any adverse reactions and actions taken to correct them, patient teaching and evidence of patient understanding, and your initials.

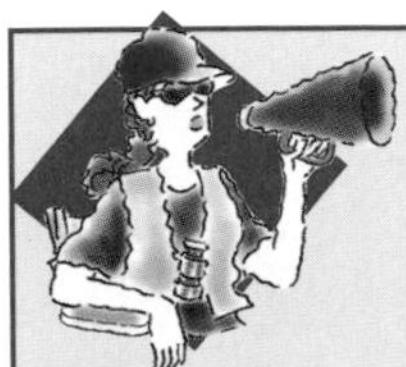

That's a wrap!

Geriatric I.V. therapy review

Physiologic changes associated with aging
Loss of some body cells, reduced metabolism, and other changes including:

Skin, hair, and nails
- Subcutaneous fat loss, dermal thinning, and decreased collagen
- Dry mucous membranes
- Decreased number and output of sweat glands
- Decreased elasticity
- Decreased vein thickness
- Decreased hair pigment, causing hair to turn gray or white; hair thinning
- Slowed nail growth, formation of longitudinal ridges; nails may also become thicker, brittle, and malformed
- Slowed wound healing
- Other possible skin conditions: senile keratosis, acrochordon, senile angiomas

Eyes and vision
- Eyes sit deeper in the orbital socket.
- Eyelids lose their elasticity, becoming baggy and wrinkled.
- Tears diminish in quantity.
- Pupil shrinks and decreased light reaches the retina.
- Night vision and depth perception diminish.

Ears and hearing
- By age 60, most adults have difficulty hearing about 4,000 Hz. (Normal range for speech recognition is 500 to 2,000 Hz.)
- Many older adults have trouble distinguishing higher-pitched consonants (*s, sh, f, ph, ch, z, t,* and *g*).
- Vision and hearing changes should be considered when preparing patient teaching.

Respiratory system
- In the upper airway, the nose enlarges from continued cartilage growth, tonsils atrophy, and tracheal deviation may occur.
- Anteroposterior chest diameter increases (may decrease chest wall mobility). Respiratory muscle degeneration and closing of some airways occur.
- Patient may have decreased maximum breathing capacity, forced vital capacity, and inspiratory reserve.

Cardiovascular system
- Heart size decreases.
- Heart muscle loses efficiency and contractile strength; fibrotic and sclerotic changes thicken heart valves, reducing their flexibility.

(continued)

Geriatric I.V. therapy review *(continued)*

- Aorta grows more rigid, causing systolic blood pressure to rise proportionately more than diastolic blood pressure.
- By age 70, many people experience a 35% decrease in cardiac output at rest.

GI system

- Diminished mucosal elasticity and reduced GI secretions alter digestion and absorption.
- GI tract motility, lower esophageal sphincter tone, and abdominal muscle strength may decrease.

Hematologic and immune systems

- Less responsive to foreign antigens such as vascular access devices
- Increased risk for health-care acquired infections and time needed for healing

Fluid balance

- Fluid reserves become limited and the total amount of body water is decreased by 6%.
- Other factors contributing to fluid volume deficit: decreased saliva, decreased thirst mechanism, electrolyte imbalances, and increased urination.
- Patient requires frequent assessments for alterations in fluid volume.

Administering I.V. therapy

- Use same principles in selecting a site as for younger patients.
- Avoid using bruised areas and areas of flexion (particularly the hands).
- Review the length and type of treatment needed, and assess whether alternative access is required.
- Carefully palpate the patient's veins.
- Tourniquet may not be necessary in many patients.
- Avoid veins that are thick and ropelike.
- Recommended disinfectants for cleaning the access site: chlorhexidine, povidone-iodine, alcohol, and 2% tincture of iodine; apply antiseptic carefully and allow the area to dry completely before inserting the catheter.
- To stabilize the vein for insertion, stretch the skin proximal to the insertion site and anchor it firmly with your nondominant hand.
- Perform venipunctures quickly and efficiently to avoid excessive bruising.
- A smaller gauge needle, such as 24G ¾″ needle may be more appropriate and easier to insert.
- If a tourniquet is used, remove it promptly to prevent bleeding through the vein wall around the infusion device.
- Secure the catheter using a catheter securement device and transparent semipermeable dressing. If appropriate, use a skin barrier and allow it to dry before securing the catheter.
- Keep the insertion site visible at all times, and insert gauze padding under the catheter to help protect skin and promote comfort.

Removing the catheter

- The same catheter can be left in place as long as no signs or symptoms of infection are present, but it should be removed as soon as possible when treatment is over or a new catheter is needed.
- Removal can be difficult, especially when the skin is very thin.
- Be careful and use an adhesive remover to help alleviate pain and prevent skin tearing.

Complications

- Most common complications include:
  - –phlebitis
  - –infiltration
  - –extravasation
  - –occlusion

Geriatric I.V. therapy review *(continued)*

–pulmonary edema
–air embolism
–speed shock.

- Carefully assess I.V. insertion site every 2 hours.
- Assess for signs and symptoms of fluid overload, hypersensitivities, and other complications on a frequent basis.

Patient teaching

- Keep in mind that older people may need more time to process and react to information, especially when learning something new and complex.
- Avoid giving long explanations, and divide sessions into short segments of information.
- Allow extra time for patient to comprehend what's been said and to answer questions; repeat information as necessary.
- If the patient speaks loudly or tilts his head when listening, assess for deafness.
- If the patient has a hearing aid, make sure he's wearing it and that it's turned on and functioning.
- Speak slowly, clearly, and in a normal tone; don't raise your voice.
- Hold teaching sessions in a quiet room.
- Read any patient teaching handouts with the patient; if possible, provide large-print handouts.
- Make sure that reading lights are properly placed and supply bright, diffused light.

Documentation

Document the following:

- date and time of the venipuncture
- type, gauge, and length of the cannula
- anatomic location of the insertion site
- length of the catheter
- number of attempts at venipuncture
- type and flow rate of the I.V. solution
- name and amount of medication in the solution (if any)
- any adverse reactions and actions taken to correct them
- patient teaching and evidence of patient understanding
- your initials.

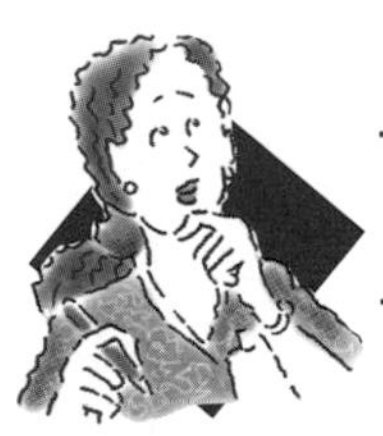

Quick quiz

1. Where should you measure skin turgor in an elderly patient?
A. Forehead
B. Forearm
C. Abdomen
D. Lower leg

Answer: A. Use the skin on the patient's forehead to test his skin turgor. This skin is less likely to have decreased elasticity.

2. The total body water in an older adult is decreased by:

A. 3%.
B. 6%.
C. 9%.
D. 12%.

Answer: B. As the body ages, its fluid reserves become limited and the total amount of body water is decreased by 6%.

3. Which skin change is characteristic of an elderly patient?

A. Decreased amount of subcutaneous fat
B. Thicker skin
C. Increased elasticity
D. Increased perspiration

Answer: A. As a person ages, his subcutaneous fat decreases and his skin tends to become thinner and less elastic. Perspiration usually decreases as well.

4. When teaching an elderly patient about I.V. therapy, which of the following considerations should the nurse keep in mind?

A. The patient probably won't want to know about his treatment.
B. Patient teaching only needs to be done once.
C. It's best to use only patient-teaching handouts.
D. It's helpful to talk slowly and be prepared to repeat information.

Answer: D. Because of the potential for sensory losses associated with aging, it's best to talk slowly and clearly to the patient and repeat information as needed.

Scoring

☆☆☆ If you answered all four questions correctly, brag all you want to your grandma! You're a first-generation geriatric I.V. therapy whiz!

☆☆ If you answered three questions correctly, not too bad. Put on your reading glasses, brush up on your age-related physiological facts, and modify your study technique. You'll do fine next time.

☆ If you answered fewer than three questions right, give yourself a break. You've only hit a few tiny wrinkles ... nothing a little reviewing, tea, and retinol can't cure.

Appendices and index

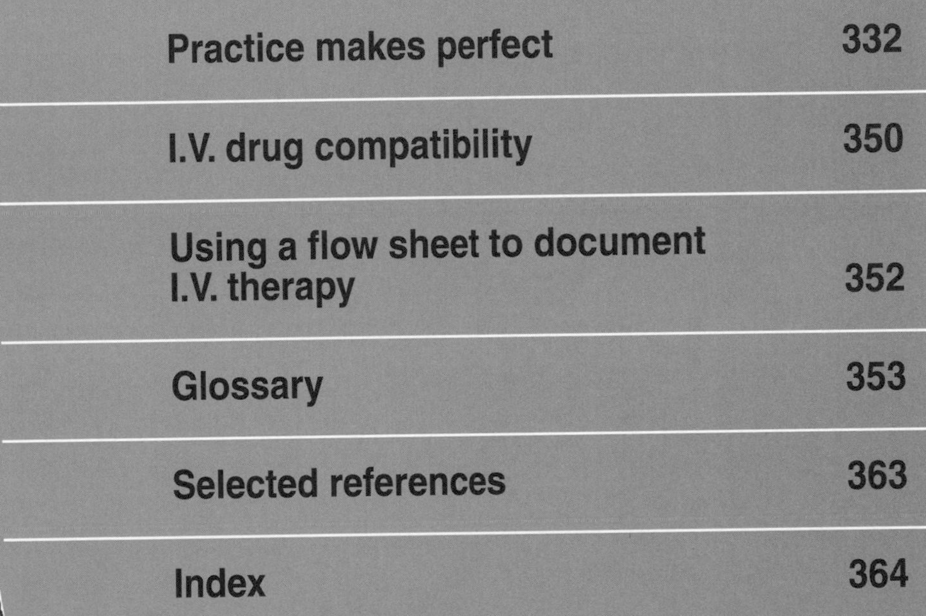

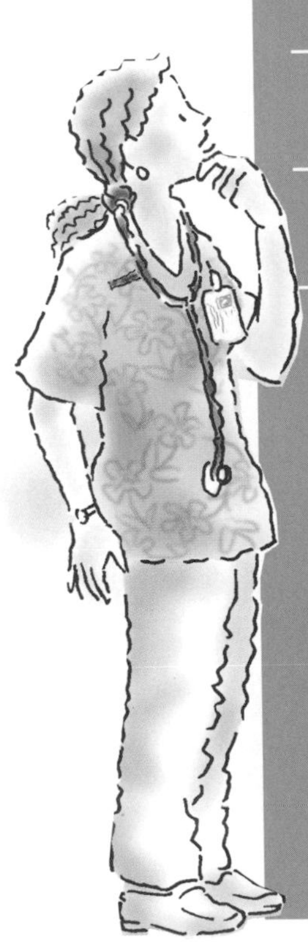

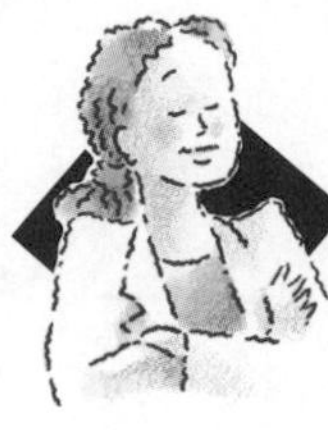

Practice makes perfect

1. A 39-year-old patient returns from the operating room after undergoing a right thoracotomy. An I.V. solution of dextrose 5% in half-normal saline solution is infusing. Which type of I.V. solution is the patient receiving?

A. Isotonic
B. Hypotonic
C. Hypertonic
D. Lactated

2. Thirst is experienced when water loss equals what percentage of body weight?

A. 2%
B. 8%
C. 10%
D. 12%

3. Which of the following electrolytes maintains cell electroneutrality?

A. Sodium
B. Magnesium
C. Chloride
D. Potassium

4. A 29-year-old patient with hepatitis is admitted to your unit with liver failure. Which type of I.V. solution may be difficult for the liver to metabolize?

A. Lactated Ringer's solution
B. Normal saline solution
C. D_5W solution
D. Parenteral nutrition

5. Which of the following statements about solutes in diffusion is accurate?

A. They move from an area with a lower concentration to an area with a higher one.
B. They ascend against the gradient of the concentration.
C. They move from an area with a higher concentration to an area with a lower one.
D. They move freely without regard to a gradient.

6. Fluid volume and concentration is regulated by the interaction of aldosterone and which other hormone?

A. ADH
B. TSH
C. LSH
D. FSH

7. Phosphorus is an electrolyte that's responsible for:
- A. maintaining cardiac muscle function.
- B. activating intracellular enzymes.
- C. maintaining serum osmolarity.
- D. maintaining bones and teeth.

8. An 89-year-old patient with a history of heart failure has an I.V. solution that's being infused through microdrip tubing. Microdrip tubing delivers how many drops per milliliter?
- A. 10 gtt
- B. 20 gtt
- C. 60 gtt
- D. 80 gtt

9. A 47-year-old patient with a history of alcohol abuse is admitted to the emergency department with dehydration. When selecting the correct setup for the I.V. administration set for this patient, what should you recall about a viscous solution?
- A. The larger the drop, the more drops per milliliter.
- B. The larger the drop, the fewer drops per milliliter.
- C. The smaller the drop, the fewer drops per milliliter.
- D. The smaller the drop, the more drops per milliliter.

10. A 74-year-old patient is receiving vancomycin through a secondary I.V. set. Which of the following devices prevents backflow of the secondary solution into the primary solution?
- A. Backcheck valve
- B. In-line filter
- C. Burette
- D. Volumetric pump

11. The practitioner orders an I.V. infusion for a patient who just entered the emergency department with complaints of severe abdominal pain. You begin preparing the equipment needed to start the infusion. At what distance should the I.V. solution be hung above the venipuncture site?
- A. 18″ (45.7 cm)
- B. 24″ (60.9 cm)
- C. 30″ (76.2 cm)
- D. 36″ (91.4 cm)

12. An 85-year-old patient with a history of abdominal aortic aneurysm resection is admitted to the emergency department with dehydration. Which of the following conditions contraindicates insertion of an I.V. catheter into his arm?
- A. Dialysis access site
- B. Previous I.V. site
- C. Nondominant arm or hand
- D. Dominant arm or hand

13. You're teaching a group of nursing students the basic principles of I.V. therapy. Which layer of a vein could you accurately say acts to allow blood cells and platelets to flow smoothly?

A. Tunica intima
B. Tunica media
C. Tunica adventitia
D. Tunica externa

14. An 18-year-old patient is admitted to your unit with seizures. Although he has an I.V. catheter in place with I.V. fluids infusing, you need to insert an intermittent infusion device for administration of phenytoin. After gathering the necessary equipment, you locate a site for insertion. Where should you place the tourniquet in proximity to the intended venipuncture site?

A. 1″ (2.5 cm) above the venipuncture site
B. 2″ (5 cm) above the venipuncture site
C. 6″ (15.2 cm) above the venipuncture site
D. 10″ (25.4 cm) above the venipuncture site

15. You need to place an I.V. catheter in a patient who's going to the operating room in the morning for repair of a fractured right hip. At what angle should you approach the vein?

A. 15 to 20 degree angle
B. 30 to 40 degree angle
C. 50 to 60 degree angle
D. 70 to 80 degree angle

16. You're caring for a patient who underwent a left thoracotomy. He has I.V. fluids infusing through a catheter in his right hand. If the semipermeable transparent dressing remains intact, when should you change the dressing?

A. Every shift
B. Every day
C. Every 2 days
D. Every week

17. A 29-year-old patient is admitted to your unit after sustaining injuries in a motor vehicle accident. He has I.V. fluids infusing in his left antecubital area. How often should you change the I.V. administration set?

A. With every bag change
B. Every 24 hours
C. Every 48 hours
D. Every 72 hours

18. After you insert an I.V. catheter in your patient, he develops itching, wheezing, tearing eyes, runny nose, and urticaria at the I.V. site. These signs and symptoms suggest:

A. nerve damage.
B. allergic reaction.
C. systemic infection.
D. infiltration.

19. A patient with acute respiratory failure requires a central venous access device for total parenteral nutrition administration. You know that central venous circulation enters the right atrium through which vein?

A. Superior vena cava
B. Cephalic vein
C. Median cubital vein
D. Jugular vein

20. A 59-year-old patient is admitted to your facility with acute abdominal pain. He's immediately taken to the operating room for an exploratory laparotomy; the test reveals inflammatory bowel disease. Postoperatively, a peripherally inserted central catheter (PICC) is inserted for administration of steroids and total parenteral nutrition. One advantage of using a PICC is that it can be used:

A. in patients with multiple venipunctures at the site.
B. in patients with scarring at the venipuncture site.
C. to accomplish long-term access to central veins.
D. without regard to the surgical site.

21. A patient has undergone numerous venipunctures for peripheral I.V. placement and now requires central venous access device placement. The practitioner chooses the subclavian approach. What's the advantage of accessing the subclavian vein?

A. Decreased risk of pneumothorax
B. High flow rate
C. Proximity to the subclavian artery
D. Decreased risk of hemothorax

22. A 23-year-old patient is admitted to your unit after sustaining a closed head injury in a motor vehicle accident. He's prescribed I.V. phenytoin, which is highly caustic to veins. When administering highly caustic I.V. medications, which veins should be avoided?

A. Internal jugular
B. Subclavian
C. Femoral
D. External jugular

23. You assist the practitioner with insertion of a central venous access device. After the catheter is inserted, the practitioner draws blood samples. What's the reason for this action?

A. To determine arterial blood gas levels
B. To determine hemoglobin levels
C. To establish baseline coagulation profiles
D. To determine venous oxygenation status

24. You're unable to access a peripheral vein in an 89-year-old patient with a hip fracture that was complicated by pneumonia. The practitioner decides that a central venous access device is necessary for this patient. He tells you that he's planning a right subclavian approach. In which position should you place the patient for insertion?

A. Semi-Fowler's
B. Trendelenburg's
C. Prone
D. Left lateral

25. A 76-year-old patient recovering from repair of a ruptured diverticulum has a central venous access device in place with total parenteral nutrition infusing. If the gauze dressing remains intact, how often should you change the dressing?

A. Every 8 hours
B. Every 24 hours
C. Every 48 hours
D. Every 72 hours

26. If the patient can't perform Valsalva's maneuver while you change the cap of a central venous access device, which of the following can serve as an alternative procedure?

A. Ask the patient to perform pursed-lip breathing.
B. Remove the cap during the inspiratory phase.
C. Have the patient breathe normally.
D. Remove the cap during the expiratory phase.

27. A 29-year-old patient who sustained a liver laceration in a motor vehicle accident has a central venous access device in place. He calls you to his room with complaints of chest pain and shortness of breath. You note that he's cyanotic and diaphoretic. Which complication associated with central venous therapy might this patient be experiencing?

A. Pneumothorax
B. Air embolism
C. Thrombosis
D. Fibrin sheath formation

28. A 37-year-old with acute leukemia has an implanted port in place. What type of needle should be used to access his implanted port?

A. Winged infusion set
B. Coring needle
C. Noncoring needle
D. Over-the-needle catheter

29. A 43-year-old patient with bladder cancer has an implanted port in place. He complains of a burning sensation and swelling in the subcutaneous tissue around the port. Which complication is he most likely experiencing?

A. Fibrin sheath formation
B. Chylothorax
C. Thrombosis
D. Extravasation

30. A patient is prescribed two medications as preoperative sedation before going to the operating room for a colon resection. You would like to administer the medications together in one syringe. In order for the drugs to be compatible in a syringe:

A. both should be opioids.
B. one should have a high pH and one a low pH.
C. they should have similar pH values.
D. they should be mixed with saline.

31. You mix two medications in a syringe and notice a precipitate. The precipitate indicates:

A. therapeutic incompatibility.
B. physical incompatibility.
C. chemical incompatibility.
D. environmental incompatibility.

32. You administer a sedative to a patient who's going to the operating room for a hernia repair. Instead of producing sedation, the medication produces excitement. Which type of reaction is the patient experiencing?

A. Hypersensitivity reaction
B. Idiosyncratic reaction
C. Cross-sensitivity reaction
D. Nonhemolytic reaction

33. The practitioner prescribes renal-dose dopamine for a patient with acute renal failure. To calculate the infusion rate, you must know the patient's weight in kilograms. Your patient weighs 186 lb. Which of the following operations will enable you to translate this weight to kilograms?

A. Divide by 1.2
B. Divide by 2.2
C. Divide by 3.4
D. Divide by 4.5

34. A patient is prescribed a drug that must be mixed in a solution for I.V. administration. When a drug and a solution are mixed:

A. the higher the concentration, the more likely it is that an incompatibility will develop.
B. concentration doesn't affect compatibility.
C. the higher the concentration, the less likely it is that an incompatibility will develop.
D. the lower the concentration, the less likely it is that an incompatibility will develop.

35. You're caring for a 92-year-old patient with fragile veins. Which infusion method places him at increased risk for developing infiltration at the I.V. site?

A. Intermittent
B. Continuous
C. Bolus
D. Primary

36. An 82-year-old patient is admitted with heart failure. Because this patient requires the delivery of a small volume of fluid, which intermittent infusion method is most appropriate?

A. Saline lock
B. Volume-control set
C. Piggyback method
D. Direct

37. Which method of continuous infusion can't be used for drugs with immediate incompatibility?

A. Secondary line
B. Piggyback line
C. Primary line
D. Volume control

38. A patient is prescribed vancomycin for treatment of a severe staphylococcal infection. The patient has a primary I.V. solution infusing. You administer the vancomycin as a secondary solution. When hanging an infusion through a secondary infusion set, the secondary solution container should be hung higher than the primary container. This is necessary:

A. because the primary container will contaminate the secondary container.
B. because the primary container will automatically flow when the secondary is empty.
C. because the secondary solution may be incompatible with the primary container.
D. because the primary container won't automatically flow when the secondary is empty.

39. A patient is receiving famotidine through a syringe pump. One advantage of using a syringe pump to administer medications is that it provides:

A. the greatest control for large-volume infusions.
B. the patient with control over his infusion.
C. the greatest control for small-volume infusions.
D. the greatest control for retrograde administration.

40. You received a report on a 65-year-old patient who underwent resection of an abdominal aortic aneurysm. The nurse told you that the patient has lactated Ringer's solution infusing at 150 ml/hour. When you enter the patient's room to perform your assessment, you note that the patient is in respiratory distress. You check his blood pressure and find that it's elevated. You also note jugular vein distention. This patient is most likely experiencing:

- A. circulatory overload.
- B. hypersensitivity.
- C. systemic infection.
- D. a hemolytic reaction.

41. You note phlebitis at the I.V. site of a patient who has been receiving I.V. fluids for the past 3 days. Phlebitis is a common complication associated with which type of I.V. solution?

- A. Low osmolarity
- B. High osmolarity
- C. Normal pH solution
- D. Isotonic

42. Erythrocytes, thrombocytes, and leukocytes, the cellular or formed elements of blood, make up about what percentage of blood volume?

- A. 35%
- B. 45%
- C. 55%
- D. 70%

43. A patient is ordered a transfusion of 1 unit of packed red blood cells (RBCs) to treat a hemoglobin (Hb) level of 8.9 g/dl. As you administer the blood, you observe the patient closely, remembering that a hemolytic reaction can occur when how much blood is infused?

- A. 10 ml
- B. 50 ml
- C. 100 ml
- D. 250 ml

44. A 52-year-old patient develops a life-threatening granulocytopenia that isn't responding to antibiotics. Which blood component might be prescribed for this patient?

- A. Leukocyte-poor red blood cells (RBCs)
- B. Platelets
- C. White blood cells (WBCs)
- D. Packed RBCs

45. An 88-year-old patient who underwent internal fixation of a fractured hip 3 days ago now has a hemoglobin level of 7.8 g/dl. The practitioner prescribes 2 units of packed red blood cells (RBCs) to run over 3 hours each. When preparing the administration set, you should:

A. piggyback blood into an existing line.
B. have normal saline solution set up in a primary line.
C. hang dextrose 5% in water as a piggyback infusion through a secondary I.V. set.
D. have the blood set up as a primary line.

46. You're administering 1 unit of packed red blood cells (RBCs) to a patient, but the infusion is running slowly. You need to use a pressure bag to speed up the infusion. As you pump up the pressure bag, you should keep in mind that hemolysis can occur if the cuff pressure exceeds:

A. 100 mm Hg.
B. 150 mm Hg
C. 200 mm Hg.
D. 300 mm Hg.

47. A patient with hemophilia A is admitted with bleeding after falling off his bicycle. Which factor, known as the *antihemophilic factor*, should be administered to this patient to control bleeding?

A. Factor VII
B. Factor VIII
C. Factor IX
D. Factor X

48. A 42-year-old with a history of alcohol abuse is admitted with upper GI bleeding. You begin a transfusion of packed red blood cells and the patient suddenly develops abdominal pain, flushing, fever, and chills. What type of transfusion reaction might this patient be experiencing?

A. Plasma protein incompatibility
B. Allergic reaction
C. Febrile reaction
D. Bacterial contamination

49. Which complication may occur as a result of the accumulation of an iron-containing pigment in a patient who received multiple transfusions?

A Hypothermia
B. Potassium intoxication
C. Hemosiderosis
D. Hyperthermia

50. Which of the following types of chemotherapy drugs has a potential for damaging tissue?

A. Irritants
B. Vesicants
C. Nonvesicants
D. Nonirritants

51. A patient who received her first dose of chemotherapy 16 hours ago develops nausea. Which type of nausea occurs within the first 24 hours of treatment?

A. Anticipatory
B. Acute
C. Delayed
D. Intermittent

52. When carbohydrates, fats, and proteins are metabolized by the body they produce:

A. energy.
B. lactose.
C. cations.
D. anions.

53. A 5-year-old is admitted to your floor with severe protein deficiency that isn't accompanied by a calorie deficit. Which type of nutritional deficiency is this child experiencing?

A. Iatrogenic protein-energy malnutrition
B. Kwashiorkor
C. Marasmus
D. Gluconeogenesis

54. An 83-year-old patient with chronic heart failure is suspected of having protein-energy malnutrition. Which laboratory finding may help diagnose this nutritional deficiency?

A. Decreased hematocrit
B. Decreased serum transferrin level
C. Decreased serum triglyceride level
D. Decreased hemoglobin level

55. The nurse is caring for a patient who's receiving I.V. therapy and had a thoracotomy 4 hours ago. The patient's record indicates that he had the following intake and output during the shift:

Intake: ½ cup of ice chips
1,000 ml LR infused I.V. in O.R.
50 ml of antibiotic infused I.V. postoperatively
1 unit (250 ml) of packed RBCs received in PACU
60 ml of NSS via NG for flush
30 ml of antacid via NG

Output: 1,000 ml of urine output
200 ml of blood from thoracic drainage system
120 ml of NG drainage

How many milliliters should the nurse document as the patient's intake?________________

56. The nurse is using an over-the-needle device to start an I.V. infusion. Identify the area where she would first see blood return.

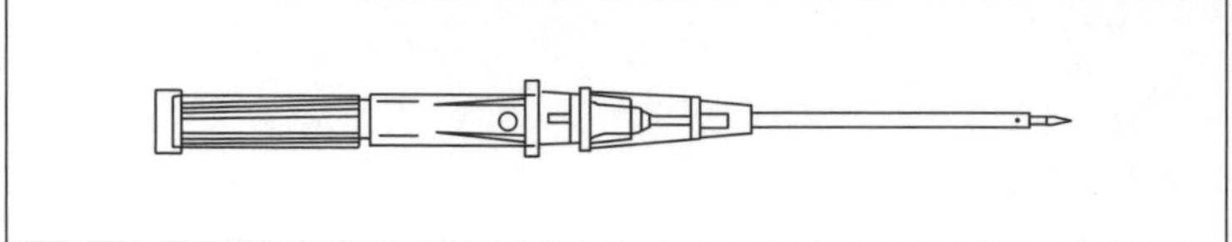

57. The nurse must calculate the flow rate for a patient with Alzheimer's disease who's experiencing dehydration. The order is for 1,000 ml of lactated Ringer's solution infused over 8 hours. The drip factor is 60 gtt/ml. How many drops per minute should the flow rate be?

____

58. The nurse is beginning I.V. therapy on a pediatric patient with Down syndrome. In what order should the nurse proceed with the following tasks?

A. Select the site.
B. Assemble and prepare equipment.
C. Explain the procedure to the patient and family.
D. Document I.V. therapy initiation.
E. Check the order.

____

59. In central venous therapy, the selection site may vary depending on which factors? Select all that apply.

A. Type of catheter
B. Patient's anatomy
C. Vessel integrity
D. Patient's gender
E. Vessel accessibility
F. Patient's age

60. The nurse is assisting a practitioner who's placing a central venous access device. In what order should the nurse perform the following tasks?

A. Monitor the patient for complications.
B Assist with insertion of the catheter.
C. Position the patient.
D. Prepare the insertion site.
E. Check to see that the consent form is signed.

____

61. Which drug administration route is most effective for quickly achieving therapeutic levels?

A. Subcutaneous
B. Intramuscular (I.M.)
C. Oral
D. Intravenous (I.V.)

62. An I.V. drug must be compatible with the solution in which it's mixed. Which solution would present the least risk of incompatibility?

A. Saline solution
B. Mannitol solution
C. Bicarbonate solution
D. Nutritional solution

63. A drug-diluent incompatibility that resulted in the formation of gas bubbles or cloudiness would be considered what type of incompatibility?

A. Chemical
B. Therapeutic
C. Iatrogenic
D. Physical

64. Hospital patients receive what amount of their medications by the I.V. route?

A. Almost one-quarter
B. Almost one-third
C. Almost one-half
D. Almost two-thirds

65. A patient who has sustained trauma lost a significant amount of blood and requires a blood transfusion. What blood component would be ordered to increase the blood volume?

A. Packed red blood cells
B. White blood cells
C. Platelets
D. Fresh frozen plasma

66. Citrate toxicity is most likely to cause which imbalance?

A. Hypercalcemia
B. Hypocalcemia
C. Potassium intoxication
D. Hemosiderosis

67. How quickly can a transfusion reaction occur after the start of the infusion?

A. 15 minutes
B. 20 minutes
C. 30 minutes
D. 60 minutes

68. Which catheter size is optimal for transfusing blood to a pediatric patient?

A. 16G
B. 18G
C. 20G
D. 24G

69. The nurse must infuse 1,000 ml of dextrose 5% in water to her patient every 12 hours. How many milliliters should be infused in 1 hour? ________________

70. The nurse notices that a patient who has been receiving I.V. therapy is developing phlebitis at the I.V. insertion site. Which of the following nursing interventions should be implemented? Select all that apply.

A. Stop the infusion and remove the device.
B. Apply warm packs.
C. Apply ice packs.
D. Elevate the limb.
E. Insert a new I.V. catheter at a new site.
F. Raise the solution container.

71. You detect signs and symptoms of an acute transfusion reaction in a patient who has been receiving packed red blood cells (RBCs). Put the following nursing interventions in order of priority for treating this reaction.

A. Infuse normal saline solution.
B. Perform a pulse and other vital signs check.
C. Stop the infusion.
D. Notify the practitioner.

____

72. To minimize the risk of a hemolytic reaction during a blood transfusion, recipient and donor blood should be tested for incompatibilities. Which tests are most important to include? Select all that apply.

A. Blood typing
B. Hemoglobin level and hematocrit
C. Rh typing
D. Cross matching
E. Platelet count
F. Direct antiglobulin

Answers

1. C. Dextrose 5% in half-normal saline solution is a hypertonic I.V. solution.

2. A. Thirst is experienced when water loss equals 2% of body weight or when osmolarity increases.

3. D. Potassium maintains cell electroneutrality.

4. A. Lactated Ringer's solution should be avoided in patients with liver disease because the liver may not be able to metabolize the lactate contained in this solution.

5. C. In diffusion, solutes move from an area with a higher concentration to an area with a lower one.

6. A. Fluid volume and concentration is regulated by the interaction of two hormones: ADH and aldosterone.

7. D. Phosphorus is an electrolyte that's responsible for maintaining bones and teeth.

8. C. Microdrip tubing delivers 60 gtt/ml.

9. B. When selecting the correct setup for I.V. administration, recall this guideline: the more viscous the solution, the larger the drop and the fewer drops per milliliter.

10. A. A backcheck valve prevents backflow of the secondary solution into the primary solution.

11. D. The I.V. bottle or bag should be hung on the I.V. pole about 36″ (91.4 cm) above the venipuncture site.

12. A. Never select a vein in an arm where a dialysis access site is placed.

13. A. The tunica intima allows blood cells and platelets to flow smoothly.

14. C. The tourniquet should be placed about 6″ (15.2 cm) above the venipuncture site.

15. A. Place the bevel up and insert the catheter into the skin at a 15 to 20 degree angle to the vein.

16. D. Unless the dressing is compromised, a transparent semipermeable I.V. dressing should be changed every 7 days.

17. D. According to Infusion Nurses Society standards, peripheral I.V. administration sets should be changed every 72 hours or as per facility policy.

18. B. Itching, wheezing, tearing eyes, runny nose, and urticaria at the I.V. site are signs of an allergic reaction.

19. A. Central venous circulation enters the right atrium through the superior or inferior vena cava.

20. C. A PICC provides long-term access to central veins.

21. B. One advantage of choosing the subclavian vein for central venous therapy is that it has a high flow rate, which reduces the risk of thrombus formation.

22. D. When administering highly caustic I.V. medications, such as phenytoin, the external jugular veins should be avoided because blood flow around the tip of the catheter may not be strong enough to sufficiently dilute the solution as it enters the vein.

23. C. After insertion of a central venous access device, blood samples are drawn to establish baseline coagulation profiles.

24. B. The patient should be placed in Trendelenburg's position before insertion of a subclavian or internal jugular vein central venous access device.

25. C. A gauze dressing should be changed every 48 hours unless it becomes moist, soiled, or loose.

26. D. If the patient can't perform Valsalva's maneuver, remove the cap during the expiratory phase of the respiratory cycle.

27. A. Chest pain, dyspnea, and cyanosis, along with decreased breath sounds on the affected side, may indicate pneumothorax, hemothorax, chylothorax, or hydrothorax.

28. C. To avoid damaging the port's silicone rubber septum, a noncoring needle should be used.

29. D. A burning sensation and swelling of the subcutaneous tissue are signs of extravasation.

30. C. Generally, drugs and solutions that are to be mixed should have similar pH values to avoid incompatibility.

31. C. Precipitation, gas bubbles, and color changes are basic signs of chemical incompatibility.

32. B. An idiosyncratic reaction to a drug is one in opposition to the drug's intended effect, such as when a tranquilizer produces excitement in a patient rather than sedation.

33. B. To convert a patient's body weight from pounds to kilograms, divide the number of pounds by 2.2 because 2.2 lb equal 1 kg.

34. A. When a drug and a solution are mixed, the higher the concentration, the more likely it is that an incompatibility will develop.

35. C. A bolus or direct injection method exerts more pressure on the vein than other methods, posing a greater risk of infiltration in patients with weak veins.

36. B. A volume-control set is used when the patient requires small volumes of fluid.

37. A. A secondary line can't be used for drugs with immediate incompatibility.

38. B. When hanging a piggyback solution, the secondary container should be hung higher than the primary container because the primary container will automatically flow when the secondary is empty.

39. C. An advantage of a syringe pump is that it provides the greatest control for small-volume infusions.

40. A. Jugular vein distention, respiratory distress, increased blood pressure, crackles, and positive fluid balance are signs of circulatory overload.

41. B. Phlebitis is associated with administration of drugs or solutions that are acidic or alkaline and those with high osmolarity.

42. B. The cellular, or formed, elements make up about 45% of blood volume and include erythrocytes, thrombocytes, and leukocytes.

43. A. A hemolytic reaction can occur with as little as 10 ml infused.

44. C. WBCs may be given to a patient with life-threatening granulocytopenia that isn't responding to antibiotics. This is especially true if the patient has positive blood cultures or a persistent fever greater than 101° F (38.3° C).

45. B. Always have sterile normal saline solution as a primary line along with the transfusion.

46. D. Don't allow the cuff to exceed 300 mm Hg because excessively high pressure can cause hemolysis and may damage the component container or rupture the blood bag.

47. B. Factor VIII, also referred to as *antihemophilic factor*, can be used to treat a patient with hemophilia A, to control bleeding associated with factor VIII deficiency, and to replace fibrinogen or factor VIII.

48. A. Signs and symptoms of a plasma protein incompatibility include flushing, urticaria, abdominal pain, chills, fever, dyspnea and wheezing, hypotension, shock, and cardiac arrest.

49. C. Hemosiderosis is caused by accumulation of an iron-containing pigment called *hemosiderin* and may be associated with red blood cell destruction in a patient who has received many transfusions.

50. B. Vesicants can cause a reaction so severe that blisters form and tissue is damaged or destroyed.

51. B. Acute nausea and vomiting occur within the first 24 hours of treatment.

52. A. When carbohydrates, fats, and proteins are metabolized by the body, they produce energy.

53. B. Kwashiorkor, which most commonly occurs in children, is a severe protein deficiency that isn't associated with a calorie deficit.

54. C. A decreased serum triglyceride level may indicate protein-energy malnutrition.

55. 1,510. The fluid intake for this patient is 120 ml (½ cup) of ice chips, 1,000 ml LR infused I.V. in O.R., 50 ml of antibiotic infused I.V. postoperatively, 1 unit (250 ml) of packed RBCs, 60 ml of NSS via NG for flush, and 30 ml of antacid via NG. Therefore, the total intake is 1,510 ml.

56. The nurse first sees blood return in the flashback area.

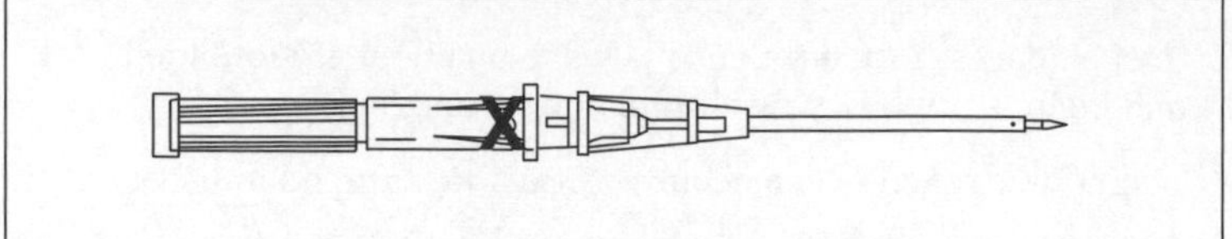

57. 125 ([1,000 ml/480 minutes] × 60 gtt/ml).

58. EBCAD. The correct sequence of events when initiating I.V. therapy is to first check the practitioner's order, assemble supplies needed and prepare equipment, explain the procedure to the patient and family (if present), select the site, and then document the procedure.

59. A, B, C, E, F. Gender isn't a consideration when selecting a site for central venous therapy.

60. ECDBA. The correct sequence of events when assisting with the insertion of a central venous access device is to first check to see that a consent form is signed, then position the patient, help prepare the insertion site, assist with insertion and, lastly, monitor for complications.

61. D. Unlike drugs that are administered orally, which take time to pass through and be absorbed by the GI system, drugs administered I.V. reach systemic circulation immediately. Because of the complexity of the musculoskeletal and integumentary systems, subcutaneous and I.M. drug administration absorption time may be erratic.

62. A. The more complex the solution, the greater the risk of incompatibility. Saline solution is the least complex of the solutions listed and has the least risk of incompatibility. All of the other substances have an increased risk of incompatibility when mixed with I.V. drugs.

63. D. A physical incompatibility occurs as a result of drug degradation and can be observed by the presence of precipitation, gas bubbles, haze, or cloudiness in the solution.

64. C. Almost one-half of the medications given to hospital patients are given by the I.V. route.

65. A. Packed red blood cells or whole blood is transfused to increase blood volume, such as with massive hemorrhage.

66. B. Citrate toxicity occurs as a result of blood being infused too rapidly. Citrate, a preservative used in blood, binds with calcium, which causes a calcium deficiency (hypocalcemia).

67. A. Signs and symptoms of a transfusion reaction can appear within 15 minutes of the start of the transfusion. Assess and monitor the patient closely according to the patient's transfusion history and your facility's policy.

68. D. A 24G catheter is optimal for administering blood to a pediatric patient.

69. 83. Divide the total volume (1,000 ml) by the number of hours required to deliver the infusion (12 hours).

70. A, B, E. When phlebitis is suspected, the appropriate order of nursing interventions should be to stop the infusion, apply warm packs, and then start a new I.V. catheter in another site.

71. CBAD. To remember the priority of nursing interventions for a transfusion reaction, think of the acronym SPIN: **S**top the infusion, **P**ulse should be assessed, **I**nfuse normal saline solution, and **N**otify the practitioner.

72. A, C, D, F. Hemoglobin level, hematocrit, and platelet count are important tests for determining need for blood or blood plasma replacements, but they aren't indicators of compatibility.

Compatibility of drugs combined in a syringe

KEY

Y = compatible for at least 30 minutes

P = provisionally compatible; give within 15 minutes

$P_{(5)}$ = provisionally compatible; give within 5 minutes

N = not compatible

* = conflicting data

(A blank space indicates no available data.)

	atropine sulfate	butorphanol tartrate	chlorpromazine HCl	cimetidine HCl	codeine phosphate	dexamethasone sodium phosphate	dimenhydrinate	diphenhydramine HCl	droperidol	fentanyl citrate	glycopyrrolate	heparin Na	hydromorphone HCl	hydroxyzine HCl	meperidine HCl	metoclopramide HCl
atropine sulfate		Y	P	Y			P	P	P	P	Y	$P_{(5)}$	Y	P*	P	P
butorphanol tartrate	Y		Y	Y			N	Y	Y	Y				Y	Y	Y
chlorpromazine HCl	P	Y		N			N	P	P	P	Y	N	Y	P	P	P
cimetidine HCl	Y	Y	N					Y	Y	Y	Y	$P_{(5)}$*	Y	Y	Y	
codeine phosphate							$P_{(5)}$				Y			Y		
dexamethasone sodium phosphate								N*			N		N*			Y
dimenhydrinate	P	N	N		$P_{(5)}$			P	P	P	N	$P_{(5)}$	Y	N	P	P
diphenhydramine HCl	P	Y	P	Y		N*	P		P	P	Y		Y	P	P	Y
droperidol	P	Y	P	Y			P	P		P	Y	N		P	P	P
fentanyl citrate	P	Y	P	Y			P	P	P			$P_{(5)}$	Y	P	P	P
glycopyrrolate	Y		Y	Y	Y	N	N	Y	Y				Y	Y	Y	
heparin Na	$P_{(5)}$		N	$P_{(5)}$*			$P_{(5)}$*		N	$P_{(5)}$			N		N	$P_{(5)}$*
hydromorphone HCl	Y		Y	Y		N*	Y	Y		Y	Y			Y		
hydroxyzine HCl	P*	Y	P	Y	Y		N	P	P	P	Y		Y		P	P
meperidine HCl	P	Y	P	Y			P	P	P	P	Y	N		P		P
metoclopramide HCl	P	Y	P			Y	P	Y	P	P		Y		P	P	
midazolam HCl	Y	Y	Y	Y			N	Y	Y	Y	Y	N	Y	Y	Y	Y
morphine sulfate	P	Y	P	Y			P	P	P	P	Y	N*		P	N	P
nalbuphine HCl	Y			Y			N	Y	Y		Y			Y		
pentazocine lactate	P	Y	P	Y			P	P	P	P	N	N	Y	P	P	P
pentobarbital Na	P*	N	N	N			N	N	N	N	N		Y	N	N	
perphenazine	Y	Y	Y	Y			Y	Y	Y	Y				Y	Y	P*
phenobarbital Na												$P_{(5)}$	N			
prochlorperazine edisylate	P	Y	P	Y			N	P	P	P	Y		N*	P	P	P
promazine HCl	P		P	Y			N	P	P	P	Y			P	P	P
promethazine HCl	P	Y	P	Y			N	P	P	P	Y	N	Y	P	P	P
ranitidine HCl	Y		N*			Y	Y	Y		Y	Y		Y	N	Y	Y
scopolamine HBr	P	Y	P	Y			P	P	P	P	Y		Y	P	P	P
secobarbital Na				N							N					
sodium bicarbonate								N			N					N
thiethylperazine maleate		Y											Y			
thiopental Na			N				N	N			N				N	

© 2010 Lippincott Williams & Wilkins

midazolam HCl	morphine sulfate	nalbuphine HCl	pentazocine lactate	pentobarbital Na	perphenazine	phenobarbital Na	prochlorperazine edisylate	promazine HCl	promethazine HCl	ranitidine HCl	scopolamine HBr	secobarbital Na	sodium bicarbonate	thiethylperazine maleate	thiopental Na	
Y	P	Y	P	P*	Y		P	P	P	Y	P					atropine sulfate
Y	Y		Y	N	Y		Y		Y		Y			Y		butorphanol tartrate
Y	P		P	N	Y		P	P	P	N*	P				N	chlorpromazine HCl
Y	Y	Y	Y	N	Y		Y	Y	Y		Y	N				cimetidine HCl
																codeine phosphate
										Y						dexamethasone sodium phosphate
N	P	N	P	N	Y		N	N	N	Y	P		N		N	dimenhydrinate
Y	P	Y	P	N	Y		P	P	P	Y	P				N	diphenhydramine HCl
Y	P	Y	P	N	Y		P	P	P		P					droperidol
Y	P		P	N	Y		P	P	P	Y	P					fentanyl citrate
Y	Y	Y	N	N			Y	Y	Y	Y	Y	N	N		N	glycopyrrolate
N	N*		N			$P_{(5)}$			N							heparin Na
Y			Y	Y		N	N*		Y	Y	Y			Y		hydromorphone HCl
Y	P	Y	P	N	Y		P	P	P	N	P					hydroxyzine HCl
Y	N		P	N	Y		P	P	P	Y	P					meperidine HCl
Y	P		P		P		P	P	P	Y	P		N			metoclopramide HCl
	Y	Y		N	N		N	Y	Y	N	Y			Y		midazolam HCl
Y			P	N*	Y		P	P	P	Y	P				N	morphine sulfate
Y				N			Y		N*	Y	Y			Y		nalbuphine HCl
	P			N	Y		P	P*	P*	Y	P					pentazocine lactate
N	N*	N	N		N		N	N	N	N	P		Y		Y	pentobarbital Na
N	Y		Y	N			Y		Y	Y	Y			N		perphenazine
										N						phenobarbital Na
N	P*	Y	P	N	Y			P	P	Y	P				N	prochlorperazine edisylate
Y	P		P*	N			P		P		P					promazine HCl
Y	P*	N*	P*	N	Y		P	P		Y	P				N	promethazine HCl
N	Y	Y	Y	N	Y	N	Y		Y		Y			Y		ranitidine HCl
Y	P	Y	P	P	Y		P	P	P	Y					Y	scopolamine HBr
																secobarbital Na
				Y											N	sodium bicarbonate
Y		Y			N					Y						thiethylperazine maleate
	N			Y			N		N		Y		N			thiopental Na

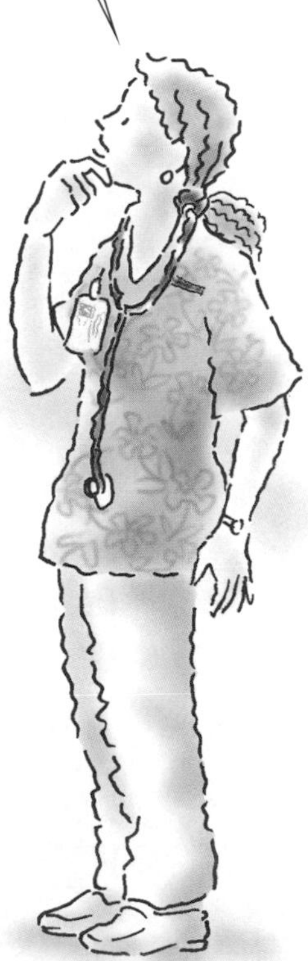

Using a flow sheet to document I.V. therapy

The sample below shows the typical features of an I.V. therapy flow sheet.

I.V. Therapy Flow Sheet

Patient: James Tolman
Diagnosis: L total hip replacement
Venipuncture limitations R arm only
Permanent access: None

INTRAVENOUS CARE COMMENT CODES C = CAP F = FILTER T= TUBING D = DRESSING								
START DATE/ TIME	INITIALS	I.V. VOLUME & SOLUTION	ADDITIVES	FLOW RATE	SITE	STOP DATE/ TIME	CHANGE	COMMENTS
6/30/09 1100	DS	1000 cc D_5W	20 meq KCL	100/hr	RFA	6/30/09 2100	T	
6/30/09 2100	JM	1000 cc D_5W	20 meq KCL	100/hr	RFA	7/1/09 0700		
7/1/09 0700	DS	1000 cc D_5W	20 meq KCL	100/hr	7/2/09 LFA		TD	

Glossary

active transport: movement of solutes from an area of lower concentration to one of higher concentration (the solutes are said to move against the concentration gradient)

add-a-line set: an I.V. administration set that can deliver intermittent secondary infusions through one or more additional Y-sites

aerosolization: dispersal of a solution into the air in an atomized form

agglutinization: clumping of red blood cells; part of the immune reaction that occurs with Rh incompatibility

air embolism: a systemic complication of I.V. therapy that occurs when air is introduced into the venous system and that includes such signs and symptoms as respiratory distress, unequal breath sounds, weak pulse, increased central venous pressure, decreased blood pressure, and loss of consciousness

albumin: a protein that can't pass through capillary walls and that draws water into the capillaries by osmosis during reabsorption

aldosterone: a hormone secreted by the adrenal cortex that regulates sodium reabsorption by the kidneys (the renin-angiotensin system responds to decreased blood flow and decreased blood pressure to stimulate aldosterone secretion)

alopecia: baldness that's partial or complete, local or general; in chemotherapy, caused by the destruction of rapidly dividing cells in the hair shaft or root

amino acids: in parenteral nutrition, nutrients that supply enough protein to replace essential amino acids, maintain protein stores, and prevent protein loss from muscle tissues

anaphylactic reaction (anaphylaxis): severe allergic reaction that may include flushing, chills, anxiety, agitation, generalized itching, palpitations, paresthesia, throbbing in the ears, wheezing, coughing, seizures, and cardiac arrest

anthropometry: an objective, noninvasive method of measuring overall body size, composition, and specific body parts that compares the patient's measurements with established standards (commonly used anthropometric measurements include height, weight, ideal body weight, body frame size, skinfold thickness, midarm circumference, and midarm muscle circumference)

antibody: an immunoglobulin molecule synthesized in response to a specific antigen

antidiuretic hormone (ADH): a hormone produced in the hypothalamus and stored in the posterior pituitary gland that responds to osmolarity and blood pressure changes and also promotes water reabsorption by the kidneys

anti-free-flow device: a device on an infusion pump that prevents inadvertent bolus infusions if the pump door is accidentally opened

antigen: a major component of blood that exists on the surface of blood cells and can initiate an immune response (a particular antigen can also induce the formation of a corresponding antibody when given to a person who doesn't normally have the antigen)

arm board: a restraining device that helps prevent unnecessary motion that could cause infiltration or inflammation when an I.V. insertion site is near a joint or in the back of the hand

arrhythmia: heart rhythm irregularity that can occur during central venous access device insertion if the catheter enters the right ventricle and irritates the cardiac muscle (arrhythmias usually abate when the catheter is withdrawn)

autotransfusion: the collection and filtration of blood from a patient and the reinfusion of that blood into the same patient

backcheck valve: a device that prevents backflow of a secondary solution into a primary solution (in a primary line with a side Y-port, a backcheck valve stops the flow from the primary line during drug infusion and returns to the primary flow after infusion)

bacterial phlebitis: painful inflammation of a vein that can occur with peripherally inserted central catheters; usually occurs after a long period of I.V. therapy

biological response modifiers: agents used in biological therapy that alter the body's response to cancer

biological safety cabinet: specialized work area for preparing chemotherapeutic drugs

blood products: the individual components that make up whole blood and are available for transfusion therapy to correct specific blood deficiencies; for example, red blood cells, plasma, platelets, granulocytes, immune globulin, albumin, and plasma protein

blood type: usually, one of the four blood types in the ABO system, including A, B, AB, and O, which is named for the antigen—A, B, both of these, or neither—that are carried on a person's red blood cells

body fluids: water and dissolved substances in the body (such as electrolytes) that help regulate body temperature, transport nutrients and gases throughout the body, carry wastes to excretion sites, and maintain cell shape

body surface area slide rule: a slide rule that's used to calculate a patient's body surface area when the patient's weight and height are known (body surface area is expressed in square meters [m^2])

butterfly needle: common name for a winged infusion set, which has flexible wings that lie flat after insertion and can be taped to the surrounding skin

capillary filtration: movement of fluid and solutes out through the capillary wall pores and into the interstitial fluid; caused by hydrostatic (or fluid) pressure and blood pressure against the walls of the capillaries

capillary reabsorption: the return of water and diffusible solutes to the capillaries that occurs when capillary blood pressure falls below colloid oncotic pressure

cell cycle: the reproductive and resting phases through which every cell, normal and malignant, passes

cellular elements: components that make up about 45% of blood volume, including erythrocytes (red blood cells [RBCs]), leukocytes (white blood cells [WBCs]), and thrombocytes (platelets); also called *formed elements;* commonly transfused cellular blood products include whole blood, packed RBCs, leukocyte-poor RBCs, WBCs, and platelets

central venous (CV) therapy: treatment in which drugs or fluids are infused directly into a major vein; used in emergencies, when a patient's peripheral veins are inaccessible, or when a patient needs infusion of a large volume of fluid, multiple infusion therapies, or long-term venous access (in CV therapy, an access device is inserted with its tip in the superior vena cava, inferior vena cava, or right atrium of the heart)

central venous pressure (CVP): an important indicator of circulatory function and the pumping ability of the right side of the heart; measured with a catheter placed in or near the right atrium

chemotherapeutic drugs: drugs used in chemotherapy that fall into categories, including alkylating agents, antimetabolites, hormones and hormone inhibitors, antibiotics, plant alkaloids, and enzymes, that are, in turn, grouped as cycle-specific (antimetabolites and plant alkaloids) and cycle-nonspecific (alkylating agents and most antibiotics); given alone or in various combinations, called *protocols*

chemotherapy: cancer treatment that requires effective delivery of a precise dose of toxic drugs and typically employs more than one drug so that each drug can target a different site or take action during a different phase of the cell cycle (the challenge is to provide a drug dose large enough to kill the greatest number of cancer cells but small enough to avoid irreversibly damaging normal tissue or causing toxicity)

chylothorax: puncture of a lymph node with leakage of lymph fluid

circulatory overload: an extremely large volume of fluid that the heart is incapable of pumping through the circulatory system (symptoms include neck vein engorgement, respiratory distress, increased blood pressure, and crackles in the lungs)

cold agglutinins: antibodies that can cause red blood cell clumping if cold blood is infused

colloid osmotic pressure: the osmotic, or pulling, force of albumin in the intravascular space that draws water into the capillaries during reabsorption

colony-stimulating factors (CSFs): biological response modifiers that regulate hematopoietic growth and differentiation; for example, hematopoietic growth factors (erythropoietin), granulocyte colony-stimulating factor, interleukin-3, macrophage colony stimulating factor, and thrombopoietin

compatibility: in transfusion therapy, typing and crossmatching the donor and recipient blood to minimize the risk of a hemolytic reaction (the most important compatibility tests include ABO blood typing, Rh typing, crossmatching, direct antiglobulin test, and antibody screening test)

complement system: a group of enzymatic proteins (in a hemolytic transfusion reaction, an antibody-antigen reaction activates the body's complement system, causing red blood cell destruction [hemolysis], which releases hemoglobin [a red blood cell component] into the bloodstream and can damage renal tubules and lead to kidney failure)

continuous delivery: in parenteral nutrition, delivery of an infusion over a 24-hour period

continuous I.V. therapy: administration of I.V. fluid over a prolonged period through a peripheral or central venous line, allowing careful regulation of drug delivery and enhancing the effectiveness of some drugs, such as lidocaine and heparin

cooling cap: in chemotherapy, a device that's used to limit superficial blood flow to the scalp during drug administration, thus partially protecting the hair follicles and limiting alopecia

cross-sensitivity: hypersensitivity to similar I.V. drugs (if a patient is hypersensitive to a particular drug, he may be hypersensitive to other chemically similar drugs)

cycle-nonspecific drugs: in chemotherapy, drugs that act independently of the cell cycle, allowing them to act on reproducing and resting cells (During a single administration of a cycle-nonspecific chemotherapeutic drug, a fixed percentage of normal and malignant cells die, while the others survive. Slower growing cancers, such as GI and pulmonary tumors, which have fewer cells undergoing division at any given moment, respond best to cycle-nonspecific drugs. Large tumors respond better to cycle-nonspecific drugs; however, once the large tumor shrinks, the practitioner may switch to a cycle-specific drug.)

cycle-specific drugs: in chemotherapy, drugs that are effective only during a specific phase of the cell cycle; designed to disrupt a specific biochemical process (When cycle-specific chemotherapy is administered, cells in the resting phase survive and eventually reproduce. Rapidly growing cancers, such as acute leukemias and lymphomas, respond best to cycle-specific chemotherapy. Generally, small tumors respond to drugs that affect deoxyribonucleic acid synthesis, especially cycle-specific drugs, because these tumors have a higher percentage of actively dividing cells than large tumors.)

cyclic delivery: in parenteral nutrition, delivery of the entire solution overnight; also used to wean a patient from total parenteral nutrition

cytokines: a type of biological response modifier—includes interferon, interleukins, tumor necrosis factor, and colony-stimulating factors

dextrose: a glucose solution that contributes most of the calories in parenteral nutrition solutions and can help maintain nitrogen balance

diffusion: movement of solutes from an area of higher concentration to one of lower concentration by passive transport (a fluid movement process that requires no energy)

diluent: a liquid used to reconstitute I.V. drugs that are supplied in powder form; for example, normal saline solution, sterile water for injection, dextrose 5% in water (some drugs should be reconstituted with diluents that contain preservatives)

direct injection: administration of a single dose (bolus) of a drug or other substance; sometimes called *I.V. push*

divalent cations: an electrolyte that carries two positively charged ions (such as Ca^{++}) (in I.V. medication therapy, a solution containing divalent cations has a higher incidence of incompatibility)

double-chambered vial: container for some drugs in which the powder form of the drug is in a lower chamber and a diluent is in an upper one with a rubber stopper on top of the vial that's pressed to dislodge the rubber plug separating the compartments, thus mixing the diluent with the drug in the bottom chamber

drip controller: device used in central venous therapy that permits infusion at low pressure; used commonly with infants and children who could suffer serious complications from high-pressure infusion

electrolyte balance: the concentration levels of intracellular and extracellular electrolytes, which are about equal when balance is maintained

electrolytes: major components of body fluids — especially sodium, potassium, calcium, chloride, phosphate, and magnesium — that are involved in fluid balance and that dissociate into ions and conduct electric current that's necessary for normal cell functioning

emetogenic (vomit-inducing) potential: likelihood that a drug or drugs may cause nausea or vomiting (For example, cisplatin has a high emetogenic potential; more than 90% of patients receiving it will experience nausea and vomiting. Bleomycin has a low potential; only 10% to 30% of patients are affected. Other factors contributing to occurrence and severity include the combination of drugs, doses and routes of administration, rates of administration, treatment schedules, and patient characteristics.)

extension tubing: small-bore tubing that can be attached to any I.V. tubing to join it to the venipuncture device, allowing I.V. tubing to be changed away from the insertion site, thereby reducing the risk of contamination

extracellular fluid (ECF): any fluid in the body that isn't contained inside the cells, including interstitial fluid, plasma, and transcellular fluid

extravasation: infiltration of irritating fluids, resulting in damage to surrounding tissues; a medical emergency

fats: in parenteral nutrition, supplied as lipid emulsions; a concentrated source of energy that prevents or corrects fatty acid deficiencies; available in several concentrations to provide 30% to 50% of a patient's daily calories

febrile reaction: a possible complication of transfusion therapy; characterized by a temperature increase of 1.8° F (1° C) with transfusion (for nonhemolytic febrile reactions), with no other known explanation and usually caused by antibodies directed against leukocytes or platelets; common in approximately 1% of transfusions within 2 hours after completion (signs and symptoms of febrile reactions include fever, chills, headache, nausea and vomiting, hypotension, chest pain, dyspnea, nonproductive cough, and malaise)

fistula: an abnormal passageway that may develop between the innominate vein and the subclavian artery due to perforation by a guide wire inserted into the vessel

flare reaction: an inflammatory response to infusion of an irritant; a local venous response with or without an accompanying skin reaction (the patient may complain of burning, pain, aching along the vein, or itching; you may observe redness surrounding the venipuncture site or along the vein path)

flow regulator: a supplemental I.V. device that ensures accurate delivery of I.V. fluids by regulating the number of milliliters delivered per hour

fluid balance: constant and approximately equal distribution of fluids between the intracellular and extracellular fluid compartments

fluid movement: the process that helps regulate fluid and electrolyte balance between the major fluid compartments and transports nutrients, waste products, and other substances into and out of cells, organs, and systems

gamma globulin: the antibody-containing portion of plasma; obtained by chemical fractionation of pooled plasma; commonly used to prevent infectious hepatitis (type A), rubella, mumps, pertussis, and tetanus

gauge: diameter of a needle

gluconeogenesis: the conversion of protein to carbohydrates for energy (essential visceral proteins [serum albumin and transferrin] and somatic body proteins [skeletal, smooth muscle, and tissue proteins] are converted to energy in starvation or severe nutrient deficiencies; when essential body proteins break down, a negative nitrogen balance results [more protein is used by the body than is taken in])

glycogenolysis: in metabolism, the mobilization and conversion of glycogen to glucose in the body

granulocytopenia: a severely low granulocyte level

Groshong catheter: a common tunneled catheter, which has a pressure-sensitive valve in the catheter tip that keeps the lumen closed when not in use and opens inward during blood aspiration and outward during blood or fluid administration, eliminating the need to flush with heparin

guide wire: a device that stiffens a catheter to ease its advancement through a vein but can damage the vein if used incorrectly

hemapheresis: collecting and removing specific blood components from blood and then returning the remaining constituents to the patient

hematocrit: the percentage of red blood cells in whole blood

hematoma: bruising at a venipuncture site as a result of bleeding in the area (symptoms include a raised dark area around the site with accompanying tenderness and an inability to advance or flush the I.V. line)

hemolytic reaction: a life-threatening reaction to transfusions that occurs as a result of incompatible ABO or Rh blood or improper blood storage

hemosiderosis: possible complication of transfusion therapy that typically results from multiple or massive transfusions; accumulation of an iron-containing pigment (hemosiderin) that causes red blood cell destruction; characterized by iron plasma level greater than 200 mg/dl

hemothorax: bleeding into the pleural cavity, a common complication of central venous catheter placement; treated with the insertion of a chest tube for draining blood

heparin: an anticoagulant

human leukocyte antigen (HLA): antigen that's essential to immunity; part of the histocompatibility system, which controls compatibility between transplant or transfusion recipients and donors (generally, the closer the HLA match between donor and recipient, the less likely the tissue or organ will be rejected)

hydrothorax: infusion of a solution into the chest

hyperglycemia: high blood glucose; a possible complication of parenteral nutrition; commonly an early warning sign of sepsis

hyperosmolar hyperglycemic nonketotic syndrome (HHNS): a possible complication of parenteral nutrition; the patient may develop confusion or lethargy, have seizures, or become comatose; hyperglycemia, dehydration, or glycosuria can also occur

hypertonic solution: a solution with higher osmolarity (concentration) than the normal range of serum (275 to 295 mOsm/L), such as dextrose 5% in half-normal saline solution, dextrose 5% in normal saline solution, and dextrose 5% in lactated Ringer's solution

hypocalcemia: calcium deficiency; signs and symptoms include tingling in the fingers, muscle cramps, nausea, vomiting, hypotension, cardiac arrhythmias, and seizures

hypoglycemia: low blood glucose; a possible complication of parenteral nutrition; signs and symptoms include sweating, shaking, and irritability

hypokalemia: low blood potassium; a possible complication of parenteral nutrition; signs and symptoms include muscle weakness, paralysis, paresthesia, and arrhythmias

hypomagnesemia: low blood magnesium; a possible complication of parenteral nutrition; patient may complain of tingling around the mouth or paresthesia in the fingers and may show signs of mental changes, hyperreflexia, tetany, and arrhythmias

hypophosphatemia: low blood phosphates; a possible complication of parenteral nutrition; patient may be irritable or weak and may have paresthesia; in extreme cases, coma and cardiac arrest can occur

hypotonic solution: a solution with lower osmolarity (concentration) than the normal range of serum (275 to 295 mOsm/L)—such as half-normal saline solution, 0.33% saline solution, or dextrose 2.5% in water—which hydrates cells while reducing fluid in the circulatory system

hypovolemic shock: shock due to loss of systemic volume; caused by internal bleeding, hemorrhage, or sepsis; signs and symptoms include increased heart rate, decreased blood pressure, mental confusion, and cool, clammy skin

iatrogenic protein-energy malnutrition: a form of malnutrition, common during hospitalization, in which a patient's nutritional status deteriorates; most common in patients hospitalized longer than 2 weeks

idiosyncratic reaction: an inherent inability to tolerate certain therapeutic chemicals (for example, a tranquilizer may cause excitation rather than sedation in a particular patient)

implanted port: a long-term central venous access device that's implanted in a pocket under the skin with an attached indwelling catheter that's tunnelled through subcutaneous tissue so the catheter tip lies in a central vein; accessed with a specially designed, noncoring needle; typically used when an external catheter isn't suitable and also used for arterial access or implanted into the epidural space, peritoneum, or pericardial or pleural cavity; usually used to deliver intermittent infusions

incompatibility: an adverse reaction to I.V. therapy that results when I.V. solutions, drugs, or blood products are mixed together (in I.V. medication therapy, the more complex the solution, the greater the risk of incompatibility; in transfusion therapy, incompatibility of donor and recipient blood can cause serious adverse effects)

inferior vena cava: a central vein (venous return from the legs enters the inferior vena cava and returns blood to the right atrium; blood enters the inferior vena cava from the legs through the femoral venous system and accessory veins of the abdomen)

infiltration: infusion of I.V. solution into surrounding tissues rather than the blood vessel; symptoms include discomfort, decreased skin temperature around the site, blanching, absent backflow of blood, and slower flow rate

infusion control device: device used to maintain precise I.V. flow rates in drops per minute or milliliters per hour (for example, clamps, controllers, volumetric pumps, and rate minders)

infusion pump: an electronic device that regulates the flow of I.V. solutions and drugs and is used when a precise flow rate is required; used in central venous (CV) therapy when positive pressure is required (for example, when solutions are administered through a CV line at low flow rates or during intra-arterial infusion)

in-line filter: a filter in the fluid pathway between the I.V. tubing and the venipuncture device that removes pathogens and particles and helps prevent air from entering the patient's vein

interferon: in chemotherapy, a type of biological response modifier subdivided into three major types (alpha, beta, and gamma) that inhibits viral replication and may also directly inhibit tumor proliferation; effective on hematologic cancers, including malignant lymphomas, cutaneous T-cell lymphoma, and chronic myelogenous leukemia as well as hairy-cell leukemia

intermittent infusion device: a device that maintains venous access in patients who must receive I.V. medications regularly or intermittently but don't require continuous infusion; commonly called a *saline* or *heparin lock* because a saline or heparin solution is flushed into it to keep the device patent

intermittent I.V. therapy: administration of a solution at set intervals for a shorter period than continuous I.V. therapy; the most common and flexible method of administering I.V. drugs

interstitial fluid (ISF): extracellular fluid that bathes all cells in the body; accounts for about 75% of extracellular fluid

intracellular fluid (ICF): fluid that's contained inside the cells of the body

intraosseous infusion: an emergency procedure for fluid resuscitation or for medication or blood infusion in children under age 6 in which an intraosseous needle is placed in the medullary cavity of a bone so that an I.V. solution can be infused directly into the cavity

intrathecal: within the spinal canal

intravenous (I.V.) therapy: treatment that involves introducing liquid solutions directly into the bloodstream

irritant: an agent that, when used locally, produces a local inflammatory reaction

isotonic solution: a solution with osmolarity that is within the range for serum (275 to 295 mOsm/L), such as lactated Ringer's solution and normal saline solution

I.V. administration set: I.V. tubing set that may be vented or unvented and may come with various features, such as ports for infusing secondary medications and filters

I.V. loop: a supplemental I.V. device made of small-bore tubing in a horseshoe shape that fits between the venipuncture device and I.V. tubing to enable the tubing to be changed away from the device and help stabilize the device

kwashiorkor: a form of malnutrition that results from severe protein deficiencies without caloric deficit; occurs most commonly in children ages 1 to 3; usually secondary to malabsorption disorders, cancer and cancer therapies, kidney disease, hypermetabolic illness, and iatrogenic causes

lipid emulsions: in parenteral nutrition, used to prevent and treat essential fatty acid deficiency and provide a major source of energy

liposome: a vehicle for transmitting a chemotherapeutic drug directly to a cancerous tumor that consists of ring-shaped layers, usually phospholipids, with a space between the lipid rings that contains an aqueous solution (drugs can be placed in the lipid layer or, if they're water-soluble, in the aqueous spaces and carried to specific tumor cells)

loading dose: preliminary dose of a medication; usually given I.V. at the start of therapy

lock: see *intermittent infusion device*

lock-out interval: a time set on a patient-controlled analgesia device during which the device can't be activated

luer-lock injection cap: a device, possibly attached to the end of an extension set, which contains a clamping mechanism to provide ready access for intermittent infusions, which reduces the discomfort of reaccessing the port and prolongs the life of the port septum by decreasing the number of needle punctures

lymphokines: in chemotherapy, a subset of cytokines that fight cancer by stimulating the production of T cells, activating the lytic (cell-destroying) mechanisms of macrophages, promoting the immigration of lymphoid cells from the bloodstream, and stimulating the release of other lymphokines, such as tumor necrosis factor and interferon gamma; examples include interleukin-1 and interleukin-2

macrodrip delivery system: an I.V. administration set that delivers a solution in large quantities at rapid rates

maintenance dose: the amount of medication a patient requires to achieve an effective therapeutic effect

marasmus: a form of malnutrition involving prolonged and gradual wasting of muscle mass and subcutaneous fat that occurs most commonly in infants, ages 6 to 18 months, and in patients with post-gastrectomy dumping syndrome, carcinomas of the mouth and esophagus, and chronic malnutrition states; caused by inadequate intake of protein, calories, and other nutrients

mechanical phlebitis: painful inflammation of a vein; possibly the most common peripherally inserted central catheter complication, which may occur during the first 24 to 72 hours after insertion; more common in left-sided insertions and when a large-gauge catheter is used

metabolic acidosis: a possible complication of parenteral nutrition that can occur if the patient develops an increased serum chloride level and a decreased serum bicarbonate level

metacarpal veins: veins located on the back of the hand, formed by the union of digital veins between the knuckles

microaggregates: small particles formed from degenerating platelets, leukocytes, and fibrin strands after a few days of blood storage that may contribute to formation of microemboli (small clots that obstruct circulation) in the lungs; can pass through a 170-micron filter (a microaggregate filter removes smaller particles but costs more and may slow the infusion rate)

microdrip delivery system: an I.V. administration set that delivers a small amount of solution with each drop and is used for pediatric patients and for adults who need small or closely regulated amounts of I.V. solution

micronutrients: in parenteral nutrition solutions, used to promote normal metabolism; also called *trace elements;* examples include zinc, copper, chromium, iodide, selenium, and manganese

midline device: an extended peripheral catheter; often incorrectly called a peripherally inserted central catheter, but its tip rests in the axillary vein rather than in the central venous circulation

mucositis: inflammation of the mucous membranes

myelosuppression: the interference with and suppression of the blood-forming stem cells in the bone marrow; a possible complication of chemotherapy

nadir: the lowest point in some series of measurements, such as white blood cell, hemoglobin, or platelet levels

necrosis: tissue death

nomogram: a table for estimating body surface area when a patient's weight and height are known

noncoring needle: implanted port needle with an angled or deflected point that slices the septum on entry, rather than coring it as a conventional needle does (when the noncoring needle is removed, the septum reseals itself)

nontunneled catheter: type of central venous access device usually designed for short-term use

nonvesicant: an agent that doesn't cause blisters

nutritional assessment: assessment of the relationship between nutrients consumed and energy expended, especially when illness or surgery compromises a patient's intake or alters his metabolic requirements; includes a dietary history, physical assessment, anthropometric measurements, and diagnostic tests

occlusion: blockage that prevents the ability to infuse fluids or flush a vein due to the accumulation of blood materials, fibrin, platelets, or incompatible infusates that causes crystallization in the lumen of the infusion device or vein

osmolarity: the concentration of a solution expressed in milliosmols of solute per liter of solution

osmosis: the passive transport of fluid across a membrane from an area of lower concentration to one of higher concentration that stops when the solute concentrations are equal

over-the-needle catheter: the most commonly used device for peripheral I.V. therapy, which consists of a plastic outer tube and an inner needle (stylet) that's removed after insertion, leaving the catheter in place

oxygen-hemoglobin affinity: the tendency of hemoglobin to hold oxygen (When oxygen's hemoglobin affinity increases, oxygen stays in the patient's bloodstream and isn't released into other tissues. Oxygen's hemoglobin affinity can increase during blood storage, causing oxygen to stay in a patient's bloodstream rather than being released into other tissues. Signs of this reaction include a depressed respiratory rate, especially in patients with chronic lung disease.)

parenteral: any route other than the GI tract by which drugs, nutrients, or other solutions may enter the body (for example, I.V., I.M., or subcutaneously)

parenteral nutrition: therapy that provides calories from dextrose and one or more nutrients that keep the body functioning; ordered when a nutritional assessment reveals a nonfunctional GI tract, increased metabolic need, or a combination of both; administered through either a peripheral or central venous infusion device; solutions may contain one or more of the following: dextrose, proteins, lipids, electrolytes, vitamins, and trace elements

passive transport: fluid movement that requires no energy and in which solutes move from an area of higher concentration to one of lower concentration (this change is called *moving down the concentration gradient* and results in an equal distribution of solutes)

patency: the state of being freely open (a patent vein is intact and without holes)

patient-controlled analgesia (PCA): treatment that allows the patient to control I.V. delivery of an analgesic (usually morphine) and maintain therapeutic serum levels (the patient uses a specialized infusion device with a timing unit that delivers a dose of an analgesic at a controlled volume)

peripheral central venous therapy: a variation of central venous therapy in which a catheter is inserted through a peripheral vein, with the catheter tip in the superior vena cava

peripherally inserted central catheter (PICC): a central venous access device that's inserted through a peripheral vein with the tip ending in the superior or inferior vena cava; generally used when patients need frequent blood transfusions or infusions of caustic drugs or solutions; especially useful if the patient doesn't have reliable routes for short-term I.V. therapy

peripheral parenteral nutrition (PPN): the delivery of nutrients through a short cannula inserted into a peripheral vein; generally provides fewer nonprotein calories than total parenteral nutrition because lower dextrose concentrations are used

phlebitis: painful inflammation along the venous path in which the cannula is placed; a common complication of I.V. therapy; signs and symptoms include redness (erythema) at the site and along the vein, puffiness over the vein, firmness on palpation, and discomfort

physiologic pump: a mechanism that's involved in the active transport of solutes; for example, the sodium-potassium pump, which moves sodium ions out of cells to the extracellular fluid and potassium ions into cells from the extracellular fluid

piggyback infusion: use of an add-a-line administration set to add an I.V. drug into a primary line

piggyback line: an adjunct or secondary I.V. line attached to a primary line to deliver medications or solutions I.V.

plasma: the liquid component of blood, which surrounds the red blood cells, accounts for about 55% of blood volume, and consists of blood's noncellular components, including water (serum), protein (albumin, globulin, and fibrinogen), lipids, electrolytes, vitamins, carbohydrates, nonprotein nitrogen compounds, bilirubin, and gases; commonly transfused plasma products include fresh frozen plasma, albumin, cryoprecipitate, and prothrombin complex; used in conjunction with plasma fractions for transfusion therapy to correct blood deficiencies, prevent disease, and control bleeding tendencies

plasma substitutes: components that lack oxygen-carrying and coagulation properties and may be used to maintain blood volume in an emergency, such as acute hemorrhage and shock; examples include synthetic volume expanders, such as dextran in saline solution, and natural volume expanders, such as plasma protein fraction and albumin

platelets: cellular elements of blood that are infused to prevent or control bleeding; may be depleted in patients with hematologic disease or those receiving antineoplastic therapy

pneumothorax: air in the thorax; the most common complication of central venous placement; signs and symptoms include chest pain, dyspnea, cyanosis, or decreased or absent breath sounds on the affected side (a thoracotomy should be performed and a chest tube inserted if pneumothorax is severe enough for intervention)

potassium intoxication: an increase in potassium levels after a transfusion that occurs because of blood cell maturation in stored blood components; may cause intestinal colic, diarrhea, muscle twitching, oliguria, renal failure, bradycardia that may proceed to cardiac arrest, and electrocardiogram changes with tall, peaked T waves

potentiate: to increase the potency of action (in chemotherapy, smaller doses of different chemotherapeutic drugs are given in combination, the drugs potentiate each other, and the tumor responds as it would to a larger dose of a single drug)

primary I.V. line: main I.V. line, usually used to deliver a continuous infusion of an I.V. solution

protein-energy malnutrition (PEM): a deficiency of protein and energy (calories); a spectrum of disorders that results from either prolonged, chronic, inadequate protein or caloric intake or high metabolic protein and energy requirements; commonly caused by cancer, GI disorders, chronic heart failure, alcoholism, and conditions causing high metabolic needs, such as burns

protocol: a description of specific steps in patient care that may describe how to administer a medication

retrograde administration: administration method that allows a medication, such as I.V. antibiotics, to be given over a 30-minute period without increasing fluid volume

rhesus (Rh) system: in blood physiology, a major blood antigen system that consists of Rh-positive and Rh-negative groups (Rh-positive blood has a variant of the Rh antigen called a *D antigen* or *D factor;*

Rh-negative blood doesn't have this antigen. A person with Rh-positive blood doesn't carry anti-Rh antibodies because they would destroy his red blood cells.)

saline lock: an intermittent infusion device that's flushed with saline

scalp tourniquet: in chemotherapy, a device that's used to limit superficial blood flow to the scalp during drug administration, thus partially protecting the hair follicles from the circulating drug and reducing the risk of alopecia

scalp vein catheter: a small-diameter, winged over-the-needle catheter; the preferred venous access device for infants and young children

sclerosis: the hardening of a tissue or vessel

secondary set: I.V. tubing and infusion attached to the primary I.V. line; usually used for the administration of I.V. medication, also called *piggyback infusion set*

sepsis: infection of tissues with disease-causing microorganisms or their toxins (Signs and symptoms of sepsis include elevated temperature, glucose in the urine [glycosuria], chills, malaise, increased white blood cells [leukocytosis], and altered level of consciousness.)

sequential system: method used to document I.V. solutions throughout therapy in which each container is numbered sequentially

speed shock: shock caused by too-rapid direct injection of a drug (most drugs must be given over a specific time period when using direct injection; to avoid speed shock, no drug should be injected in less than 1 minute, unless the order specifically requires it or the patient is in cardiac or respiratory arrest)

stomatitis: inflammation of the mouth; in chemotherapy, painful mouth ulcers apparent 3 to 7 days after treatment begins, with symptoms ranging from mild to severe (accompanying pain can lead to malnutrition and fluid and electrolyte imbalance if the patient can't chew and swallow adequate food and fluid; treatment includes scrupulous oral hygiene and topical anesthetic mixtures)

superior vena cava: a central vein (Venous return from the head, neck, and arms enters the superior vena cava before flowing into the right atrium. Blood enters the superior vena cava mainly through the subclavian, jugular, and innominate veins of the head, neck, and arms.)

syringe pump: a type of pump that's especially useful for giving intermittent I.V. medications to pediatric patients because it gives the greatest control over small-volume infusions; used with syringe sizes from 1 to 60 ml using low-volume tubing

T-connector: a supplemental I.V. device that's attached to I.V. tubing and into which another I.V. needle can be inserted, allowing simultaneous administration of fluids and drugs; also used as an intermittent infusion device

tension pneumothorax: type of pneumothorax in which air leaks into the lungs but can't escape, causing pressure in the lungs and eventually leading to lung collapse; a medical emergency in which the patient exhibits signs of acute respiratory distress, asymmetrical chest wall movement and, possibly, a tracheal shift away from the midline (a chest tube must be inserted immediately, before respiratory and cardiac decompensation occur)

thrombocytopenia: blood platelet depletion

thrombogenic: a device or process that may cause or lead to thrombosis formation

thrombophlebitis: inflammation of the vein due to the formation of a blood clot

thrombosis: the development of a thrombus (blood clot)

time tape: a tape or preprinted strip marked in 1-hour increments; attached to an I.V. container and used to check the infusion rate

titration: gradual addition of a component to a solution that ends when no more of the component can be consumed by reaction in the solution (with I.V. therapy, you can accurately titrate medication doses by adjusting the concentration of the infusate and the administration rate)

total nutrient admixture (TNA): daily allotments of total parenteral nutrition solution, including lipids and other parenteral solution components; commonly given in a single, 3-L bag; also called *3:1 solution*

total parenteral nutrition (TPN): delivery of nutrients through a central line and usually through the subclavian vein with the tip of the catheter in the superior vena cava; usually indicated when parenteral nutrition is needed for more than 5 days

tourniquet: commonly, a soft rubber band 2″ (5 cm) wide that encircles a limb and traps blood in the veins by applying enough pressure to impede the venous flow

toxicity: the quality of being poisonous

transcellular fluids: a form of extracellular fluid that includes cerebrospinal fluid, lymph, and fluids in such spaces as the pleural and abdominal cavities

transfusion reaction: adverse reaction to transfusion therapy, the most severe of which is a hemolytic reaction, which destroys red blood cells and may become life-threatening; signs include fever, chills, rigors, headache, and nausea

transfusion therapy: the introduction of whole blood or blood components directly into the bloodstream; used mainly to restore and maintain blood volume, improve the oxygen-carrying capacity of blood, replace deficient blood components, or improve coagulation

treatment cycle: in chemotherapy, repeated drug doses, usually over several days, that's considered a single course of chemotherapy and is repeated on a cyclic basis, usually every 3 to 4 weeks; carefully planned so normal cells can regenerate (most patients require at least three treatment cycles before they show any beneficial response)

Trendelenburg's position: position in which the head is low and the body and legs are on an inclined plane; used in central venous catheter insertion to distend neck and thoracic veins, thereby making them more visible and accessible

tumor resistance: the ability of a tumor to withstand the effects of chemotherapeutic drugs, either initially during treatment or developed after treatment

tunneled central venous catheter: central venous catheter with a cuff (usually made of Dacron) that encourages tissue growth at the exit site to anchor the catheter; designed for long-term use and usually made of silicone, which minimizes irritation or damage to the vein lining

universal donor: a person with group O blood, which lacks both A and B antigens and can be transfused in limited amounts in an emergency to any patient — regardless of the recipient's blood type — with little risk of adverse reaction

universal recipient: a person with AB blood type, which has neither anti-A nor anti-B antibodies; may receive A, B, AB, or O blood

urokinase: a fibrinolytic agent used to dissolve clots

urticaria: a vascular reaction of the skin characterized by the eruption of hives and severe itching

Valsalva's maneuver: a maneuver involving forced exhalation that a patient can perform to help prevent air embolism whenever the catheter is open to the air; especially important when the patient is taking care of a catheter at home

vasoconstriction: narrowing of the lumen of a blood vessel

vasovagal reaction: sudden collapse of a vein during venipuncture, possibly caused by vasospasm due to anxiety or pain

vein dissection: a seldom-used way to access a peripheral vein in which a small incision is made in the vein to insert a plastic catheter that can remain in place for several days

venogram: radiographic examination of a vein filled with contrast medium; performed before catheter insertion to check the status of blood vessels, especially if the catheter is intended for long-term use

vesicant: an agent that causes or forms blisters

volume-control set: an I.V. administration set that's used to deliver small, precise amounts of fluids and medications and that may be attached directly to the venipuncture device or connected as a secondary infusion device at a Y-site

washed cells: blood from which 80% of the plasma is removed; rinsed with a special solution that removes white blood cells and platelets (for example, leukocyte-poor red blood cells)

winged infusion set: an infusion set that has flexible wings that lie flat after insertion and can be taped to the surrounding skin; also called *butterfly needle*

Y-site: a secondary injection port on an I.V. administration set that allows separate or simultaneous infusion of two compatible solutions

Selected references

American Association of Blood Banks. *Standards for Blood Banks and Transfusion Services*, 25th ed. Bethesda, Md.: AABB, 2008.

American Red Cross. *Practice Guidelines for Blood Transfusion: A Compilation from Recent Peer-Reviewed Literature.* Washington, D.C.: American National Red Cross, 2002.

Brown, K., et al. *Chemotherapy and Biotherapy Guidelines and Recommendations for Practice*, 2nd ed. Pittsburgh: Oncology Nursing Society, 2005.

Brungs, S.M., and Render, M.L. "Using Evidence-based Practice to Reduce Central Line Infections," *Clinical Journal of Oncology Nursing* 10(6):723–25, December 2006.

Centers for Disease Control and Prevention. "Guidelines for the Prevention of Intravascular Catheter-related Infections," *MMWR* 51(RR-10):1–26, August 2002.

Hadaway, L.C. "Tips for Using Implanted Ports Safely," *Nursing2006* 36(8):66–67, August 2006.

Higgins, P.A., et al. "Assessing Nutritional Status in Critically Ill Adult Patients," *American Journal of Critical Care* 15(2):166-76, March 2006.

"Infusion Nursing Standards of Practice," *Journal of Infusion Nursing* 29(1S), January–February 2006.

Kasper, D., et al., eds. *Harrison's Principles of Internal Medicine*, 16th ed. New York: McGraw-Hill Book Co., 2005.

Lynn-McHale Wiegand, D.J., and Carlson, K.K., eds. AACN *Procedure Manual for Critical Care*, 5th ed. Philadelphia: W.B. Saunders Co., 2005.

Masoorli, S. "Legal Issues Related to Vascular Access Devices and Infusion Therapy," *Journal of Infusion Nursing* 28(3 Suppl):S18-21; quiz S33–6, May–June 2006.

Mimoz, O., et al. "Chlorhexidine-based Antiseptic Solution vs. Alcohol-based Povidone-Iodine for Central Venous Catheter Care," *Archives of Internal Medicine* 167(19):2066–2072, October 2007.

Nettina, S. *The Lippincott Manual of Nursing Practice*, 9th ed. Philadelphia: Lippincott Williams & Wilkins, 2010.

Nursing2010 Drug Handbook, 30th ed. Ambler, Pa.: Lippincott Williams & Wilkins, 2010.

Oncology Nursing Society. *Access Device Guidelines: Recommendations for Nursing Practice and Education*, 2nd ed. Pittsburgh: Oncology Nursing Society, 2004.

Richardson, D.K. "Vascular Access Nursing: A Review of Flushing Solutions and Injection Caps," *Journal of Association of Vascular Access* 12(2):74–84, Summer 2007.

Sabbadini, G., et al. "Managing Heart Failure in the Very Old," *Aging Health* 2(2):253–75, April 2006.

Taylor, C., et al. *Fundamentals of Nursing: The Art and Science of Nursing Care*, 6th ed. Philadelphia: Lippincott Williams & Wilkins, 2008.

Warren, D.K., et al. "A Multicenter Intervention to Prevent Catheter-associated Bloodstream Infections," *Infection Control and Hospital Epidemiology* 27(7):662–69, July 2006.

Weinstein, S. *Plumer's Principles & Practice of Intravenous Therapy*, 8th ed. Philadelphia: Lippincott Williams & Wilkins, 2007.

Index

A

B

i refers to an illustration; t refers to a table; **boldface** indicates color pages.

i refers to an illustration; t refers to a table; **boldface** indicates color pages.

i refers to an illustration; t refers to a table; **boldface** indicates color pages.

IJ

i refers to an illustration; t refers to a table; **boldface** indicates color pages.

O

PQ

R

i refers to an illustration; t refers to a table; **boldface** indicates color pages.

RRS1207